From Surviving To Thriving:

Navigating the First Year of Professional Nursing Practice

Judy Boychuk Duchscher RN, PhD

Published by: *Nursing The Future*, PO Box 22058, RPO Wildwood,
Saskatoon SK, Canada, S7H 5P1

Printed in Canada by Saskatoon Fastprint
2938 Millar Avenue
Saskatoon, Saskatchewan
S7K 5X7
Canada

Layout design by Ken Cahill
K21 Graphics & Printing
226 Wrigley Crescent
Saskatoon, Saskatchewan
S7M 4Y4
Canada

Cover Design by Karenna Boychuk
Graphic Designer
www.kewbdesign.com

Library and Archives Canada Catalogue-In-Publication Data
Duchscher, Judy E.B./Nursing The Future

ISBN 978-0-9877783-1-4

SECOND EDITION
1st Print January 2012 (Canadian Nursing Students Association 2012 AGM)
2nd Print February 2012 (Editorial Revisions) – Print for Purchase
3rd Printing April 2012 (Editorial Revisions)

TO PURCHASE BOOK GO TO
www. nursingthefuture.ca

Table of Contents

Dedication

This book is dedicated to all new nursing graduates and their devoted supporters for fueling the flame of caring, compassionate and committed competence that sustains the nursing profession.

Acknowledgements

I would like to thank all the family, friends and colleagues who have sustained me through the stages of conceiving, developing and building this theory of transition. While we all recognize the rudimentary need FOR support, what we do not always see clearly is how those whom we support hold US up.

My life changed when I began this journey in 1996. Along the way, I have had the absolute privilege of working with numerous new graduates who have not just blessed me with their insights, but have led me to a professional 'place' where I know, without question, I *belong*. How ironic….given that *belonging* is the primary developmental objective of a newly graduated professional nurse. Perhaps it is simply a basic human need.

To my new graduate and student leadership team across Canada—quite simply, I owe you the latter years of my working life. You have nurtured my body by modeling for me how to rest, you have sustained my energy by renewing my faith in the power of the nursing collective, you have expanded my mind by challenging my assumptions and demanding reason and rationale for all I purport, you have balanced my life by reminding me how to work AND play (even *together* ☺), and you have touched my soul with your unfailing commitment to our future. I have never quite known how to thank you for the amazing gift you have been to me. I hope that hearing your 'voice' and seeing your early nursing experiences reflected in the words of this publication will, at least in part, compensate you for the sacrifice, risk and generous energy you have devoted to this work. Perhaps above all, I hope that you feel commensurately honored for the creativity, passion, creative intellect and faith you consistently demonstrate for this profession. I believe in ALL of you. Remember that you ARE the future. Without you we are but rafts afloat with neither oars to steer nor handles to hold—caught up in rapids that are as unforgiving as they are invigorating.

To my mentors, too abundant in collective spirit to do justice to individually—you know who you are—who have shown me 'a way through the woods', oftentimes equipping me with tools I didn't even know I would need to forge my own path. Often, without my knowledge, you positioned yourselves behind me to catch me when I fell; walked ahead of me so I could see HOW you climbed and, when the brush was thick, cleared the way for me; stood by my side when the climb was particularly challenging so I could gain strength and courage from your presence; and surrounded me with your loving spirit when I inevitably and necessarily had to 'go it alone'. When I think of you, I am reminded of the words of Bernard of Chartres—a 12th century French philosopher and scholar—who said that *"we are like dwarfs on the shoulders of giants, so that we can see more than they, and things at a greater distance, not by virtue of any sharpness of sight on our part, or any physical distinction, but because we are carried high and raised up by their giant size."*

To my 'funny' brothers (Brian and Ron Boychuk of the 'Chuckle Bros' http://www.chucklebros.com/) for showing me how the use of humor can save us from the often relentless and confining clutch of 'life' – OURSELVES! I can see now how you provided our family with needed relief during life's darker moments and for that I am truly grateful. Your continued support of my life, my work, and the painful but necessary growth these often demand of us, has been critical to my development. I treasure your unique influences in my life more every day.

To my parents, who demonstrated tremendous patience and sacrifice in their struggles to provide both vision and sight to a curious child with strong convictions. Mom, thank you for doing all you could with everything you had. Dad, I have grown to love the ache that missing you brings.

Intentionally I end with gratitude for you, Eldon. Your Divinely appointed presence in my life has allowed me to understand and fulfill my God directed purpose. You are my partner in every way—my lighthouse when dense fog clouds my vision, my reach when things seem beyond me, my strength when I have grown unusually weary, my spirit when circumstances leave me feeling hopeless and my island when the waves of life threaten to drown me. I cannot imagine my life without you. Thank you for sharing both your strength and vulnerability with me. You have taught me how to love and what it means to be loved. That knowledge has transformed my life.

To He who Divinely appoints my life. . . .in everything I do, I hope to honor you.

Special Mentions

Hillary Clinton had it right when she said '*It takes a village*'. BEING MENTORED MATTERS!!!! I cannot imagine how I might have written a cogent word that carried any hope of international impact without the tremendous support of my treasured colleagues around the globe.

It is appropriate to '*start at the very beginning*' of my graduate journey, during which I was Blessed to cross paths with the following outstanding teachers, researchers and scholars: *Dr. Karen Wright, Dr. Norma Stewart, Dr. Gail Laing and Dr. Debra Morgan (MN Studies—University of Saskatchewan, Canada); Dr. Joanne Profetto-McGrath, Dr. Olive Yonge and Dr. Flo Myrick (PhD Studies—University of Alberta, Canada)*. It is humbling now to reflect on the time I spent in their protected embrace as a young graduate and then doctoral student. I have often thought of the lessons they took the time and energy to teach me, despite being steeped in their own rigorous work and demanding schedules. As Joanne once said (actually it was more than once), '*It took TWO to supervise YOU Judy!* John Bunyon was credited with a notable quote, befitting my feelings toward these mentors: "*You have not lived until you have done something for someone who can never repay you.*"

Lynn Digney Davis, Chief Nursing Officer of the Saskatchewan Ministry of Health Nursing Secretariat is the epitome of a new graduate nurse champion! Lynn received Nursing The Future's inaugural *Torch Award* for excellence in nursing leadership in recognition of her outstanding commitment to the advancement of new nurse issues. Without fail, Lynn has found a way to fund NTF annually, allowing us to take yet another step in supporting grads not only in her province but across North America. Nursing owes you a debt of gratitude Lynn, and I owe you so much more.

Dr. Marlene Kramer, whose work in the 1960s pioneered this field of study, graciously honored my request to write the '*Foreword*' for this book. It is truly difficult to express my gratitude for this act of support and for the lifetime of contributions she has made, and continues to make, to our global nursing community. Thank you, Marlene, for supporting me as I joined your journey to give voice to the newest members of our discipline..

Dr. Patricia Benner's seminal body of work in the evolutionary skill acquisition and knowledge development continuum of practicing nurses changed our world in the 1980s. Her most recent publication, *Educating Nurses: A Call for Radical Transformation*[1] has drawn our attention to the need for a reorientation in nursing curricula commensurate with our professional vision. Through this call to action, Dr. Benner invites us all to share in advancing nursing education, research and practice. Her willingness to support this body of work, and to graciously support my ongoing desire to pave a new way for the newest members of our profession, is truly humbling and inspiring.

[1]Benner, P., Stutphen, M., Leonard, V., Day, L. (2011). *Educating nurses: A call for radical transformation*. San Francisco: Jossey-Bass

I remember the first time I had the pleasure of meeting *Dr. Marilyn Oermann*. It was in Saskatoon, Saskatchewan during her visit to the University of Saskatchewan to work with our faculty on advancing our clinical education platforms. I was driving her to the airport and we stopped for lunch at a local hotel. In one hour, I felt more encouraged in my scholarly journey than I had in years prior. I have kept in touch with Marilyn for 10 years now and her support has never wavered....the spark of her positive nature and her professional encouragement have lit many a dark path for me over the years. Thank you Marilyn, over many miles and years, for '*being there*'.

Dr. Leanne Cowin came into my life in 2001 with the gift of her collegiality. Since that time, she has reached out to me as a mentor, colleague and friend on more occasions than I could possibly count. Leanne has supported and promoted my message about new graduate transition whenever, wherever and to whomever she could. She has successfully traversed our geographical distance in typical 'Auzzie' style—with remarkable humor, humility, transparency, challenge, critique and above all acceptance. You have no equal in my books, Leanne.

Finally, I would be remiss if I did not acknowledge my tremendously supportive colleagues in the *Faculty of Nursing at the University of Calgary*. Dean Dr. Dianne Tapp leads an outstanding and growing team of nurse educators, practitioners, administrators and researchers who are leaving a deep and enduring legacy for our profession. I am consistently impressed with the breadth and scope of their reach in our community and feel privileged to practice amongst them.

Editorial Review Board

I extend my heartfelt gratitude and profound respect to the following colleagues for their editorial contributions to this book:

Christina Cossette, RN, BScN
NTF Professional Development Coordinator
Direct Care—Foothills Hospital
Calgary, Alberta
Canada

Sarah Covino, BScN(s)
4th Year Nursing Student
Lakehead University
Thunderbay, ON
Canada

Noorin Darvesh, BScN(s)
NTF Antigonish Bridge Club Coordinator
3rd Year Nursing Student
Saint Francis Xavier University
Antigonish, Nova Scotia
Canada

Heather Dickie, RN, BScN
NTF Nova Scotia Provincial Chair
Direct Care—IWK Health Centre
Neonatal Intensive Care Unit
Halifax, Nova Scotia
Canada

Meredith Dignan, RN, BScN
NTF Halifax Chapter Coordinator
Direct Care—IWK Health Centre
Halifax, Nova Scotia
Canada

Lisa Doepker, RN, BScN
NTF Sustaining Member
Direct Care—Royal University Hospital
Saskatoon, Saskatchewan
Canada

Jennifer Dolliver, LPN
NTF Halifax LPN New Graduate Liaison
Direct Care—IWK Health Centre
Halifax, Nova Scotia
Canada

Lorisa Earnshaw, RN, BScN
NTF e-Newsletter Chief Editor
Direct Care—All Nations' Healing Hospital
Fort Qu'Appelle, Saskatchewan
Canada

Angela Espejo, RN, BScN, MN(s)
Graduate Student
NTF Social Networking Coordinator
Edmonton, Alberta
Canada

Jodi Foley, RN, BScN
NTF Board of Directors
Direct Care—Regina General Hospital
Regina, Saskatchewan
Canada

Thomas Froh, RN, BScN, ENC(c), CCN
NTF Sustaining Member
Direct Care—Regina General Hospital
Regina, Saskatchewan
Canada

Kandis Harris, RN, BScN, MN(s)
NTF National Leadership Director
NTF Board of Directors
Direct Care—Cardiac Step Down Unit
Regina, Saskatchewan
Canada

Chantal Kachur, RN, BScN
NTF Sustaining Member
Direct Care—Royal University Hospital
Saskatoon, Saskatchewan
Canada

Sophia Lepore, RN, BScN
NTF Edmonton RN Graduate Liaison
Direct Care—Sturgeon Community Hospital
Edmonton, Alberta
Canada

Annie Lucas, BScN(s)
NTF Saskatoon Chapter Leader
NTF Student Liaison
2nd Year Nursing Student
University of Saskatchewan
Saskatoon, Saskatchewan
Canada

Courtney McCool, RN, BScN
NTF Bridge Club Coordinator
Direct Care—IWK Health Center
Halifax, Nova Scotia
Canada

Donnie MacDonald, BScN(s)
NTF Antigonish Chapter Coordinator
3rd Year Nursing Student
Saint Francis Xavier University
Antigonish, Nova Scotia
Canada

Victoria Murray, BScN(s)
NTF Antigonish New Graduate Liaison
3rd Year Nursing Student
Saint Francis Xavier University
Antigonish, Nova Scotia
Canada

Nicole Nanowski, RN, BScN
NTF Edmonton Bridge Club Coordinator
Direct Care—University of Alberta Hospital
Edmonton, Alberta
Canada

Phuong Nguyen, RN BScN
NTF Halifax Bridge Club Coordinator
Direct Care—Capital District Health Authority
Halifax, Nova Scotia
Canada

Anna-Marie Offiah, RN, BScN, MN(c)
NTF Board of Directors
Staff Health/Immunization Nurse
All Nations Healing Hospital
Fort Qu'Appelle, Saskatchewan
Canada

Denyne Park, BScN(s)
NTF RN Student Liaison
3rd Year Nursing Student
Dalhousie University
Halifax, Nova Scotia
Canada

Jennifer Parsonage, RN, BScN (Distinction)
Chapter Coordinator, NTF Edmonton
Perioperative RN—Orthopedic Surgery Centre
Edmonton, Alberta
Canada

Brock Paterson, BSc, RN, BScN
NTF Halifax RN New Graduate Liaison
Direct Care—Capital District Health Authority
Halifax, Nova Scotia
Canada

Ruhina Rana, RN, BSN, BA
Heart Centre—Providence Health Care
Vancouver, BC
Canada

Carlena Scriven, RN, BScN
NTF National Registrar
NTF Sustaining Member
Direct Care—Labor and Delivery
Royal University Hospital
Saskatoon, Saskatchewan
Canada

Krista Smith, RN, BScN, MN(s)
NTF Cape Breton New Graduate Liaison
Direct Care—Cape Breton Regional Health Authority
Sydney, Nova Scotia
Canada

International Editorial Review Board

Jeanne Besner, C.M., PhD, RN
Director—JFB Workforce Consulting Ltd.
Calgary, Alberta
Canada

Janis Brown, RN, MN
Senior Policy Analyst
Department of Health and Wellness
Halifax, NS
Canada

Roni Clubb, RN, BSN, MSA
Faculty—Practical Nursing Program
Saskatchewan Institute of Applied Science and Technology
Wascana Campus
Regina, SK
Canada

Lisa Covey, RN, BScN
Nurse Educator—Practice Support
Professional Practice
Capital District Health Authority
Halifax, NS
Canada

Lynn Digney Davis, MN, RN(NP)
Chief Nursing Officer
Saskatchewan Ministry of Health
Nursing Secretariat/Workforce Planning Branch
Regina, Saskatchewan
Canada

Valerie Eden, RN, BN, MDE
Director
Registered Nurses Professional Development Centre
Halifax, Nova Scotia
Canada

Carol Ewashen, RN PhD
Associate Professor—Faculty of Nursing
University of Calgary
Calgary, Alberta
Canada

Julie Fraser, RN, BSN, IIWCC, MN
Clinical Nurse Specialist
Home Health
Fraserhealth Regional Health Authority
British Columbia
Canada

Lorna Guse, RN, PhD
Professor of Nursing—University of Manitoba
Winnipeg, MB
Canada

Bernadette Julian, RN, BScN, BACS, BEd
Faculty Practical Nursing
Nova Scotia Community College
Sydney, Nova Scotia
Canada

Jo-Ann Lapointe McKenzie, RN, MN
Chief Nursing Officer
Deer Lodge Centre
Winnipeg, Manitoba
Canada

Pat Lewis-Vandenbrink, RN, BN
Manager, PCU 102, ET Therapy Clinic
ACESS Program
Foothills Medical Centre
Calgary, Alberta
Canada

Rosalee Longmoore, RN
Executive Director
Saskatchewan Union of Nurses
Regina, Saskatchewan
Canada

Tracy L. Lust, RN, BSN, MA
Quality and Safety Leader
Surgery and Neurosciences Program
BC Children's Hospital
Vancouver, BC
Canada

Leanne MacKeen, RN, BScN
Professional Practice Liaison
Chief of Nursing Office
IWK Health Centre
Halifax, NS
Canada

Ann Mann, RN, MN
Executive Director/ Registrar
College of Licensed Practical Nurses of Nova Scotia (CLPNNS)
Halifax, NS
Canada

Linda Nelson, RN, BSN
Clinical Nurse Educator
Fraser Health Authority
British, Columbia
Canada

Susan Page, RN, BSN, MSA
Faculty—Practical Nursing Program
Saskatchewan Institute of Applied Science and Technology
Wascana Campus
Regina, SK
Canada

Nicole Pitre, RN, PhD
Faculty of Nursing
University of Alberta
Edmonton, Alberta
Canada

Janet Rankin, RN, PhD
Faculty of Nursing
University of Calgary
Calgary, Alberta
Canada

Tilda Shalof, RN, BScN, CNCC(C)
Staff Nurse, Toronto General Hospital
Medical-Surgical ICU
Toronto, Ontario
Canada

Judith Shamian, RN, PhD
President—Canadian Nurses Association
President and CEO—Victoria Order of Nurses
Ottawa, ON
Canada

Linda Silas, RN, BScN
President
Canadian Federation of Nurses Unions
Ottawa, ON
Canada

Cindy Smith, RN, BScN, MN
Associate Dean
Nursing Division—Regina Campus
Saskatchewan Institute of Applied Science and Technology
Regina, SK
Canada

Heather K. Spence Laschinger, RN, PhD, FAAN, FCAHS
Distinguished Professor
Arthur Labatt Family Nursing Research Chair
Health Human Resource Optimization
Faculty of Health Sciences
University of Western Ontario
London, Ontario
Canada

Pamela Thorsteinsson, RN, BSN, MHS
Director
Professional Practice - Nursing
Fraserhealth
British Columbia
Canada

Kathy Wilson, RN, MN, PhD
Associate Professor
Interim Assistant Dean Graduate and Advanced RN Studies
University of New Brunswick
Fredericton, NB
Canada

United States

Kelly Adams, MSN, RN, PCCN
Doctoral Student & Teaching Assistant
Michigan State University College of Nursing
East Lansing, Michigan
USA

Patricia E. Benner, RN, PhD, FAAN
Professor Emerita
Former Thelma Shobe Endowed Chair in Ethics and Spirituality
Dept. of Social and Behavioral Sciences
Joint Appointment, Dept. of Physiological Nursing
University of California, San Francisco
USA

Ellen Ceppetelli, RN, MSN, CNL
Adjunct Professor
Dartmouth Medical School & The University of Vermont School of Nursing
Hanover, New Hampshire
USA

Patricia A. Duclos-Miller, MS, RN, NE-BC
Professor
Capital Community College
Hartford, Connecticut
USA

Doris Edwards, RN, EdD
Dean Of Nursing Emerita
Capital University
Columbus, Ohio
USA

Marlene Kramer, PhD, RN, FAAN
Professor and Chair, Adult/Geriatric Health Division
School of Nursing
The University of North Carolina at Chapel Hill
Chapel Hill, North Carolina
USA

Renee Norberg, MPA, BSN, MSN, RN-BC
Manager, Education Department
Advocate Good Shepherd Hospital
Barrington, IL
USA

Marilyn H. Oermann, PhD, RN, FAAN, ANEF
Professor and Chair, Adult/Geriatric Health Division
School of Nursing
The University of North Carolina at Chapel Hill
Chapel Hill, North Carolina
USA

Debra Pilling Hastings, PhD, RN-BC, CNOR
Director of Continuing Nursing Education
Dartmouth Hitchcock
Lebanon, New Hampshire
USA

Kendra Varner, BSN, MSN, RN-BC
Assistant Professor / Kettering College
Nurse Residency Program Co-facilitator / Grandview-Southview Medical Centers
Dayton, Ohio
USA

Australia

Leanne Cowin, RN, PhD
Head of Program, Master of Nursing
School of Nursing & Midwifery
University of Western Sydney
New South Wales
Australia

Jayne Hartwig, RN, BN, Grad Dip Nursing (Nurse Ed) Grad Cert Health (Paeds)
Nurse Education Facilitator - Transition to Professional Practice
Women's and Children's Health Network
North Adelaide, South Australia
Australia

Anne Hofmeyer, RN, MPHC, PhD
Program Director: Higher Degrees by Research
School of Nursing and Midwifery
University of South Australia
Adelaide, South Australia
Australia

Christine Holliday, RM, RN, BN
Midwifery Education Facilitator - Transition to Professional Practice
Women's and Children's Health Network
North Adelaide, South Australia
Australia

Karen White, RN, BEd (Adult and Vocational), Cert IV Training and Assessment, MRCNA, ITD Accred.
Acting Director
Centre for Nursing & Midwifery Education & Research
Coordinator, Transition to Professional Practice Program (RN)
Flinders Medical Centre
Southern Adelaide Local Health Network
Bedford Park, South Australia

United Kingdom

Lynn Basford, RN, PhD
Retired Dean and Professor of Nursing and Health Sciences
Education and Research Consultant
Energy Medicine Practitioner
Basford Associates
Whitwell, Notts
UK

Preface

From Surviving to Thriving – Navigating the First Year of Professional Nursing Practice was originally published in 2006 through my organization *Nursing the Future* ©, selling over 5000 copies in Canada, the US and Australia from 2006-2011. In 2007, I completed my doctoral dissertation on the experience of professional role transition for the newly graduated nurse; this constituted my 4th serial study (3 qualitative studies of my own and the retrospective analysis of qualitative data from a study by Dr. Leanne Cowin in Australia) in this substantive area of research. At that point, I felt confident that my evolving findings had generated a grounded theory of transition for new nurses that I could stand behind . While the 1st Edition of this guide provided a solid framework to guide both new nurses and those who support them, it lacked the detail contained within my Stages of Transition © and Transition Shock © theoretical constructs and the strategies that arose both out of my research and through my work and consultation with thousands of novice and experienced nurses, managers and educators who seek to support new nursing graduates in professional role transition. These additional insights are offered in this 3rd Edition.

The response of the professional community to my work has inspired me to create a program of research that will further examine the professional role transition of new nurses and extend those insights to other disciplines. As of the writing of this 3rd Edition, I am leading one study exploring the experience of professional role transition for Accelerated Degree Nurses (prior non-nursing degree graduates) and another study of male nurses making their initial transition to professional nursing practice. As well, I am a Co-Investigator on a research team led by Dr. Janet Rankin (University of Calgary) to understand how the social construction of the contemporary nursing workplace influences the new graduate's initial experience of nursing practice. Finally, alongside Dr. Jane Lemaire (Medicine) and Dr. Jean Wallace (Sociology) from the University of Calgary, I am exploring how physicians newly licensed for independent practice experience their initial professional role transition.

Once again, I have been truly blessed to work with a devoted team of new graduate nursing leaders, all of whom have assisted me to build this resource for you. I would like to acknowledge their tremendous work in supporting their colleagues in transition and being champions for the facilitation of a healthy professional role transition

[1]It is important to note that while my initial 4 studies were conducted with Registered Nurses in acute-care practice areas, this book and its contents have been exhaustively vetted by Practical Nurses in a variety of positions including student, new practitioner, practical nurse educators and managers. While the majority of new nurses (of all scopes) continue to make their initial transition to professional practice in acute-care, I took significant steps to ensure this book was edited by new nurses whose experiences of transition included rural, community and public health practice settings.

for new practitioners of nursing. It is with the deepest gratitude that I acknowledge **Kandis Harris RN, BScN, MN(s)**, the **National Leadership Director** for *Nursing The Future* along with my thoroughly outstanding ***NTF New Graduate Leadership Team*** for the inspiration they have offered me for the past 12 years. Working with these young leaders has transformed me and allowed me to be all that I can be as a nursing leader. I am humbled to include myself among these brilliant minds, enduring spirits and compassionate souls. Finally, I have been blessed by the committed support of numerous professional and personal mentors throughout my 32 year career. **The 2nd Edition International Editorial Review Board** includes many of those supporters and I am eternally grateful for the guidance and encouragement they offered me as I wrote this book.

Directly as a result of the selfless cumulative efforts of over 100 grassroots leaders, NTF continues to support nursing's newest professionals as they strive to sustain their professional values at a time when everyone is being asked to 'do more with less', practice to a standard that honors the experiences of the patients, families and communities they serve, and fulfill their dual—and oftentimes competing—desire for a dynamic, challenging professional career and a quality personal life. We say it can be done—but we all need support to do it.

I challenge you to take what is offered in this resource and use it to challenge, confirm, validate, sustain or advance your experience AS a new graduate or your work WITH new graduates. I encourage my senior colleagues to look around them for that new nurse who is in need of encouragement, support and your experienced perspective. Equally, ***I remind all new graduates reading this book*** to be aware of the growing force of support that is yours if you can find the courage within to grab hold of the out-stretched hand. We must ALL be within reach of the 'other' in order to create something stronger—in order to be more tomorrow than we are today. This is the legacy we are all privileged to leave.

The future is built by giving the next generation reason to hope.....

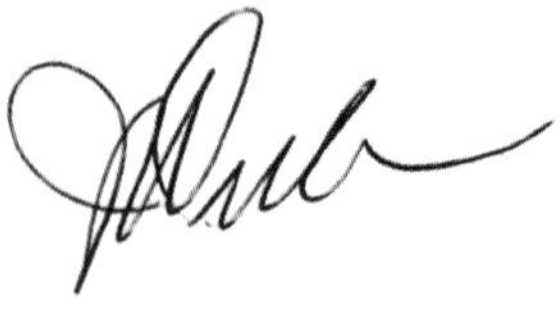

Judy E. Boychuk Duchscher RN, PhD
Founder and Executive Director
Nursing The Future ©
www.nursingthefuture.ca

Introduction

This book offers new nursing graduates, experienced nurses, managers and educators a basis for understanding the issues inherent in making the transition from nursing student to professional practicing nurse in the contemporary healthcare climate. Please note that this book was written to reflect the collective experiences of new graduates and students from Canada, the United States, the United Kingdom and Australia. If a component of the text does NOT resonate with your geographical context, please keep this in mind. It was my intent that the book be as inclusive as possible without appearing biased to any one geographical location. I hope this is your experience in reading it.

The content in this book was reviewed by the NTF Canada Leadership Team, as well as numerous nursing students, newly graduated and experienced nurses and nursing leaders throughout North America, Australia and the United Kingdom. The knowledge used to develop and evolve the *Transition Shock* © model and the *Stages of Transition* © theory that frame this publication exists as part of the ongoing research and study program of Dr. Judy Boychuk Duchscher. The anecdotal evidence that substantiates these stages and the suggested strategies for a successful transition that are contained within this resource have evolved out of the experiences of new nursing graduates. A debt of gratitude is owed to the many new nurses who have contributed to our understanding of the struggles and triumphs experienced while making the transition to professional nursing practice.

This book has been licensed to Nursing The Future© by Dr. Boychuk Duchscher for limited production and distribution. Funds from the sale of these books are committed to providing resources and initiatives that support the professional role transition of new nurses and to developing new nursing leadership capacity.

Published by Nursing The Future© 2012

How Will This Book Help You?

This 'survival guide' (as my new grad leaders like to refer to it) will accompany you through the first 12 months of your journey into professional nursing practice. We know (because we've been there!) that there will be ups and downs during this initial year, but remember that you are NEVER ALONE. The numerous colleagues who have gone before you now embrace you with words of wisdom, smiles of encouragement and the outreached hand of support. *Nursing The Future* and all of your new graduate and experienced colleagues, both in this organization and within your new practice settings, will be there for you any time you need them. Yes, there will be times of loneliness, painstaking growth and personal, as well as professional, change. But this will be balanced by many moments of comforting familiarity and thrilling success. You will learn that you can't have one without the other - that when you are up to your eyeballs in one (either screaming YIKES or yelling YIPPEE), the other is on the horizon…and so it goes.

The book is divided into chapters: *Chapter 1* provides an overview of the process of transition and offers you insights to consider PRIOR to graduating as a professional nurse. *Chapter 2* introduces you to Transition Shock and walks you through the elements that both influence and are influenced by your initial entry into professional practice. This comprehensive section emphasizes the wholistic nature of transition and talks about why many graduates feel a sense of 'shock' when taking on the full weight of their professional nursing role for the 1st time. Unlike the extensive emphasis it assumes in this publication, thankfully this phase of transition is relatively short-lived ☺ and may be significantly muted for those who have strong supports during this time, have previous familiarity with the workplace in which they are transitioning, or whose life experience has afforded them perspective on relationships, work and the process of transition.

Once over this initial 'hump', the remaining elements of the 1st Stage of Transition—DOING NURSING—unfold within about 4 months after orientation is complete and the new nurse is 'on their own'. *Chapter 3* outlines this *1st Stage of Transition* as a time of recognizing and accepting that life is different now that you are a practicing nurse. This is a time of focus for the new practitioner; doing what is required of you as a fully responsible and accountable nurse and 'getting through your shift without killing anyone' (not really, but this is how it feels…) is your primary objective. *Chapter 4* follows with an overview of the *2nd Stage of Transition—BEING* A NURSE—during which time there is an evolution in your perceptions of what nursing is and you strive to make sense of what has changed for you. This third chapter offers guidance on how you can reconcile what nursing 'is' with what you thought it 'was' and, perhaps more importantly, what you want it 'to be'. We want you to know that you are not alone in what you are feeling or experiencing – contrary to the evidence that may overwhelm you during that 2nd Stage, YOU ARE NOT GOING CRAZY!

The *3rd Stage of Transition*—KNOWING NURSING—or *Chapter 5* of the book, accompanies you on what has by this point (we hope) become your 'accepted' career. It speaks about how you, now a more seasoned professional with an idea of what you want, can move forward in nursing while also moving nursing forward. It draws attention to the new perspectives you are gaining about healthcare as a system, and offers you ideas on how to pursue the path in nursing that can develop you professionally and satisfy you personally.

In **TEXT INSERTS enclosed with shaded boxes** I have interspersed 'famous' quotations—some are intended to give you a much needed emotional break and some are intended to simply give you pause. As well, there are narratives (verbatim text from my research) that you will find in **indented text with double quotation marks and italics**. these are the words of new graduates JUST LIKE YOU who faced what you are facing and shared their experiences with me; now I am sharing them with you. Standards related to research ethics prohibit me from sharing the names of the individual/s from whom these narratives originate.

Each chapter culminates in a 'review' section at the end that is situated in summative commentary that highlights what I believe you:

1) NEED TO KNOW

2) NEED TO THINK ABOUT

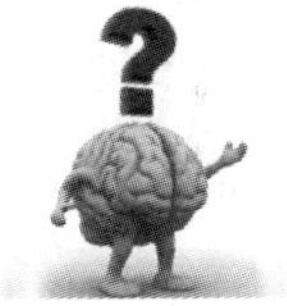

3) NEED TO DO

Finally, there are numerous and extensive **APPENDICES** at the back of the book that offer tips on how to find the professional role that matches your aspirations and inclinations, strategies to cope with the first 12 months of your professional role transition and resources that can assist you to advance both your career and the profession.

We offer you this resource with the hope that it might help you to feel more understood and less overwhelmed.

So let's begin.....

Foreword
Dr. Marlene Kramer

Years ago, when Judy first introduced herself to me, she recounted her journey to secure a copy of my now-archived book *Reality Shock: Why Nurses Leave Nursing*. She talked about spending months scouring the bookshelves of her 'senior' colleagues and searching 'used' bookstores for a copy without success. I thought to myself, this nurse researcher is really serious about pursuing the work I had started on examining the trials and perils of new graduate nurses in their initial professional practice experience. Since then, I have tracked the progress and evolution of Judy's research and am honored that she asked me to write the foreword for this book.

Nursing is the planned, scientific alteration of patients' *internal* and *external* environments with the intent of placing them in the best possible situation for the laws of nature to act, thereby facilitating the healing process. Nightingale's definition of nursing, based on the "environment as alterable medium" theory, served as a platform for two Institute of Medicine (IOM) reports that have captivated and revolutionized the health care industry and professions. The first IOM report, published in 1999 was entitled: *To Err is Human*, and described healthcare in US hospitals as unsafe, citing as many as a million people injured and 98,000 dying annually as a result of medical errors. (Subsequent studies in multiple countries suggest that the above statistics may have been largely underestimated). The 2003 IOM report, *Keeping Patients Safe: Transforming the Work Environment of Nurses* followed up on the initial report with identified solutions to environmental problems that threatened patient safety by affecting nurses and nursing care, and challenged the health care industry and professions to improve work environments of nurses. Most recently, the IOM has published a third report, *The Future of Nursing: Leading Change, Advancing Health* (2011) which emphasizes the close ties between nursing work and patient outcomes, recommending advancement in the education, practice preparation and utilization of nurses across all scopes of practice. Interestingly, the foreward pages of this latest report quote Goethe: *"Knowing is not enough; we must apply. Willing is not enough; we must do"*. I believe Dr. Duchscher's book represents a living example of this vision as she makes the journey of professional role transition for new nurses 'come alive'. Judy not only offers the newest members of our profession insights on what to 'do' to optimize this journey for themselves, but affords those of us who seek to support them a framework by which to do so.

Patient, family, clinical and organizational situations and interactions constitute the *external* environments of practicing nurses while the physical and emotional stress, loss of self-confidence and reduced self-esteem that result from the differences between the concept of nursing they learn in school and the concept of nursing demanded of them in hospital nursing practice constitute the nurse's internal environment. My extensive research of *magnet* environments clearly demonstrates that the external environments within which nurses practice strongly influence their internal environments. Although professional practice environments impact performance of all nurses and health care professionals, they have a profound effect on new graduates' tolerance, motivation and ability to engage in safe practice. Structured support—usually in the form of Nurse Residency or Transition Facilitation Programs—that utilize evidence-informed approaches to alter both the *internal* and *external* environments may well be the most effective way to enhance the new graduate nurse's role performance, provide job and professional practice satisfaction, and halt the flight of these aspiring professionals from the bedside and from the nursing profession.

My work in the 1960s was the first to explore the concept of *reality shock* in newly graduated nurses. Using reflective learning seminars, I sought to counter the negative socialization effects of the workplace on these newly graduated nurses' *internal environments*. The four decades that have transpired since my original work have given way to tremendous change in our healthcare systems, particularly in hospital practice where most new graduates start out. Dr. Duchscher, in her work, has emphasized the direct and interactive impact of the external environment on new (or aspirant) professional nurses.

In this new book, written specifically for newly graduated nurses transitioning from academia to their first employed professional practice experience, Dr. Duchscher summarizes the results of her 12 years of research. Through her direct observation of new graduates in clinical practice situations, countless interviews and focus groups, years of undergraduate teaching, and most recently through her experiences mentoring hundreds of new graduate leaders as part of her non-profit new graduate support network *Nursing The Future*, Dr. Duchscher has built a grounded theory that describes the *journey* of transition. This much needed explication is an outstanding contribution to our understanding of the difficulties and joys nurse graduates experience in their first year of practice. Of prime importance is that Dr. Duchscher's work focuses on new graduates' *external* as well as *internal* practice environments. Her theory is intended to help the new nurse gain 'insight' into the structures and processes that underlie the challenges they might be experiencing, while providing them with initiatives and approaches that can be used to alter BOTH of these environments.

A word to new graduates: This is not a dull, dry textbook. As you travel with Dr. Duchscher through your transition journey, you will encounter a delightful and very practical mix of theoretical concepts, enlivened and illustrated by quoted excerpts from practicing new graduates, light-hearted humor, as well as by parenthetical author feelings and comments. The very unusual first person insertion of the author's experiences and comments offered by Dr. Duchscher not only brings her concepts to life, but creates a feeling of 'oneness' between new nurses everywhere and the author.

Through the understanding and subsequent framing of new graduates' lived experiences, others who read this book will be in a position to assist newcomers to cope with the alterations of their internal environments while assisting them to adjust to, and perhaps even change, the structures and processes in their external environments. Through a deep understanding of the transition journey lived by new grads, experienced nurses, clinical coaches, preceptors and mentors can facilitate the socialization and professionalization processes needed to support these aspiring professionals, their professional practice and the quality of care offered to the communities that nurses serve.

Marlene Kramer, PhD, RN, FAAN

About the Foreword Author:

Dr. Marlene Kramer received her BSN from St. Louis University in 1953, her MSN from Case-Western Reserve University (1958), and her PhD in education/sociology from Stanford University (1966). While at Stanford, she had the opportunity to study with Dr. Leon Festinger, father of the Cognitive Dissonance Theory that has become the major theory providing direction for coping with the "expectation-reality generated stress" encountered by nurses and other health care professionals in initial positions post graduation. She has held a variety of positions in Nursing Service and has been a member of the faculty of three Schools of Nursing: University of California in San Francisco, University of Connecticut, and University of Nevada, Reno where she was the first occupant of the Orvis Chair in Nursing Research. In the late 1960's, Dr. Kramer tested the effects of an *Anticipatory Socialization Program* during academia, the first stage of professional socialization, on senior nursing students' role conceptions. This study led to the publication in 1974 of her seminal work *Reality Shock: Why Nurses Leave Nursing*. From 1974 to 1979, Dr. Kramer received the first federally (US) funded research grant focused on empirical testing of programs designed to alleviate Reality Shock and assist new graduate nurses in making the transition from academia to acute care practice. This series of studies tested the effect of Reflective Seminars, Bicultural and Conflict Resolution training on new graduate nurses' transition into practice, and resulted in two publications—*Path to Biculturalism* (1977) and *Coping with Reality Shock* (1979).

For the next 20 years, Dr. Kramer's research focused on nurses' work environments and the effect that these have on nurses' productivity, satisfaction with the work of nursing, and retention. The birth of the *Magnet Hospital* concept in the early 80's provided the opportunity to conduct this extensive program of research in institutions of Excellence. Since 2000, Dr. Kramer and her colleagues at *Health Science Research Associates* have conducted a series of 8 studies in which they have identified 9 essential structures and 8 essential work processes that produce productive, healthy work environments and desired patient and nurse outcomes. Her current research program focuses on the impact of healthy work environments and Nurse Residency Programs on new graduate transition and integration into practice.

Student Nurse to Professional 101

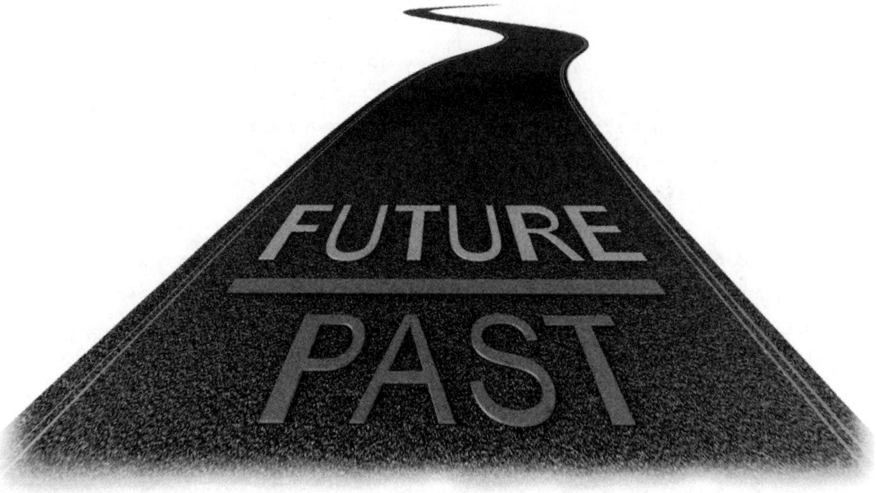

Welcome To Nursing!

Accepting your 1st role as a professional nurse is the beginning of the next phase of *'the rest of your life'*! Isn't that how the saying goes? It is, without a doubt, one of the most exciting times of your life!!! Having said that, I'll bet there is also a place, deep in the pit of your stomach, that turns at the thought of graduating—that feels nervous and strangely anxious about what's ahead. That is likely because you are not entirely sure what it will be like to practice as a 'real' nurse and you may not know who you will be working with, if you will be able to work well together, or even if you will find the work you are looking for. You may not really have a good sense of what will be expected of you as a new nurse, what unit or institution you will be employed by, how working as a professional will be different from working as a student. This guide is intended to respond to these concerns with insight about this experience AND to offer you hope and support as you make your way into the profession of nursing.

> ***I attribute my success to this – I never gave or took any excuse.***
>
> ***- Florence Nightingale***

> *"It would be nice to sort of be able to talk with [someone] to say 'is this where you're at or am I really not getting this' or 'okay this is normal and this is how we sort of go about this'. I worry that [other] new grads usually by this point are functioning completely independently and effectively and efficiently and I'm sort of back here stumbling through the motions."*

Anytime someone makes a 'change' from what they know to what they don't know or are not completely familiar with, they experience a transition—a journey from what **was** to what **is**. It is not so much the actual CHANGE (motivating event or 'catalyst') that challenges us, but the process of MAKING THE CHANGE. *Transitions* are considered passages or movements from one state or condition to another and they can profoundly influence and alter the lives of the individuals involved as well as their significant others (friends, family and co-workers). Transitions usually begin with events that create instability and make change necessary—graduating as a nurse and moving from being a nursing student to being a fully responsible professional nurse IS such an event.

> *"It hasn't sunken in yet actually. Like I was amazed the other day because I took my shoes to work and I could actually leave them there. Like I have a locker and I can leave my stuff there and it's hard to get used to the fact that this is kind of a permanent thing. That it's not a 4 month rotation or four week rotation or a three month rotation or whatever."*

Making the transition from being a student to being a 'real' nurse is rewarding and exciting. At the same time however, it can be frightening, lonely and overwhelming as the realization dawns that you are responsible for what happens with the patients under your care, and that you are essentially 'on your own'.

> *"I like to think of myself as a competent [person]. I do like to think that I do have some degree of competence. Now going into this profession, one shift is never like the other. You have to be prepared for whatever can be thrown at you and like I've told my co-workers, for me it seems like whenever it rains, it pours for me meaning that when one thing goes wrong or one admission comes in, I get three. And it's almost like it's harping on my confidence a little bit right now. It's kind of breaking it down and I've never felt like that before so maybe I'm questioning this position I'm thinking to myself 'can I do this'? And that's new for me 'cause[1] up to this point it has been 'how am I going to do this'? Now it's 'CAN I do this at all'?"*

We want you to know that you are NOT alone – that every other nursing student who has ever graduated goes through a similar process of adjustment. Have patience and know that you WILL get through this experience and you will become the professional nurse you have always wanted to be.

> ***Whatever my individual desires were to be free, I was not alone. There were many others who felt the same way.***
>
> ***-Rosa Parks***

But let's not get too far ahead of ourselves. As Julie Andrews' character Maria sang in *The Sound of Music*, "Let's start at the very beginning....a very good place to start"!

Prior to Graduating

> *"You know they talked a lot about it in school and I always thought 'Uh, whatever'. I thought you know that's common sense but it's not really when you think about it... Like they did ask us questions in school about 'OK, you have this patient, this patient, this patient. Who do you go to first?' Those kinds of questions. And I just thought she's [faculty] the meanest woman in the whole world. She just wants to trick us! But you know what? I think we needed more of that cause you need that once you're there. I think that's why I found her a difficult teacher is cause she's teaching you things that you really needed to know. You needed to know those things to be on the ward and to be by yourself and it just seemed like a lot when you were in that class. You thought, 'Oh like you ask too hard questions'. We shouldn't be knowing these things but you should and I'm glad that she did talk about things. Like she did talk about someone*

[1]In North America, the word '*cause* acts as an abbreviation of the word 'because'. The Australian equivalent would be 'coz'.

coming with this and this, what do you think their diagnosis is going to be. And you know she wanted you to analyze the situation and through that know what steps you should take and I never really realized it then but now I'm like 'Oh'. If only I'd paid attention to what she was saying to me."

My research, the numerous conversations I have had with leading scholars on the subject of nursing and my lengthy experience teaching nursing and working with newly graduated nurses has taught me that the process of 'socialization' into the profession begins LONG BEFORE you enroll in a nursing education program. For instance, can you tell me you haven't seen episodes of 'ER', 'Scrubs', 'Grey's Anatomy' or 'Nurse Jackie' before or during your education? And we all know that these shows give people impressions about what nursing IS

School is learning things you don't want to know, surrounded by people you wish you didn't know, while working toward a future you don't know will ever come.

-Dave Kellett

and what nurses DO. We also know, and you have likely learned over time, that not all of these impressions are accurate. Some students go into nursing because they have experience with a family member who is a nurse and they admire that individual for the work they do, or even just 'like' them personally and associate who they ARE with what they DO. Some students have had experiences with the healthcare system prior to entering school, either as a young patient or as the family member of someone struggling with a health challenge—they see a role for themselves in making a difference in the lives of individuals in need. Finally, there are the encounters with experienced nurses that you have throughout your education; some of those encounters have likely inspired you to be better than you currently are, while some may have made you wish you had never started......these experiences are not new, nor unique to the nursing profession. Sad to say, but human nature can, on occasion, be strangely disappointing.

"Disappointed I would say is the biggest thing because you have an expectation that you're going to graduate and become a nurse. You're going to buy a nice house. You're going to drive a nice car. You know everything's going to be dandy and then you get out and you have a bunch of older nurses that it feels like they hate you, you know, where they're ready to run you off the floor you know. You realize that you owe $40,000.00 in student loans and you can't get your new house. You can't get your new car. You know, it's a disappointment."

Some people reasonably assume the healthcare system will always need nurses and further, that employability as a nurse is a relatively timeless certainty. And finally, some individuals (like me!) see nursing as a rewarding, dynamic, flexible, mobile career that can take you ANYWHERE and allow you to do almost ANYTHING (my experience tells me that's TRUE!). All of these experiences breed expectations and they don't call them 'lasting impressions' for nothing!

A novel is balanced between a few true impressions and a multitude of false ones that make up most of what we call life.
-Saul Bellow

So, chances are there were very personal reasons that grounded your decision to enter nursing. Those reasons may well have influenced:

1) what you chose to study (the subjects you wrote about in your papers for instance);
2) the area of practice you are seeking as a professional (hospital, community, or public health);
3) how you see your role in relation to other healthcare providers (how nurses relate to other healthcare providers and the relative autonomy, respect and acknowledgment they are afforded); and
4) how you 'want' to practice in relationship to your patients, the communities you serve and the profession as a whole (hands on direct care, nursing education, research or administration for instance).

It is important that BEFORE YOU GRADUATE you take time to explore the reasons why you wanted to be a nurse in the first place, how those reasons might have changed and how your reasons might be challenged or supported by the roles you anticipate assuming as a practitioner in the 'real' world. This reflection will help you to prepare to practice in an area that is compatible with those expectations. Case in point—if you enjoy working in high intensity, rapidly changing situations you may want to choose a busy medical-surgical hospital unit as your initial practice experience. Conversely, if you like to teach, work to develop programs and initiatives or provide international healthcare relief, you may want to consider a community, public or international placement. As well, this kind of self-knowledge can alert you to the potential incompatibility of your goals and expectations with the jobs for which you are applying. For instance, if you enjoy rapidly changing situations but you have a history of a stress-induced ailment, you may want to choose an initial practice context that has lower stress, or you may want to consider casual or part-time work in acute-care after graduation so you can control your hours and workload intensity during your initial adjustment to a professional practice role.

We shall not cease from exploration. And the end of all our exploring will be to arrive where we started and know the place for the first time.
-T.S.Eliot

"Well maybe because when you're a student, you know you've like a maximum of three people to take care of ever as a nursing student, and then you come out and you've got ten. Like ten is a big difference you know, and plus, on top of that, like those three you care for from what 7:00 in the morning till 2:00 in the afternoon, you barely make it to post-conference. Now I'm working shifts with ten other nurses and as students you really helped each other out like you know you've

been friends. You've been together for four years and now I get out to the unit and nobody wants to help me it seems like and yeah, it's different. It's just so different. By the end of the day I can't even think straight or stand up anymore. It's just I've been run off my feet every day."

Despite these suggestions, the reality is that you might not always HAVE a choice about where you work initially. While you may want to work in surgical acute-care or public health initially, the positions available to you may be in long-term care or medicine. Or, there may be personal circumstances (a desire to stay close to family, children or a spouse) in your life that require you to remain in the area where you graduated, limiting your options for employment. You may also feel anxious about leaving your education-based hospital experience behind too soon AND the acute-care job market may be more open to novice practitioners than other agencies (more experienced nurses often seek the less *physically* demanding work found in homecare, community or public health). So despite the anxieties that come with acute-care nursing, you may choose to 'start' your professional career there, branching out later in your career to community, public or home health positions. Remember—this is a CAREER and you WILL get where you want to go—it just might not be immediately!

Regardless of WHERE you choose to nurse at the start of your career, or WHAT role you take on as a new nurse, there are certain elements of BECOMING a nurse that are common to the vast majority of graduates.

He knows nothing; and he thinks he knows everything. That points clearly to a political career.

-George Bernard Shaw

What's the Deal with Transition?

"I might as well start by telling you that it's the hardest thing I've ever had to do was to make the transition from going to school to practicing in the real world. Everyone told me everything is going to come together. But that's something I have learned – I had to experience it for myself."

As we talked about above, the transition from being a student to being a fully responsible, accountable, professionally practicing nurse is one of the most anticipated moments of a person's career. The fact that we are formally 'ending' one phase of our professional socialization and moving into another assumes a certain degree of change—changing roles, responsibilities, relationships and knowledge. With these changes come additional or different pressures, expectations and challenges. It is what you have prepared for throughout your education, but when it actually happens, it often hits you like a wet towel across the face.

> *"Hmm. Strange. I don't really feel like I am done [school]. Like I walked to work one morning and as I was walking I was thinking 'I'm getting paid to do this' cause it was like I was still in clinical and you know like I know it's different. I mean there's a little bit of financial freedom now, which is nice. I can actually do things that I enjoy. But yeah it's very strange to all of a sudden be done and it's like the thing is, I found this especially when we first got out of school. You build up for years and there's this huge excitement of graduating and then you have your first shift and your first you know all these firsts. All at once."*

Newly graduated nurses usually begin the process of professional role transition once they formally leave the safe and predictable confinement of their nursing education program. In fact, some have described the 1st year of professional nursing practice as 'an obstacle course,' with the graduate experiencing their work as overwhelming, primarily because of expectations of employers (and graduates themselves) that they will 'hit the ground running'. There may be individuals with whom you work who do not appreciate, or have clearly forgotten, the struggles of starting out as a new professional. These individuals may give you the impression that you should be functioning more like a experienced nurse rather than at the level of a graduate nurse.

> ***A love for humanity came over me, and watered and fertilized the fields of my inner world which had been lying fallow, and this love of humanity vented itself in a vast compassion.***
> ***-Georg Brandes***

> *"I feel like yes I am ready. I've been through my school. If there's something I don't know, I have all the textbooks. I have people to ask. I mean I know that there's so much learning yet and it's still to come and that I'll feel more comfortable with more experience. But at a new grad level I'm ready. You know I can work as a new graduate."*

As a new grad, you recognize that things are 'different', but you may not yet be sure exactly what that means. To begin, you may be experiencing total and independent responsibility for your own life for the first time, managing your own money and caring for your own home (complete with cleaning, laundry and shoveling walks ☺). You may be paying your own rent or mortgage now, maybe paying off the loans you accumulated during your education, and trying to figure out how you are going to pay your VISA with your MASTERCARD so you can afford that long-anticipated vacation that doubles as a reward for all your hard work in school!

> *"Well I think that it's just a lot of what people tell me—you know like 'You're done school', or 'welcome into the real world.' Like that's always what I've heard and I just think 'Yeah like now I have to start paying those bills and I have to start paying back that student loan' and you know like things can start moving now."*

Perhaps you are looking to live apart from friends who have served as your roommates throughout college or university. If nursing is your 2nd professional diploma or degree, you may have children or a spouse (or perhaps aging parents) who have been 'patient' with your absence the past couple of years and now expect you to be there for and with them. It doesn't take long for you to begin to wonder what happened to the 'time off' from life's stresses that the end of this long study period was expected to produce!

> *"I really didn't think it was going to be that different. But it was a big change going from a student to actually having to be there doing things. It is a big change and it's really overwhelming. Kind of like you know happy about it one minute and bawling about it the next. You're just not sure what to think."*

All of these issues bring with them unexpected, and perhaps even disappointing, reminders that life is complicated—that hard work doesn't always 'pay off' immediately, or even in the way that we thought it would, or think it should. It's a strange juxtaposition—graduating and getting back into your 'real' life—it has its joys AND its challenges. Now, just managing your relationships with, and responsibilities to, family, friends and significant others while trying to navigate a work schedule, get to know new colleagues, re-establish a personal life, figure out who you ARE when you aren't studying and understand what it means to BE a professional nurse consumes your energy and time—you just exchanged one set of challenges for what almost seem like GREATER challenges!!

We're not lost! We're just locationally challenged.

-John Ford

> *"I just find for me, I'm not at the point where I'm confident in my abilities yet and I feel like I just want somebody to reassure me that 'Yes, that's right Barb' You can do that'. It's like a continual. It's always and it's in almost everything. I feel like I just want to know that my clinical judgments, my clinical assessments, that they're correct. That I'm not missing something and that because I want to be competent and safe....I just want to make sure. It's like back to the word scary like it's just kind of scary to be making those decisions."*

> *"I am feeling increasingly confident in my nursing abilities everyday but feeling like I am failing at life. Graduating was supposed to mean I was going to get my life back but I can't seem to find the balance. I work and sleep, and everything else seems so hard to incorporate."*

TAKE A BREATH.......you'll land on your feet!!! This is simply a period of time where you are learning how to balance the personal with the professional as you explore the new dimensions of your life separate from being a student.

What Factors Influence a New Nurse's Transition Experience?

My research has consistently revealed that new nurses leave their basic nursing program with the ability to apply a critically thoughtful and reflective approach to their practice as nurses, but within weeks of being introduced into the 'real' world, their practice becomes more about *doing* than *knowing*. While this often corrects itself over time, there are factors contributing to this 'back peddling' in the new graduate's initial few months of practice:

1) the majority of graduates transition into professional practice through the dynamic, fast-paced and relatively unforgiving environment of acute-care;
2) acute-care patients are more clinically complex and generally sicker than ever;
3) the care resources available to nurses have not kept pace with the demands of nursing work;
4) new nurses are not entirely prepared to work in 'teams', therefore their comfort level with and knowledge of task delegation, supervision of unlicensed staff and workload collaboration with nursing and allied health colleagues is extremely limited;
5) students are not consistently expected to integrate population health indices in their patient/client care (i.e. the majority of acute-care admissions are geriatric patients yet the issues related to gerontology—for instance the propensity for dehydration in the elderly—are not comprehensively considered in the daily care planning of the aged acute-care admission);
6) the education of nurses has advanced in the direction of a primary health care focus, while the environment within which new practitioners work remains based upon a biomedical 'illness' model of care that focuses nursing work on '*doing*' rather than '*knowing*'; AND
7) the varying scopes of practice of nurses, and the emphasis on power rather than value sets nurses up to compete rather than collaborate on ways to optimize the care of their patients.

The nursing profession expects much from its members. I have always been an acute-care practitioner (except for several stints up north and some community development projects) and have worked as both a direct-care nurse and a clinical educator. I would always tell my students that nursing in acute-care will ask you for everything you have; then when you feel you have given everything you could possibly give, it will turn around and ask for more. I can completely appreciate how difficult it is for the experienced practitioner to sustain their passion and energy AND instill hope in others while working in a system that:

- calls their employees in for overtime on a daily basis;
- is unable to adequately or consistently honor their requests for days off even after those requests have been approved and their plans secured;
- maintains a census requiring nurses to care for 'clients' who are consistently more complex, admitted with multiple, chronic co-morbid conditions, as well as socioeconomic and psychosocial challenges that make caring for them exceedingly complicated and consuming;
- requires vulnerable individuals to be admitted to hallways, closets or abandoned supply rooms due to bed shortages;
- does not always ask nurses what they think about a new staffing schedule or care delivery model before implementing it; AND
- fails to support leaders who, despite their tremendous sacrifices, feel powerless to affect change that can advance the profession toward its agenda to 'heal the nation'.

I lived in similar times as a new graduate, but life has gotten increasingly layered as the world has evolved. And so it is with our healthcare system.

> ***Insanity in individuals is something rare – but in groups, parties, nations, and epochs, it is the rule.***
>
> ***-Friedrich Nietzsche***

It's complicated……

In part perhaps because of their own challenges coping with a system within which they have long worked, some of your disenfranchised colleagues (nurses and physicians) reinforce the idea that in order to 'fit in' you must simply 'get the job done' within the existing institutional and socio-cultural traditions of the workplace. Sometimes complacency is just easier than banging your head against a wall in an attempt to 'make change'. As a new nurse, you may get subtle messages to 'keep your head down and your nose to the grindstone'. In other words, FOCUS ON GETTING YOUR WORK DONE ON TIME regardless of the patient or family issues that distract you or require you to change the priorities of your day. Though it is your responsibility to question the rationale behind what you do as a nurse, and the focus SHOULD BE our patients, families and communities, workplaces are cultural, political and social communities of their own. It may appear initially as if to align yourself with your new workplace means you must simply do things the way they've always been done, and refrain from challenging established routines or protocols. In fact, there may be subtle but important 'rewards' for this relative conformity—acceptance by your colleagues.

Finding that balance between what you believe SHOULD be happening and what IS happening is sometimes difficult to negotiate. You need to be careful not to be seen as presumptuous and pretentious by over-criticizing what you see without first seeking to understand WHY things might be the way they are. As much as a particular practice might not make sense to YOU, try to remember that it made sense to SOMEONE at some point. While it may be that times have changed and this way of doing things is no longer effective or even SAFE, it might also be that this WORKS at some level that you simply don't understand. It is always advised that you INVESTIGATE the details surrounding a situation before suggesting it should be otherwise if long term change is really what you are trying to accomplish.

To be honest, one is wise to be cautious during ANY new employment period; a relative truth is that nursing care decisions are not always explicit (i.e. easy to determine, able to be prescribed or 'taught'). You will want to tread the fertile ground of nursing practice with caution when you begin, as there is a certain reverence for what has come before. In a profession that is so critically dependent on experiential knowledge, complex judgment and advanced decision making, the practitioner cannot quickly or easily learn what it means to be an 'expert'. While relatively 'simple' situations may be approached prescriptively (by the strict application of existing knowledge 'blueprints'), more often than not, the human experience and expression of illness is complex, multidimensional and 'grey'. *Theory*, while unquestionably essential to framing nursing practice, is wholly inadequate when faced with a threat to human health, be it individual, community or population. It takes significant experience in a variety of contexts to evolve theoretical 'knowledge' into nursing 'know-how'. In other words, it takes time to develop expert nursing practice and if you're anything like I was as a new graduate, you may not have much patience as you move forward with your plans to CHANGE THE WORLD!

> *"Probably even two weeks after I started—just 'You're having a bad day.' Nothing's going right. Everyone's crabby and you go home and you're thinking, 'Why did I choose this profession?' And then I'll phone my mom, who's been a nurse for 30 years, and she'll tell me 'You know you'll have good days and you'll have bad days and you know you're just having a bad day', so I gotta remember that. But yeah there's been a few days when I'm thinking, 'why did I pick this because it's just so stressful at times you just can't win with anyone. Nobody's happy and nobody's pain is relieved'. But then there's days that remind you that it's worth it."*

HOLD ON TIGHT everyone....this first ride can feel more like a rollercoaster than a merry-go-round!

Transition Shock

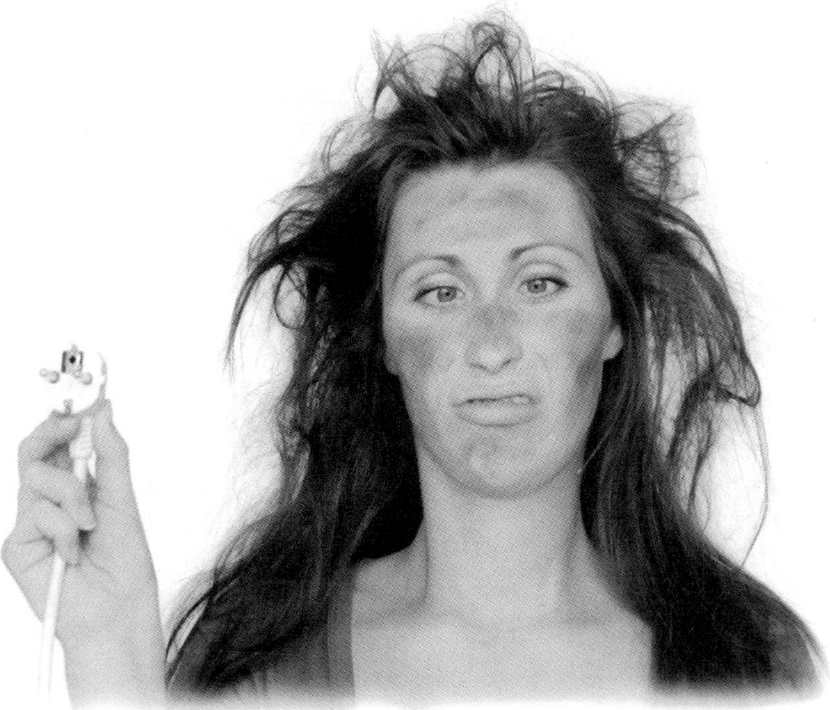

A Shock to the System

> *"And then you get there and you have a patient who has gone bad and you're like 'this is just too much for me. I don't want to come back tomorrow.' You just have one bad day and you're like, 'I never want to go back there again. I can't do this. No one should have passed me in nursing. I'm not good enough to be doing this'. And then you talk to someone. They're like 'you know tomorrow will be better. Go back and it will be fine'. I was talking to RN's that have been there for 6 months to a year, and they still have those days and even up to 4 years they've been there. I think you're always going to have some of those days that are just bad and you just want to go home and cry. But you just have to forget about it and start the next day new."*

Transition Shock© is the term I have coined to embody the elements of the new nurse's initial entry (the first 1-2 months after orientation) into the workplace. I chose this term because it best captures EVERYTHING related to roles, responsibilities, relationships and knowledge that both motivate and mediate the intensity and duration of a graduate's earliest experiences as a nurse.

> *"I might as well start by telling you what I felt when I first started because I've kind of come to the conclusion that it's the hardest thing I've ever had to do was to make the transition from going to school to practicing in the real world. Everyone told me everything is going to come together. But that's something that I have learned....no one could tell me what was going to happen. It's something that I had to experience for myself...."*

My work with transition shock builds and expands on Dr. Marlene Kramer's[1] theory of 'reality shock' from the 1960's by demonstrating that the new nurse engaging in a professional practice role for the first time is confronted with a broad range and scope of changes that are both expressions and catalysts of the experience of transition.

How these changes affect each new nurse (YOU) is influenced by:

1) how familiar, expected or anticipated and consistent the levels of responsibility and accountability are in your new job when compared to what you learned in your education;
2) how extensively you were afforded insight into these expectations during your education, how 'quickly' you are asked to take on increasingly complex and risk-intensive situations;

[1]Kramer, M. (1974). *Reality shock: Why nurses leave nursing.* St. Louis: C. V. Mosby.

3) how much support you are given as you navigate the early days of your new roles and responsibilities;
4) your level of developmental 'maturity' or life experience; AND
5) any prior nursing practice experience you have had (LPN/RN/Enrolled Nurse), including being an employed student nurse in the area where you are now working.

Further to this, new nurses are often expected to apply clinical knowledge to practice situations with which they may have little or no experience, or that may not 'look like' the situations they learned theoretically.

> *"Well it's a lot of responsibility and the ward I work—the nurse-patient ratio it's quite heavy. There's quite a variety of conditions that we see so it takes time to know a little bit about everything. Because I'd never been there as a student, I felt it was really hard to get familiar with things and it's intimidating at times and you know you're making decisions that you really don't feel comfortable making or you know you're not sure if you're correct in the decisions you're making."*

An impressive finding throughout my research has been the 'surprise' expressed by new nurses as they are faced with the challenges of transitioning into a professional workplace role. The predominance of this feeling in a graduate nurse should inform us that we have somehow failed to either adequately prepare senior students for the reality of the transition experience **and/or** not put in place the supports necessary to ensure a gradual, smooth and tenable entry into the 'real' world of practice.

> ***Democracy is a process by which the people are free to choose who will get the blame when something goes wrong.***
>
> ***-Lawrence Peter***

This is not about laying blame on either the education OR the healthcare employer systems. It is about sharing responsibility and accountability for preparing, orientating, transitioning, integrating and stabilizing the future practitioners upon which the healthcare system is completely reliant—YOU!

I have come to believe that it is not possible, nor desirable, to expect that the process of moving from school to professional work will be uneventful; this period encompasses tremendous growth for a new professional and with such significant growth necessarily comes struggle. Transition shock speaks to the extent of the initial struggle (anywhere from 2 weeks-2 months) to adjust to a new reality. While the experience changes over time (we will talk more about the stages of transition later) and individuals express their experience varyingly, I have identified the 'initial' professional role transition for the new nurse as extending for approximately 12 months following orientation. This is not to imply that there is ever really an 'end' to the growth and development of a professional nurse. As Dr. Patricia Benner[2] has so clearly outlined, nurses continue to progress through skill and knowledge acquisition stages throughout their career. The task for both you and those who support you is to determine what you can anticipate during the different stages of transition, what can and cannot be done to reduce the unnecessary difficulty in this process, and what strategies can be created or implemented to remove the obstacles to a successful professional transition, or support you through the rough spots that most graduates describe.

> ***Support the strong, give courage to the timid, remind the indifferent, and warn the opposed.***
>
> ***-Whitney M. Young, Jr***

Let's Talk *SHOCK*

There are two critical issues that feed into the experience of transition shock. The ***first issue*** is that professional nursing practice is NOT as simple as the application of theory to 'text book' clinical events (that are oh, so rare….). Rather, the development of proficient practice habits results from: 1) the subtle integration of theory into varied practice experiences, 2) the maturation of one's political, economic, organizational, cultural and socio-developmental insight, 3) the know-how that comes with collaboratively consulting with other nurses and healthcare professionals during the course of a day, and 4) the expertise that settles in as one both observes and participates in practice over time.

> *"Probably organizing your day. Like you have much different responsibilities [as a practicing nurse]. Like prioritizing who you're going to go see first. Why you're going to go see them first. What things you need to get done first. What things can wait…I would say that would be my issue just like making decisions on how you know this person is a little more sick. We'll deal with this now and so-and-so can wait to get up in the chair because it's not really important right now. So then you just figure out what needs to be done right now and what can wait 20 minutes or whatever."*

> *"Like when I'm working on a unit without an assist or an aide, if you don't get, you know, so-and-so bathed until 3:00 in the afternoon, as long as it gets done today like that's fine, you know. It's stuff like that. You know you get your meds out on time. You have certain things that they expect you to get out on time as per schedule obviously but the other stuff is very flexible. Like I would come in at 7:30 and check in on everybody and get my vitals done and get all my a.m. meds given and I sit there for a minute and I go 'Okay, I have a minute to*

[2]Benner, P. (1984). *From novice to expert: Excellence and power in clinical nursing practice.* Menlo Park, CA: Addison-Wesley.

breathe.' Maybe I should be charting'. And then all of a sudden... bang... call bells are ringing and doctors are writing orders and blah, blah, blah, and the next thing you know it's 10:00 and you have to do the next a.m. meds and 'Oh, I didn't get any of that charting done yet and I still haven't listened to so-and-so's lungs'." How do you go about determining which of these things you really need to do? For instance, if a physician came in and wrote some orders or needed to chat with you and you hadn't yet listened to someone's chest that you were concerned about, how would you go about making that decision?"

The ***second issue*** related to the transition shock experience is that it is not JUST a professional experience. The response to a major change like your initial integration into a professional role affects the WHOLE of you: it is intellectual, physical, social, cultural, developmental, spiritual, emotional and economic. While it is commonly accepted that there will be an adjustment when making a significant change in one's life such as the initial integration into professional practice, what is often underestimated is the degree of pervasiveness of this experience. If it were JUST a 'theory-practice gap', then the adjustment would be relatively linear—get more experience and you're set!

There are several elemental aspects of transitioning from student to professional that new graduates commonly describe as part of their experience and which I have seen as correlating with the intensity and duration of transition shock – you judge whether or not they apply to your situation:

1) As a new nurse, you want your workplace colleagues to respect and embrace what you have to offer as a professional and you want to be 'accepted' as a competent practitioner—it is a basic human need to belong or 'fit in';
2) There are financial, physical, emotional and relational stressors that accumulate over the years as you complete your education;
3) You may not be completely aware of the socio-cultural nuances of the workplace into which you are transitioning and therefore may not know who wields what kind of power in your new social structure;
4) Your confidence is often fragile during the initial months of your transition;
5) Most graduates have accumulated debt during school so getting and KEEPING A JOB is relatively high on the priority list;
6) Work in nursing is an 'ebbs and tides' kind of thing; sometimes employers are bending over backwards for you to work and sometimes you have to think quite creatively about how you can grow 'nursing' skills and aptitudes doing something OTHER than nursing until the job market opens up again...but it ALWAYS DOES;
7) The theory you have learned intellectually does not always translate easily into all possible ways that human illness can express itself; AND
8) New nurses care very much that their practice is safe.....

In short, like I said before, it's COMPLICATED!!!! Making the transition to professional practice can feel as though you walked out of your education and into some sort of MAN-wHOLE that someone forgot to cover!

SOCIO-DEVELOPMENTAL

- Changing social structures
- Role uncertainty & unfamiliarity
- Inadequate & insufficient guidance/assistance
- Professional culture naiveté
- Intra-interdisciplinary relations
- Intergenerational dynamics
- Leadership & delegation skills lacking
- Oppressively hierarchical work structure
- Evolving self - separation from dependent role
- Loss of known supports
- Insufficient exposure to role models

EMOTIONAL

- Labile nature of emotions
- Emotions variable in origin
- Intense and overwhelming feelings
- Extreme sensitivities
- Seeking validation and reassurance
- Seeking familiar protective nurturing
- Require positive reinforcement
- Fears of failure or incompetence
- Fears of disappointing family/friends/colleagues
- Loss of control
- Lack of support
- Emotions fed by w'hole' experience

TRANSITION SHOCK

- Theory-Practice incongruence
- Witnessed practice improprieties
- Lack of knowledge on role transition
- Lack of awareness regarding graduate roles and responsibilities
- Limited practice aspect/pattern recognition
- Limited tacit/practical knowledge
- Practice inconsistency/unpredictability
- Limited decision making and clinical judgment capacity
- Organizational naiveté
- Professional role-relations immaturity
- Limited performance feedback

INTELLECTUAL

- Relentless and terminal physical, emotional, intellectual exhaustion
- Energy consumed to conceal feelings and transition responses
- Physical demands of acute-care
- Unaccustomed to full shift presence (minimal time off unit), full shift rotation (36-48 hour work week), or shift turnovers
- Emotional extremes
- Maladjustments to shift-work
- Sleeplessness – active dreaming
- Poor nutrition and lack of exercise
- Change in social habits and routine

PHYSICAL

Transition as a w'HOLE' ©

Just Before The Earth Moves

Prior to the onset of the transition shock experience there are often feelings of elation, excitement and anticipation; after all, you have worked so hard and sacrificed so much to get to this point. We are often somewhat idealistic during our educational preparation. As a nursing educator, I can't imagine teaching you only what nursing IS without teaching you what it COULD BE. Having said that, I think it is my sense that the greater the anticipation of being able to enact ALL the values that you held dear in your education, the more susceptible you are to the range, overwhelming intensity and labile nature of the experience of professional role transition. The degree to which you experience transition shock, and the relative skills you have to manage that experience, depend to a large degree on previous life experience, the maturity of your coping skills, how quickly you are expected to get 'up to speed', the degree and nature of the support that exists in your new workplace, and how DIFFERENT the world of work is from what you experienced as a nursing student.

It was not uncommon in my research, nor is it in my ongoing work with nursing students and new graduates, to hear them using words, phrases or expressions such as 'terrified' and 'scared to death' when referring to their transition experience.

> *"As a student moving into the 'real world' in a few short months, I have recently (during the past month) become scared, anxious, and hesitant regarding graduation. It has occurred to me that it will be the first time I will encounter this degree of responsibility, accountability, and change."*

New graduates claim that relentless anxieties are routine during the initial weeks of being on their own (usually after orientation is complete and they are given the full weight of responsibility for a nursing workload). It is 'normal' for you to have some anxieties around your ability to perform with confidence and competence as a new graduate, and it is normal for you to be unsure about how to interact with new colleagues. I also believe that how you experience your introduction to professional nursing work significantly influences how you come to view your professional capacity, the path you feel you CAN take in nursing and the confidence with which you deal with the evolving stages of professional role transition. The workplace where you first experience nursing as a fully accountable professional nurse is critical to your progression – **so think about this as you begin.**

> *"I think we're just trying to put everything together of what we learned in school and trying to think back on things and... you go through a lot of, 'Should I do this, should I not be doing this, should I go back to school'...I found I was very hard on myself. Very critical of what I was doing and wanted to quit a few times. I think it really makes a difference on where you start and how your experience is at that time. It changes your opinion of nursing."*

For many newly graduated nurses, the experience of transition shock feels 'like I just jumped into the deep end of the pool'. While we assume that ALL graduating nurses are **prepared** to practice as beginning nurses (that IS the purpose of the rigorous evaluative expectations of your educational colleges and the reason for your national qualifying examination), some new nurses (like other new professionals) are not **ready** to jump into their practice with both feet.

> *"I think you're trying to understand who you are as a nurse in those first 6 months... I think you discover which kind of nurse you want to be like cause you see others and you try and follow somebody that you want to see as a role model."*

For many, there is a lack of awareness regarding the toll this initial transition may take on their personal energy and time, and on their evolving professional identity. Although most graduates anticipate some adjustments to their professional work situation as they leave school and move into practice, prior to this transition you probably rarely doubted your choice of career nor did you likely question the investment of the years of study that were required of you. No doubt, you expected to be met by a welcoming collegial environment and afforded a workload that is challenging but achievable; more an extension of the roles and responsibilities you have grown accustomed to as a senior student. It is common for new nurses to anticipate the thrill of actualizing the professional role to which they have earned a title, and it is also normal to expect a certain level of recognition for the knowledge you have acquired and the commitment you have already made to the profession. These are very reasonable expectations.

> *"You know all of those feelings are just overwhelming you and you don't know what's going on, you just have too many feelings. But now that...we're all calm and doing okay, now we can look back and see all the stuff that we've done and learned."*

What I would like to do now is to review the experience of transition shock, offering some insights into why the experience plays out the way it does. You may relate to all or just some of the elements of the experience and likely at varying levels of intensity when compared to your fellow colleagues going through this transition. I can tell you that the experience of transition shock is not linear, and not necessarily similar in the way it is expressed or managed from person to person. I can also tell you that the personal and professional adjustments of this period have been found to affect graduates most intensely in the first 1–4 months post-orientation (the time after which workplace orientation processes and additional induction learning has taken place and after the new nurse had been teamed up with a senior qualified nurse for the purposes of learning expected routines, roles and responsibilities). I would anticipate the adjustments to vary according to your own personal history, coping mechanisms, support systems, co-existing life issues and stress resilience levels.

> ***Any transition serious enough to alter your definition of self will require not just small adjustments in your way of living and thinking, but a full-on metamorphosis.***
>
> ***-Martha Beck***

Foundational Elements of Professional Role Transition for New Nurses

There are intersecting foundational elements that feed into your initial experience in the workplace: 1) stability, 2) predictability, 3) familiarity, 4) consistency and 5) success. It is important to say at the outset that the underlying issue here is 'control' – having an environment that is stable, predictable, familiar and consistent that in turn allows one to feel successful speaks to our innate desire to control what happens to us, including when it happens, how it happens, and with whom. These elements, when in 'order' put us in the driver's seat of our own life. The challenge with a major change like professional role transition is that much of what is happening is outside of our control—leaving us stranded on this island of uncertainty—and we consume a lot of our energy just trying to get things BACK to 'normal'. Often our limited knowledge of what is ahead translates into 'let's get things back to the way they WERE' as we recognize this former way of being and know how to cope with it—it's comfortable. But, often without realizing it, doing just that prevents us from moving ahead to what is beyond that which we currently know, making it hard for us to accept, adjust, adapt, and ultimately grow.

I hope now you can see why it is SO important to understand the foundational elements that feed into a new nurse's sense of control—success in making a healthy professional role transition with the least amount of resistance DEPENDS on this knowledge!

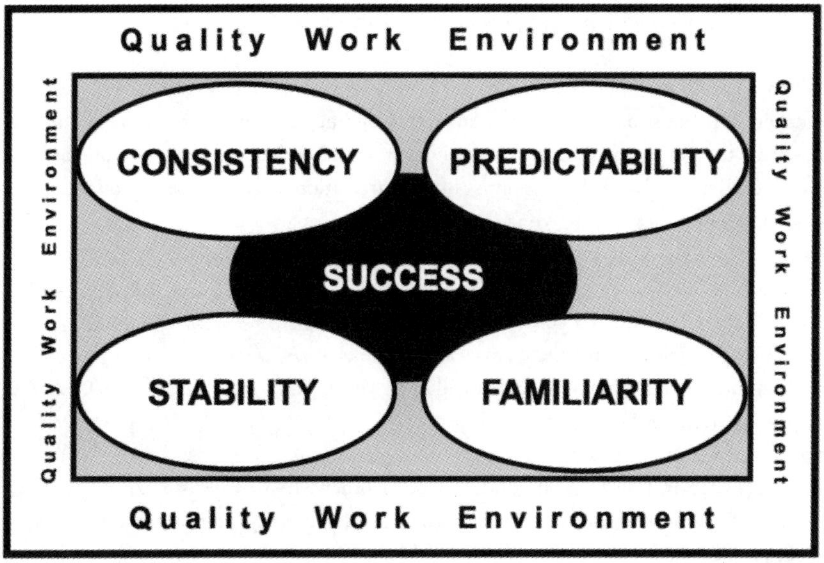

Quality Workplace Factors for New Nursing Graduates©

So, let's talk about each of these elements as they relate to how you evolve as a new nurse. Strategies to address some of the issues related to these elements will be waiting for you at the end of the chapter!!

STABILITY, as used here, refers to how steady the circumstances and situations are for you during your transition experience; essentially, stability refers to that which is unlikely to change or 'deteriorate'. If we think about you as a PERSONAL being, this translates into having a POST-GRADUATION life that you recognize as similar to what life was like BEFORE your transition to professional practice took place. Now, there are individuals who thrive on chaos (hhhhmmmm, well, I don't really know too many who truly thrive on chaos outside of the fact that it can be motivating and exhilarating for limited periods of time and may be familiar if one was exposed to chaos a lot as a child....) and therefore they may have more well developed skills to cope with instability in their life. But **stability** is the quest of the human 'being'—it is a fundamental feature of 'homeostasis', which even from a purely bio-physiological perspective is something all humans seek. I mean, seriously, have you been to an amusement park lately? The roller coaster is an AWESOME ride—it's exciting and scary in a safe sort of way. But I couldn't stay on it all day—I want to get my feet back on the ground or the shifts in equilibrium just disorientate and nauseate me.

> *"My 1st 6 months were horrible. Absolutely horrible....it was just the whole confidence, being in a new place,...not knowing what to do as a nurse cause I'm just starting out and just the situations that I don't know—that you get put into and you're not confident and you don't know what you're doing."*

When it comes to your LIFE, you might want to spend some time thinking about how stable your current life situation is as you enter this significant change. If you are a student about to graduate, you might want to think about how many decisions you can 'put off' until you have experienced the initial 6 months of your transition so that those personal changes don't contribute unnecessarily to your transition stress. When you are considering all the changes you are anticipating, remember that POSITIVE changes are still changes—moving, purchasing a home or car, getting married. While these are clearly exciting and wonderful events in your life that will bring you much joy, remember that they will also consume your energy and contribute to 'instability' in your life. Just keep in mind that if you CAN delay other MAJOR decisions until you have been working for at least 6 months, it will allow you to conserve needed energy that may get you through the initial stress of this life change.

> ***If the people who made the decision were the people who also bore the consequences of the decisions, perhaps better decisions would be the result.***
> ***-John Abrams***

Now, as for the change that you can't control......life has its way with us more often than not and controlling change is not always possible. Sometimes you simply have to roll with it. In such cases, simply being aware that you ARE experiencing instability in your relationships, your financial situation, your living arrangements or other areas of your life will be a step toward managing your stress during transition.

So what about you as a PROFESSIONAL—how do you manage the level of stability in the workplace? The factors feeding instability in the workplace are less likely to be 'in your court' as they say – you may not have as much control over these factors, but you DO have *some* control over whether or not you choose to be employed there and ultimately, we all have control over how we RESPOND to what is happening around us.

To begin, **ASK QUESTIONS!!!!** For instance, when you meet key individuals with whom you may be working in the near future (and you should ALWAYS meet with the manager, the clinical educator and several nurses—senior and junior—in the area to which you are seriously considering working), think about questions you might ask them:

- how many nurses have left in the past year and for what reasons;
- what kinds of staffing levels do they maintain (what is the nurse-patient ratio, how often are nurses called in on overtime and how much sick time does the unit manage on a weekly basis);
- how long is the average length of stay for patients on this unit/in this health center;
- on average, what is the 'census' of the unit (how many beds are full on average each day OR how many clients will I be expected to visit each day and what is the region/ part of the city I will be responsible for OR how many programs will I be given responsibility for);
- what is the level of acuity of the patients (how SICK are the patients on the unit—how is that measured and if patients deteriorate over the course of a shift, what adjustments need to be made for this change in the workload of the nurse);
- what kinds of social activities do they organize for their staff (how 'social' the staff are often tells you a lot about how 'happy' they are working there – even high workloads can be managed if staff work together and enjoy each other);
- how much time does the manager spend interacting with staff;
- what are the opportunities for continuing education (when was the last educational session for nurses, how many attended, were they replaced to attend the session, and what was the session about);
- do they employ support staff (housekeeping, unit clerks, porters) after 4pm;
- do people enjoy working there (are there 'humor boards' or cartoons scattered about the unit/workplace, do they have a social committee and when is the last event they organized);
- what does a typical day look like for a nurse in this workplace;

- on average how many breaks do the nurses *actually* take each day; AND
- how do staff collaborate on the provision of care (how do Registered Nurses and Licensed or Registered Practical Nurses[3]/Certified Nurses Aides discuss and distribute the care required from their team during a shift.

These questions can be asked as you meet with different people in your workplace (remember to pose varying questions to nurses on the unit—not just the manager, educator, coordinator or charge nurse). Another strategy is to ask similar questions to different people and see if the responses vary. These questions can give you insight into how 'stable' the unit is to which you are thinking about going. It is not necessarily that what you hear will STOP you from going to that unit (TRUST ME – there are pros and cons to EVERY place of employment and there is NO workplace Nirvana!!), but the answers might prepare you for some of the checks and balances you will need to put in place for yourself during your transition to that workplace.

I need to make a comment at this point about the 'clinical' stability of the patient demographic you choose to care for as a new nurse. My research in the emergency department was particularly enlightening for me around this. New nurses, though often highly intellectually competent and skilled, have had very little experience witnessing acute decompensating patterns of change in patients that are associated with high levels of risk (likelihood of catastrophic outcome). The new nurse's ability to recognize subtle changes in a patient's clinical condition is significantly limited by their inexperience (remember at the beginning of the book when I was talking about the fact that MOST nursing knowledge comes from dealing with increasingly complex situations over time—as they say, "there's nothing like experience").

> *"Some of the new grads have come to me now and said, 'I don't know what we were thinking, we don't even know where we are as nurses and here we are in an emergency department where you're expected to know and do and anticipate', and like they said they're so tired of learning they just want to catch up to what they've learnt instead of cramming all of this information in and not really being able to digest it....It's such a different focus, emergency though you know....it's just their [new grads] problem solving skills aren't there. They get stuck and they can't move forward. And they're not able to change quick."*

This lack or absence of 'tacit' knowledge may render the patients, new practitioners and their colleagues vulnerable. If you add to this mix the highly **unpredictable** (rapidly changing situations that cannot be anticipated), **unfamiliar** (the potential for numerous clinical conditions being presented), **inconsistent** (the variation in clinical presentations of a given condition) and **emotionally charged** (patients whose health may be threatened or families

[3] Practical Nurses are variably referenced as Licensed or Registered, according to geographical location. For the purposes of clarity, this nursing scope of practice will be referred to dually as Licensed/Registered Practical Nurse or as LPN/RPN in this publication. Specific reference will be made to Enrolled Nurses and Registered Psychiatric Nurses when appropriate.

who are often in crisis) context of high acuity practice areas such as the emergency room and critical care, you have a potentially **volatile** environment with a high risk for an unhealthy, ineffective and potentially unsafe transition.

While there are always exceptions to the rule, my experience as a critical care nurse who started in ICU after only one year of nursing experience, and my research and work with numerous new graduates inspires me to caution others regarding the practice of hiring new graduates into high acuity environments (particularly emergency) right out of school. The stability of the patient population you are going to care for as a new nurse is very important to your professional development.

> *"I just found it interesting that one of the new grads said that one of her co-workers upstairs…got to spend the whole year and learn who she was as a nurse and that was something that the new grads in emerg didn't get to do. She said you get to mature as a nurse for that 1st year as to who you are and what it is you really want to do with all this knowledge…get to learn about yourself as a nurse."*

> *"I could see us hiring them as new grads and then not setting foot in our department for 6 months to a year…Send them out to different areas to work for 4-6 weeks as a buddy and just learn the process and MI's and what kind of care there is.…Send them to neurology and get them used to seeing…normal to abnormal or abnormal back to normal…and getting that kind of ground under them."*

Remember that your **primary task** as a new practitioner is to **develop** (NOTE TO SELF: this does not say **'HAVE'**):

- a strong base of organizational skills, time management competence;
- foundational skills in the assessment of the 'normal—abnormal' continuum (be that clinical pathophysiology or community and relational dynamics);
- the capacity to prioritize and delegate;
- cultural and social knowledge related to working on *a* team and working with *this* team;
- an understanding of how expectations of a graduate nurse differ from those of a senior student;
- the ability to balance your personal and professional life (or actually FIND your personal life again….);
- the flexibility to navigate the circadian and lifestyle flux that is synonymous with shift work; AND
- an understanding of how to collaborate and consult with allied health professions (physicians, social workers, physiotherapists, etc.).

AND to do so in a *relatively safe environment* (that means personally AND professionally safe).

PREDICTABILITY for a new graduate is concerned with their ability to know:

1) ***WHAT*** they will do (what level of performance is expected of me now that I am a graduate nurse; what do I need to 'do' in this role; am I comfortable enough with those in charge to be able to tell them when I am in 'over my head');
2) ***WHERE*** they will do it (where am I working; am I going to the same workplace every shift or floating to multiple units; if I have to start as a casual[4] employee how can I get enough hours without exposing myself to too many unfamiliar workplaces);
3) ***WHEN*** they will do it (am I working 8-hour or 12-hour shifts; what is the rotation; when 'this' happens [a code, a death, a distraught patient, a diagnosis of an STI[5] , a suicide in the community] how do I respond);
4) with ***WHOM*** they will do it (who will I be working with, who do I go to if I have questions, who can fire me, who can I trust); and
5) ***HOW*** they will do it (what are the differences between what I did as a student and what is expected of me now as a graduate nurse, what will I do if I come up against something I have never done before.

To be honest, the WHY doesn't enter the picture that much during this initial stage of transition (Stage 1)—for most new graduates, 'WHY' can be too complex and potentially threatening, leading to places that are inconsistent with a new graduate's primary developmental objective—finding a place where they fit and belong. Asking 'why', at the BEST of times, can be defensively or reactively received by others (particularly if those other individuals don't know the answer either but feel like they should) and has the potential to inadvertently expose to others that the new nurse 'doesn't know'.

> *"Because we're still focusing on the skill and the assessment. I don't think ahead, like I can't. I can think of certain things, but I don't think, 'Oh this person may have this going on inside'. Like it's hard for me to think that way when I'm concentrating on just getting them set up and oxygen and everything."*

Asking WHY will come later so don't beat yourself up if you feel like a taskmaster initially—your feet will grow to fit your shoes and you get to leave those shoes in your own private locker ☺. The key is to find someone or someplace where it is safe for you to ask the 'why's' that come out of your practice, even if that is not at work (i.e. perhaps it will be with a peer colleague over lunch or your nursing mentor over a beer).

> *"You know, because they've seen it, they've been there, they know, they've seen thousands of things and I don't have those gut instincts. I have a few, but not like*

[4]The position of a *casual* nurse is variably referred to as *relief, per diem*, or sometimes *agency* nurse. This term is used to identify a nurse who is NOT on a line or in a permanent or part-time position, but comes in to relieve staff during illnesses or vacation.
[5]Sexually transmitted infection (STI)

> *they do....It's like asking a person who's never seen a cat before to pick out a cat. So you trust people with the experience and the gut feeling. There's been times when I wish I had that feeling about a patient."*

The challenge of **FAMILIARITY** for the new nurse is that **LITTLE** is familiar. Familiarity evokes a sense of: *'I've seen **THIS** before'* and perhaps even *'...and I know EXACTLY what to do about it'!!*

NOT the usual mantra of the newly graduated nurse ☺

If you were privileged to be employed as a senior student or spend your final practicum (or CAPSTONE[6] experience) on the unit or in the practice context where you intend to work as a graduate nurse, the enhanced *familiarity* that results from these experiences may significantly influence your transition stress. Even knowing WHERE to get what you need to do your work is a relief of transition stress (i.e. where the STI kits are in the clinic or where the special bags of N/S with 20meqK+/L are located on the unit).

> ***No man can climb out beyond the limitations of his own character.***
>
> ***-John Morley***

Knowing WHO is WHO (you know what I mean—who is *really* in charge) in the practice area is very helpful. While I know many new graduates who experience phenomenal collegiality with their senior counterparts as newcomers, there are equal numbers who are quickly introduced to, or warned about those individuals to 'avoid' because they 'eat' new nurses..... A new workplace is a bit like a minefield—you obviously need to keep moving but no one tells you where the mines are planted (sometimes even THEY don't know) and not all mines have obvious triggers that you can see before they explode.

Floating[7], or being part of a team of nurses who work on different units depending on the staffing needs of those units, is often presented as an employment option for new nurses.While at first glance it may seem like the ideal place to 'get experience', you must remember that the experience you get is often less predictable (you often do not know what unit you are going to until you arrive that day), less consistent (as a float nurse you can easily be on one unit your first shift and a different unit the next shift), and less familiar. Because you rarely float to the same unit each day, the chances that you will work with the same staff each shift is unlikely, reducing your ability to get to know them, the patient population, the unit-specific routines or even the way supplies are organized. While the patient population on the various units you

[6]CAPSTONE refers to a senior nursing practicum where there is a clear intent to facilitate the students' ability to bring together the parts of their nursing program learning into a 'whole' by 'consolidating' theory into practice just prior to graduation (also called transition, immersion or consolidation courses).

[7]Also referred to as *Nursing Resource/Relief Team* or *Agency Nursing*

go to as a float nurse might be relatively stable, this staffing arrangement does not allow for the fundamental practice, professional or developmental needs of newly graduated nurse.

> *"I was originally in the float pool, that's how I started out nursing, floating between four or five different units in the hospital. Now I'm on one unit and I'm actually on the unit where I started, where I had my fourth year practicum…so I mean, I, it's a comfortableness there. I think being known and getting to know the staff is a huge thing for adaptability [as a new nurse]. Um, like that questionnaire…on what is the one thing that made your transition easy…and I would have to say that would probably be just knowing the staff before going in."*

IF this is the only option available to you as a grad, see if you can negotiate a start (orientation followed by several months of work) on only 2 float units; get orientated and work for a period of time in each and THEN add on additional units **slowly**. In these cases it really is critical that you have an individual on every shift that you feel safe going to with questions or to ask for assistance.

It is in the area of familiarity that nursing residency/internship programs (also sometimes called a Graduate Nurse Program, a Transition to Professional Practice Program or a Transition Facilitation Program) or less formal staffing arrangements are able to impact significantly on a transition experience. Programs vary but generally these 'extended orientation' programs provide you with support for around 6-12 months with the intent to gradually 'introduce' you into the work expectations of a fully functioning, accountable and responsible nurse (according to your scope of practice). There are different models but many programs try to balance 'theory', or the learning of work and practice environment expectations, with actual 'work' assignments given to the new nurse on a daily basis. Supernumerary staffing means that you work WITH patients and your colleagues without being given an actual ASSIGNMENT. The advantage of this is that you can move around your new environment, taking advantage of various learning experiences, getting to know your colleagues and the patient demographic without the stress of predetermined workload expectations. Most residency, internship or graduate nurse programs have a component of supernumerary staffing embedded into their structure—but the way they roll out the program and for how long differs between institutions. It is most certainly worth discussing with the manager during your recruitment interview.

Mentorship or preceptorship programs constitute another approach to 'familiarizing' you with your roles and responsibilities as a new nurse. The concept of *mentor* usually encompasses a longer-term, more 'personally professional' relationship between a novice and experienced nurse. Conversely, the role of *preceptor* is often associated with the transferring of *skill* knowledge and therefore is often used in the context of a pairing between a nursing student and their senior nursing guide. Having said that, *preceptors* can also be expert clinical nurses who are buddied[8] with a new nurse for the purposes of teaching them about the roles, routines and responsibilities related to their new workplace. Along those lines, it is thought that individuals can be 'assigned' a preceptor, while a mentor is someone you choose because this relationship requires more of a personal connection between mentor and mentee. The tenure of mentorship and preceptorship programs is usually determined by the manager or educator where you are to be employed and may vary anywhere between 3 weeks and about 6 months. While a preceptor often comes to their role with a focus on helping you develop your 'skill' as a new nurse, mentors more commonly extend themselves beyond that which you 'need to know' to assist you to access social, cultural, relational and professional knowledge and opportunities as your career develops.

> ***If you want to build a ship, don't herd people together to collect wood and don't assign them tasks or work, but teach them to long for the endless immensity of the sea.***
>
> ***-Antoine de Saint-Exupery***

It is important to note that a formal transition program is different than an 'orientation', the latter referring more to a relatively narrow and usually more limited and brief introduction to the **INSTITUTION/CENTER** and **GENERAL AREA OF PRACTICE** where you will be working. Often consisting of anywhere from several days to a couple of weeks, an orientation usually includes an introduction to the basics of being an 'employee' such as getting paid, accessing employee benefits, documenting your nursing care or responding to a fire; kind of the 'nuts and bolts' of the workplace. A **'general'** orientation (about the hospital/healthcare center/institution) is usually followed by a **'practice specific'** or '**nursing**' orientation that informs you about the unique aspects of working on a particular unit/community center/clinic that you will need to know to function on a day-to-day basis. Remember that some workplaces simply have an ORIENTATION, while others have a more layered approach to familiarizing the new nurse to their workplace (transition facilitation, graduate nurse program, mentorship or preceptorship, internship or residency)—you should find out what YOUR employer has to offer as this may contribute to your decision to accept the offer of a position.

CONSISTENCY.....aaahhhhhh, yes. This is the experience of being exposed to a similarly presenting event/situation/concept/idea that AFFORDS you a level of familiarity and predictability. From a purely logical perspective, consistency is defined as that which does not contain contradictions.

---

[8]'BUDDIES' are essentially 'experienced' nurses (well, more experienced than YOU), with whom you are formally connected for a day or a set of shifts, who can 'show you the ropes'. Depending on the place of work, these individuals may or may not be given a workload reduction to compensate for the time they need to 'teach' you. Preceptors are often individuals in the workplace who are considered clinical or practice EXPERTS and may be chosen more for their practice expertise than for their personality or disposition. Those with whom you are partnered for emotional support and reassurance would more likely be considered 'mentors' and may or may NOT be the same individual as your preceptor.

> ***POTENTIAL INCONSISTENCY #1****—while you have been educated and prepared to provide broad and comprehensive nursing care to patients, families and communities, the practice environment is more often than not constructed to ensure efficiency and productivity over effectiveness and quality optimization.*

Oh dear……this is a definite hurdle for the new graduate.

Let's start with the pre-graduate assumption that as a professional you will have the time, energy and opportunity to practice 'caring, compassionate and competent' nursing. YOU WILL!!! But if you don't feel you can do that initially, **be patient.** Upon entry to practice, your time and energy are consumed by trying to **KEEP YOUR HEAD ABOVE WATER** as you:

1) *adjust* to the changes in your personal and professional life;
2) *accommodate* differences between what you learned about nursing in school and what you see being done in practice;
3) *perform* the multitude of skills required of you without revealing your feelings of anxiety and self-perceptions of inadequacy; AND
4) *learn* everything you need to know about your practice that you couldn't be taught in school.

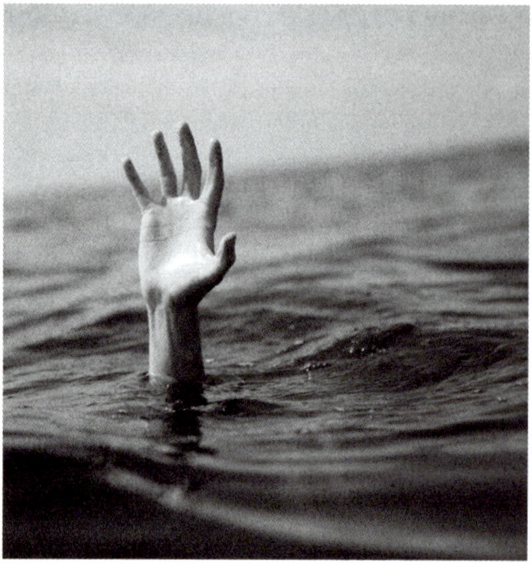

YIKES – now that's intense!!!!

The bottom line is that new graduates sometimes feel it is **reasonable** to expect to:

- manage a nursing workload that even senior nurses struggle with (e.g. it is *REASONABLE* to manage about 4 patients/nurse in acute-care);

- help out colleagues in an equal work exchange (you do this for me and I will do that for you);
- be there to console, care for and educate patients and families desperately struggling with their own life transition;
- provide a comprehensive and holistic, but perhaps premature, discharge for a patient whose life has been unequivocally altered by a massive stroke and who is returning to a life for which neither he nor his family are prepared, and for which there is minimal homecare and community support;
- navigate the unavoidable relational conflicts that plague any work environment;
- deal with the 'minor' emergencies that naturally interrupt a nurse's daily routine; AND
- complete all of this **ON TIME and without any sign of a struggle......**

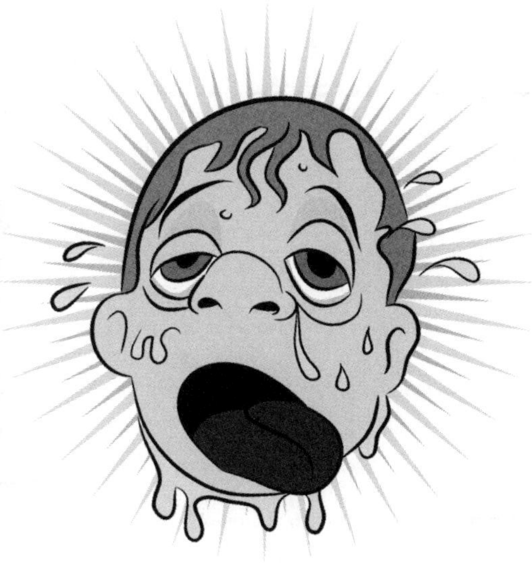

PHEW!!!!!!! If this is YOU, chances are **HIGH** that you will experience a significant amount of transition stress. My point is that **IT SIMPLY ISN'T REALISTIC** for you or for others to have this expectation. That's why we call it a **TRANSITION!!!** It takes time and experience to become a proficient practitioner within a dynamic and intense workplace.

"I think we're just trying to put everything together of what you learned in school and trying to think back on things and… you go through a lot of, 'should I do this, should I not be doing this, should I go back to school'…I found I was very hard on myself. Very critical of what I was doing and wanted to quit a few times. I think it really makes a difference on where you start and how your experience is at that time. It changes your opinion of nursing."

> ***POTENTIAL INCONSISTENCY #2***—*while the intent of all healthcare institutions is to deliver evidence-based high quality healthcare, they are required to do so within budgets that are influenced by many competing sociopolitical and economic factors. This means that there will often be tension between the ethics-based value-driven motivations of healthcare providers and the fiscal and human resource limitations of the healthcare system. Particularly in a democratic capitalist society such as ours, this tension serves as an indicator of how well we are maintaining the balance between what 'should be' and what 'is'. Having said that, the realities of how this tension plays out 'on the ground' is an education all its own; one that usually doesn't start until we feel the full weight of it in our own professional practice.*

In line with the first inconsistency is the fact that your education may have appropriately (though arguably idealistically) framed 'quality nursing care' as:

> *the critically reflective assessment, diagnosis, planning, implementation and evaluation of measures that optimize the biophysical, emotional, psychosocial, spiritual and cultural needs of the patient, family and community under your care.*

Some of you may wonder, *"Why would my education prepare me to practice with all these 'ideals', only to have me thrown in to a 'real' situation that does NOT reflect all, or sometimes ANY of these ideals"?*

That is a tough one….but as a nursing educator AND a direct care nurse I have come to believe that my knowledge of what CAN or SHOULD be the standard of practice to which I aspire allows me perspective—if what I see, and how I am encouraged to practice as a nurse does NOT meet that standard then it is my professional obligation to work TOWARD changes that can ELEVATE the standard of practice. If I was taught the BARE MINIMUM and encouraged to ACCEPT what IS without questioning it or seeking to advance something more, there would be little hope that the profession would ever see anything different. There are GOOD reasons for idealism—and there is a place where you will likely come to 'rest', somewhere between the current reality and the ideal that you have come to expect. Finding that place without jeopardizing your practice ethics is your goal as a new nurse.

It is worth remembering that the institution within which you work has political, economic and institutional demands that require attention. Financial and human resources are finite. Increasing healthcare costs combined with years of fiscal 'belt- tightening' make the limitations in spending by many institutions necessary, prudent and sometimes even acceptable.

Nurses, as advocates of quality care and proponents of the inclusive self determination of those being cared FOR, often struggle under the weight of a bureaucracy whose own functional sustainability rests on its ability to conserve resources and control costs.

Situations that delay flow-through or impede 'input-output' in one part of the healthcare system generally mean additional resources will need to be consumed in another part of the system to compensate. For example:

1) patients may be unable to be discharged out of hospital to the community because of inaccessible homecare, lack of funds or inadequate social support networks;
2) acute-care may become a temporary 'home' to long-term care clients due to financial cuts to chronic-care residences that promote a 'buckling' in the census of patients in hospitals; OR
3) escalating public health, chronic illness or mental health issues in the community can 'push back' against the acute-care discharge process, delaying the normal flow-through of patients and ultimately fostering the inappropriate utilization of resources.

These are examples of the ongoing 'tension' of healthcare administration. As a recent graduate and therefore a relative newcomer to the healthcare landscape, you are particularly vulnerable to narrow interpretations of 'situational' events that are actually part of an exceedingly complex but interwoven sequence of 'systems' issues. Your understandably limited perspective may originate from a lack of experience with the healthcare system's multidimensionality and can render you extremely frustrated when change that you believe NEEDS to happen DOESN'T happen. This is NOT to say that you must bear the entire brunt of this conflict by completely readjusting your lens—it may mean that when you DO feel overwhelming frustration within a system that seems nonsensical, you might benefit by connecting with a knowledgeable colleague who can help you wade through the mud and the muck of the situation to find whatever shiny coins lay hidden beneath.

Having said ALL THAT.....there are times when practice patterns of nurses simply deteriorate over time. The reasons for this are often complex but here are a few possibilities:

1) *learned* helplessness (if you beat your head against a wall of resistance for long enough, or feel your questions about, or suggestions for, changes to the conditions of your work fail to motivate any response, sometimes you just give up trying);
2) *chronic complacency* (if what you contribute isn't valued then you may begin to question how much you are willing to contribute);

3) *devaluing of nurses' work* (to influence professional issues, nurses need to be at the decision making table when it comes to issues that directly impact their work);
4) *exhaustion* (nursing work is physical, intellectual, emotional, relational and political, and everyone is being asked to 'do more with less'); AND
5) differences in the *meaning of our work* (viewing one's work as a career that can make a difference in the world or viewing work as a job that pays the bills and puts my children through school....or more likely something in the middle).

I do believe that the slow and steady changes to the practice standards of nurses is rarely maliciously intended—a nurse doesn't go to work thinking, "*Today, I am going to strive to be the worst nurse a patient/colleague/family/community could ever encounter*"!!! Or in the middle of their career say *'I want to practice below all the standards I held when I graduated'*. Things happen insidiously most times—maybe I start by cutting an inconsequential corner, benignly bantering about another colleague, or holding on to assumptions about people that I have not clarified, confirmed, witnessed or critically examined. And maybe I forgot, or never really knew, how to infuse strategies into my practice that could warn me that I was *'slipping'* or surround myself with people who could remind me of the nurse I said I wanted to be.

> *"I can remember learning the principles of sterile technique in school. Our instructor had our partner monitoring us for any contamination of our sterile field. Now I'm standing here watching an experienced nurse pull off a dressing with no gloves, and slap another dressing back on the incision without even cleaning it, and I don't say anything."*

NOTHING justifies bullying or aggression by professionals against one another (also referred to as *'lateral aggression'* or *'horizontal violence'*) or unethical and substandard professional practice. But we cannot change others—we can only be the best WE can be. and perhaps model something different. Look around you and decide what standard of practice YOU want to sustain and put in checks and balances for yourself to monitor your practice over time. And remember, we ALL have an ethical obligation (or said another way, we are all legally bound by our professional ethics) to report UNSAFE practice. If you have seen substandard care provided by your colleagues, no matter HOW senior they are, talk with someone you can trust to strategize on ways to bring this to their attention before they do something they will regret or hurt someone.

> ***A great leader needs to love and respect people, and he needs to be comfortable with himself and with the world. He also needs to be able to forgive himself and others. In other words, a leader needs grace.***
>
> ***- Leo Hindery Jr.***

POTENTIAL INCONSISTENCY #3—*when you graduate from an educational program that encourages independent critical thinking, it is a bit disconcerting to find yourself relatively DEPENDENT on the experienced nurses around you. There is this sense that you SHOULD be independent—you think others are expecting you to perform independently and this is what you often expect of yourself. Confusion reigns when you quickly come to realize that so much of what you are doing and seeing is NEW. The inconsistency is between what you THINK people expect of you, what you expected of yourself before graduating, and the recognition and acceptance of your own limitations as a new practitioner.*

With respect to your 'thinking' during the early stages of transition, it is important to remember that you may **NOT** always be expressing your true thinking **CAPACITY** initially as much as you may be revealing the natural limitations in your thinking **CAPABILITY** during what is a very stressful time in your professional development. Remember, you are thinking about many things during your transition—clinical scenarios you have never seen before, changes in your personal life, additional professional responsibilities, increased performance expectations, pressures of accountability and the potential for and implications of error—to name just a few.

GO EASY ON THE SELF CRITICISM – it takes a long time to become an expert!

Now there may be individuals around you who will give you the impression that you are not functioning to specifications—that you should know more, that your education was inadequate, or that if you had paid more attention in class you wouldn't be in this pickle ☺. But there are just as many who would suggest that if you were oriented longer, had a more committed mentor or a 12-month residency program you would not experience the stress of transition. No doubt there are shreds of truth to all of these claims. But those who play the blame game, pitting your education against your workplace, do little to solve the problem.

Transition to professional practice continues to exist today in a similar fashion to when Dr. Marlene Kramer talked about reality shock in the 1970s largely because *THERE IS NO NIRVANA*. From an educational perspective, no nursing program worth its salt would educate students for what the workplace is really like without also preparing them to elevate the standards to which we are able to practice as nurses. That is the objective of a rigorous nursing education. Conversely, there are FEW workplaces whose orientation, transition facilitation, staff integration strategies and practice environments could live up to the ideals represented by the largely 'theoretical' foundations of nursing education. The IDEAL, in either nursing education or the healthcare system, simply doesn't exist, though 'magnet care environments'[9] strive to achieve optimum practice contexts for nurses. That is not to say that the majority of healthcare systems OR the educational program from which you graduated are failures if they have not achieved this level of excellence, but rather that 'excellence' is a continuum and most educational programs and health institutions/centers fall somewhere in the middle—there is room for improvement but they are doing what they can with the resources they have. In the end, we are all obligated to push the boundaries of what we are capable of in order to produce a contemporary context of nursing education, clinical practice and healthcare delivery that is everything it CAN be.

SUCCESS for a new nurse is not that mysterious and, to be honest, it is similar to that sought by all nurses. You want to leave work MOST DAYS having:

- **not killed anyone** ☺;
- **learned** something new;
- **contributed** something significant;
- **fulfilled** the needs of the majority of those under your care;
- **enjoyed** a sense of cohesion with the physician, nursing and allied health colleagues you work alongside;
- **functioned** collaboratively with those you have called upon to assist in the plan of care;
- **been empowered** by your leadership to make decisions appropriate to your level of knowledge, skill and experience; AND
- **been supported** to create and advance new ideas that optimize the level of nursing practice in your healthcare community.

The difference with a newly graduated nurse is that 'being successful' is critical to a healthy and progressive movement through the various stages of early professional development. Unlike their more experienced colleagues, new nurses don't have the well-honed skills that allow them to easily navigate (or recover from) threats to their as yet fragile sense of professional identity. I would suggest it takes at least a year to mature one's construct of what a nurse is, what a

[9] The American Nurses Credentialing Center (ANCC) MAGNET RECOGNITION PROGRAM® is characterized by practice environments in which nurses work with other nurses who are clinically competent; nurse-physician communication and work is collegial/collaborative; interdisciplinary relationships are promoted and facilitated; autonomy and clinical decision making in nursing practice is supported; nurse managers are supportive; nurses control their own practice; there is support for foundational and ongoing education; staffing is adequate; and nurses work in a culture where concern for patients is paramount (see also Kramer M, Schmalenberg C. [2002]. Essentials of magnetism. In McClure ML, Hinshaw AS, eds. *Magnet Hospitals Revisited: Attraction and Retention of Professional Nurses*. Washington, DC: American Nurses Association, p. 25-59.)

nurse does, how a nurse interacts with colleagues and where nursing fits on the professional continuum and within the overall healthcare 'machine'. As much as I would like to say it no longer exists, there remains a hierarchy in healthcare and naming it is a starting point for determining how to function *within* it, while simultaneously considering how you can *change* it where necessary. Failing to provide the new professional with a graduated, success-oriented initiation to practice is 'preparing them for failure'. My experience with new nurses over the years, and with senior nurses wounded by their early professional experiences, tells me that the successful introduction of a newly graduated nurse into the profession is FOUNDATIONAL to the success of the profession as a whole.

A final word about progress—**SMALL STEPS WIN THE RACE!!!!!!!!!** A professional career is a marathon, not a sprint. You CAN be and WILL be that expert practitioner you came into nursing wanting to be, but expertise takes time, struggle and painstaking growth. Beverly Sills reminds us "*there are no shortcuts to any place worth going.*"

Try to stay grounded in the **fundamental** objectives of a newly graduated nurse:

- Gaining a sense of the **roles and responsibilities** of a graduate nurse;
- Creating a **workload organizational system** that works for you;
- Learning how to **manage your time** within a workload of GRADUALLY increased complexity;
- Learning the **routines** of your workplace;
- Seeing and experiencing a variety of **'normal' and 'abnormal' situations** under contained conditions;
- **Debriefing** with a trusted experienced colleague, nursing educator, or mentor about clinical situations to gain a depth of understanding of 'clinical patterns' and the relationships between those patterns and the judgments that arise out of them;
- Gaining confidence in **performing** the fundamental skills required of a nurse in the setting where you work (the competencies of an expert nurse are not singular 'skills' or 'tasks' performed in isolation, but a complex and layered portfolio of roles and responsibilities enacted in an infinitely varied set of sequences and combinations and under dynamic, fluid and often intense and risk-laden conditions);
- **Assessing** patients or practice situations of increasing complexity and varying levels of stability;
- Learning how to work **ON** a team—and learning **ABOUT** your team;
- Getting to know the **dynamics of your workplace**—what is 'nursing' to your colleagues and how is nursing valued within your institution and community;
- Gaining a **balance** between your personal and professional life;
- **Learning who you ARE** when you are not consumed by studying and academic deadlines; AND
- Learning to have **FUN** again!

At this point, it is worth reinforcing the need to SLOWLY INCREASE the level of clinical complexity, intensity and scope of your nursing practice. Success is not as likely if you are placed in situations that are beyond your capacity—this practice could be unnecessarily counterproductive in the long run. While it may be tempting to jump into clinical practice areas that are demanding and high paced, your practice is best served with a strong foundation and strategic approach to growing your nursing skill and experiential knowledge prior to engaging in high level and critical impact decision making and clinical problem solving under conditions of duress. IF you are interested in high acuity practice (for example ICU or ER), meet with the manager or educator in that practice area and determine the skills, knowledge and experience that would best prepare you for that career path (See Appendix *Working in High Acuity*). Advance your skill portfolio and consider making the first step toward that career after a year of 'getting your feet wet'. **MAKE A CAREER PLAN** that lands you in the area you really want to be within 2 years post-graduation and you will enter that area with a much greater sense of confidence, competence and clarity.

There is a final element that I did NOT include in the overall schemata but that I would like to make note of here. At the risk of being redundant, that element is **FREQUENCY, FREQUENCY, FREQUENCY.** The more OFTEN you are exposed to stable, predictable, familiar and consistent elements in your personal and professional life immediately after you graduate, and the more gradually you advance the complexity, intensity and scope of your practice by monitoring your developing competence and confidence, the more likely you are to successfully progress THROUGH transition shock, and subsequently through the anticipated stages of professional role transition.

Categories of Influence in the Experience of Transition

Through my research I have been able to generate 4 core categories that I suggest influence, and are influenced by, the professional role transition of the new nurse. I have identified these core categories as: 1) ***roles***, 2) ***relationships***, 3) ***responsibilities***, and 4) ***knowledge***. I am choosing to talk about these four categories within the transition shock phase of your experience because I believe that WHICHEVER of these core categories, or elements within them, afford you the **LEAST amount of stability, predictability, familiarity and consistency** are areas in which you may want to FOCUS your coping STRATEGIES. If you can understand what is or what might challenge your transition experience, you will be more likely to successfully resolve the challenges and minimize the intensity and duration of your transition shock experience.

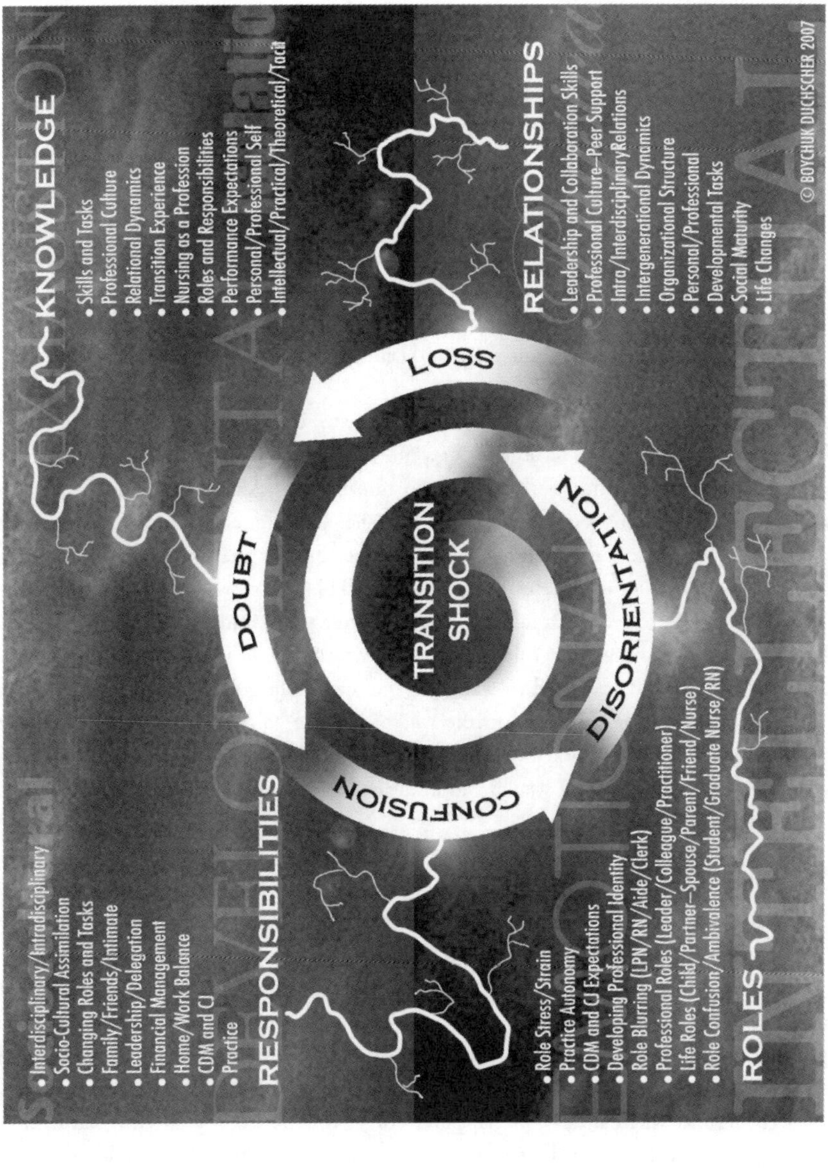
TRANSITION SHOCK
DOUBT
LOSS
DISORIENTATION
CONFUSION
KNOWLEDGE
• Skills and Tasks
• Professional Culture
• Relational Dynamics
• Transition Experience
• Nursing as a Profession
• Roles and Responsibilities
• Performance Expectations
• Personal/Professional Self
• Intellectual/Practical/Theoretical/Tacit
RELATIONSHIPS
• Leadership and Collaboration Skills
• Professional Culture—Peer Support
• Intra/InterdisciplinaryRelations
• Intergenerational Dynamics
• Organizational Structure
• Personal/Professional
• Developmental Tasks
• Social Maturity
• Life Changes
RESPONSIBILITIES
• Interdisciplinary/Intradisciplinary
• Socio-Cultural Assimilation
• Changing Roles and Tasks
• Family/Friends/Intimate
• Leadership/Delegation
• Financial Management
• Home/Work Balance
• CDM and CJ
• Practice
ROLES
• Role Stress/Strain
• Practice Autonomy
• CDM and CJ Expectations
• Developing Professional Identity
• Role Blurring (LPN/RN/Aide/Clerk)
• Professional Roles (Leader/Colleague/Practitioner)
• Life Roles (Child/Partner–Spouse/Parent/Friend/Nurse)
• Role Confusion/Ambivalence (Student/Graduate Nurse/RN)
© BOYCHUK DUCHSCHER 2007

Roles. As a new nurse, you can't help but notice a subtle but distinct change in your overall role from one of dependent learner to one of independent practitioner and interdependent collaborator. While you may have enacted some of your professional 'roles' as a student (care provider, advocate, counselor, teacher to name a few), the change in accountability and responsibility for the process and outcome of those same roles as you enter the world of professional practice can alter your perception of them. They can take on a relative 'unfamiliarity' that is surprising to a lot of graduates—things you did with relative ease prior to graduating 'look' different through the lens of your new credentialing. Suddenly (and sometimes VERY suddenly), the safety net of faculty or preceptorial collaboration and consultation is no longer available and even the permission not to know because 'I'm a student' is no longer an acceptable fall back (although 'I'm a grad nurse' can have a similar effect during those months prior to national licensure). The weight of the ultimate responsibility can strangely alter your perceptions and interpretations of situations that are really quite similar to those you dealt with as a student. This contributes to role stress and can weigh heavily on you.

Role stress turns into role strain when you are unable to reconcile for yourself or others what role you are assuming (are you a student or a professional nurse). I recall a graduate who had previous experience as a unit clerk, porter and nurses aide—ALL on the unit to which she was planning to transition. As she was completing her senior nursing practicum in that unit, there was significant role **confusion** not only for her but for the unit staff who continued to consult her for issues that were more about the OTHER roles she had assumed and not commensurate with her role as a nursing student. While still a student, she pursued a creative solution of distinguishing what role she was engaging in by wearing colored uniforms (for example a red uniform indicated to staff that she was in the role of a nursing student and a white uniform indicated she was in the role of a nurse's aide). By virtue of this creative strategy the graduate prevented role stress from extending to role strain. The staff became accustomed to her categorizing system and in the end her transition was relatively uneventful. Hey, whatever WORKS!!!!

It is possible that you could experience something similar if you practiced as a Licensed/ Registered Practical Nurse or Enrolled Nurse (UK) in a particular practice area and then return there as a Registered Nurse—the point is that if your 'formal' title, and therefore your ROLE changes you should expect a period of adjustment for you and those you work with. This includes those of you who might have worked as a nursing student, or had educational experiences on the unit to which you are now transitioning. It is not uncommon, and I suppose not unexpected, for your nursing colleagues to feel somewhat 'familiar' with you because you have been 'around' them already; perhaps even forget you are a new grad. This can lend itself to unrealistic expectations on the part of the staff and is something that should be discussed (YOU might have to bring it up!) during the first several days of your new role. The best approach is good communication and transparency, particularly with those you are working alongside, as to what roles and responsibilities you are assuming at any given time. Patience with yourself and others will put you ahead of the game as well ☺.

I believe that students who experience a capstone practicum on the unit to which they will be transitioning, or who take employment in that unit prior to graduating as a new nurse can significantly reduce overall transition shock. Having said that, there is something quite phenomenal and unexpected that occurs for even those graduates the nurses with whom they worked collaboratively as a senior student (maybe even just a short week ago) appear to treat them differently. Sometimes your status as a new nurse in the eyes of your experienced colleagues is ENHANCED and the new role feels empowering, while sometimes the more senior nurses' expectations rise more RAPIDLY than the confidence you have in your new position, rendering you vulnerable to feelings of inadequacy and incompetence. My research was not clear on this, but it was consistent—something changed. It is hard to know if this 'change' was in the receptivity of senior co-workers to the new nurses' altered role designation, or if the change was in the self-perceptions of the graduates themselves; but an adjustment to new role expectations was necessary by all. Along these lines, the challenge of returning to a unit where you were previously a senior student may result in staff expecting you to know more than other new graduates and assuming that you require less orientation or transition support. This may not be a fair assumption and I encourage you to discuss this potential issue with your manager, educator and practice area manager prior to employment.

Finally, the roles you will be assuming in this newest chapter of your life are as PERSONAL as they are PROFESSIONAL. The fact is that family (parents, spouses, children) and friends KNOW you graduated and now THEY have changing expectations of you. It might be something as simple as no longer being able to 'escape' the clutches of unwanted social invitations by saying 'I have to study' ☺ or something as complex as trying to explain to your 4 year old daughter how your mind, body and soul have been depleted by the past 3 years of school and that you need to rest awhile; your child who simply wants your attention believes all that celebrating that occurred for graduation was reason to believe YOU'RE BACK!!!!

I recently had someone approach me to ask if I was going to write a professional role transition guide for the family and friends of new graduates!!! I actually thought that was quite an insightful query as graduates sometimes forget that they are not necessarily the only ones who 'graduated' from this chapter in their lives. Those who have 'stuck by you' during the challenging times are ALSO experiencing a transition of sorts—it may be that they have 'buffered' aspects of their own lives in order to give you space to study, or 'put off' advancements they have wanted to pursue in order to be the stabilizing force you required during your education. It may even be that they sacrificed material purchases or the even more precious commodity of 'time', in order that you could pursue your dream.

I am NOT suggesting that these individuals have a malicious intent….but if aspects of your life (and the lives of those around you) had to undergo change to accommodate this educational 'hiatus' then it is really only reasonable for there to be some expectation that it will change 'back' to the way they were BEFORE you took your education 'break'. BRACE YOURSELF for this possibility. First of all, as the saying goes, 'you can never go back'….

and this educational experience has likely changed you fundamentally. It is hard to imagine watching life being born and ending; seeing for yourself how the homeless navigate the streets at night; holding a heart in your hands (literally); or playing a game with your 10 year old pediatric oncology patient while his chemo is running and NOT find your perspective about life transformed. Be prepared for the experience of re-entering a life that looks different than it did before you started school. Friends you had before may not understand why or how you've changed and your relationships with them may need some tweaking. Sadly, there may be relationships that you will simply outgrow and you may find yourself needing to move on. As much as you have gained during your education, there is a sense of loss as well—knowing this gives you permission to grieve what you have left behind as you move forward with the next chapter of your life. For parents to whom you now owe money in student loans, spouses whose social lives have been a series of lonely nights, children who have been inordinately patient with your 'neglectful absence', and friends who 'put up' with your theorizing and stories of calamity, sacrifice and growing pains simply WANT YOU BACK. You can't blame them! Their demands on your now 'free' time may be premature for where you are actually at emotionally, physically and socially. You may find it stressful and challenging in the early months after graduation as you come to realize that the next level of your education has just begun and it is taking more out of you than you originally thought it would.

If you can, sit down with those individuals in your life and explain beforehand what they can expect from you as a newly graduated professional nurse (and perhaps in the years to come you can give them my *Professional Role Transition Support Guide for People Who Love Their Nursing Graduate And Want Them Back).* Outline for them the challenges you may be facing over the initial 12 months so that you might stem the tide of expectation at least for the first stage of your transition (up to 4 months post orientation). In the end, you may simply have to apologize for your 'absence' and let it go; many graduates say that friends and family simply don't understand what they are going through during the initial transition to practice.

Spending time with other new graduates (come and find us at www.nursingthefuture.ca or access a regional or local new nurse support network where you work) may take on an important role in sustaining your sense of normalcy and reminding you that it's not just YOU that is experiencing this disconnect! Hey, you might even be able to swap strategies that can help you cope with misinformed but well-meaning supporters!

Responsibilities. This is a big one! If there is anything that knocks a new graduate off their 'axis' it is likely the sense of responsibility they feel as a new practitioner. The awareness that you are now RESPONSIBLE for the judgments that arise from the application of your knowledge, the decisions that arise from those judgments, and the impact and influence of the outcomes of your judgments and decisions on people's LIVES, can initially feel overwhelming. It is something you get accustomed to but it takes time. That is often the reason why, even in areas that you felt confident in as a senior student, there is a relative DROP in confidence as a practicing nurse. The weight of responsibility can cloud your vision such that what was previously quite comfortable and familiar to you becomes partially or sometimes completely unrecognizable. Like when your patient requires a top up of morphine for 7/10 pain and you have to give him an intramuscular injection because his PCA (that's patient-controlled-analgesia for those of you who have been in a community placement for the last year ☺) is interstitial and you know you need to get his pain under control before you can start another line—and you need to ACT NOW! Somehow your skill proficiency in IM injections—and you were the recipient of the *North American Intramuscular Injection Excellence Award* for heaven's sake—is UNAVAILABLE to you now and you are shaking as you draw up the medication because you know the patient's wife will want to be present while you administer it and you think she will clearly see how incompetent you are (not that you actually ARE incompetent, but that is how you FEEL)!

> *"Some things go so fast though I can't even process them....Like it's so fast that I can't even process some stuff and it takes like 5 or 6 times to catch it all. It's just going so fast."*

You know what? You'll give the injection after which you will come back to the nursing station and sit down because the post-adrenaline jitters are upon you, and you will realize that you AND your patient (AND his wife) are FINE! And the next time you have to deal with a similar situation it will be much easier. And so it goes......this is the experiential knowledge that is nursing practice in the 'real' world.

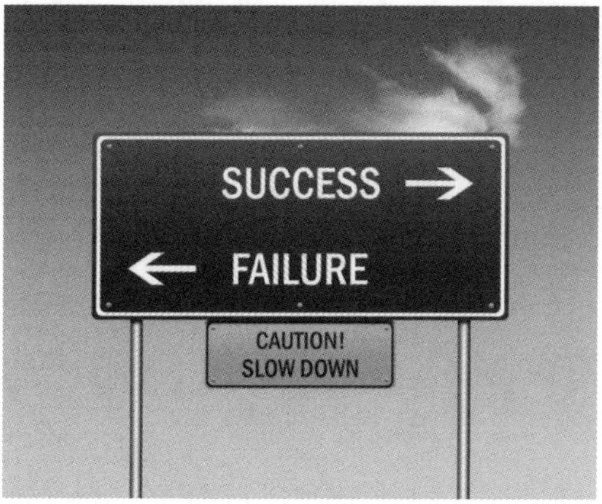

Now the responsibilities related to your performance at work are only one piece of this puzzle. Other responsibilities that new professionals are often dealing with include, but may not be limited to:

1) **Developmental responsibilities**
   a. moving out of home;
   b. managing finances for the first time;
   c. learning how to live independently from family;
   d. making major purchases (cars, homes); AND
   e. figuring out how to pay for them ☺.
2) **Relational responsibilities**
   a. marriage;
   b. divorce (it is amazing how one major change gives way to another);

   c. establishment of new friend/colleague relationships with co-workers that includes understanding which relationships fit the different positions on that continuum;
   d. navigating relationships with authority figures (what do managers, educators and charge nurses want);
   e. understanding what it means to have a 'relationship' with patients and their families (boundaries related to self vs other, friend vs patient, nurse vs gendered being); AND
   f. navigating the future of long-standing friendships to which you are NOT bonded professionally (friends who cringe when you talk about what you do on a daily basis).

3) **Work responsibilities**
   a. completing routines and tasks on time (many which you have never experienced prior to employment such as transcribing physician orders, administering intravenous narcotics or chemotherapy, intracranial pressure or hemodynamic monitoring, sexually transmitted infection notification);
   b. communicating certain information to the 'right' people while NOT communicating certain information to the 'wrong' people (socially constructed power structures); AND
   c. learning which decisions and judgments are appropriate for a new graduate level of knowledge and when consultations with senior nursing staff or physicians are necessary.

4) Learning about and enacting **professional responsibilities**
   a. involvement in professional associations and unions (rights vs obligations of the profession);
   b. knowledge of and respect for unit culture and power/authority hierarchy (who to go to about what);
   c. intra-disciplinary relationships (working collaboratively with varying scopes of practice within the nursing discipline);
   d. generational dynamics (how to approach a baby boomer about a change you think needs to be made, or how to delegate to an Xer);
   e. interdisciplinary collaboration (when to consult pharmacy, physiotherapy or social work); AND
   f. leadership, collaboration and delegation/assignment (learning who on your team is capable of doing what, how to assign tasks to more established nurses who ask if you need help, how to share a workload by collaborating with your nurse partners for that day, or how to delegate to an unlicensed healthcare worker who is 20 years your senior).

Relationships. The relationships nurses engage in with one another both determine and reveal the 'culture' of the nursing profession. They say that one can learn much about a society by the way it treats its most vulnerable members. With this in mind, many would claim that nursing has some work to do…

A significant challenge to 'belonging' is that it is often determined not by ourselves, but by OTHERS (those individuals with whom we seek to belong). The need to fit IN to a social structure assumes acceptance by the 'other'—and that is not completely within the control of the individual looking to fit in. Unless of course, that person doesn't CARE if they fit—in which case the concept of belonging is somewhat mute.

So assuming that the newly graduated nurse WANTS to fit in (HELLO!!! Of course you do!!!), there is a degree of vulnerability involved in that objective. How far will a new nurse go to be accepted by the individuals who represent their professional 'social structure'? The answer is sometimes quite far…..which speaks less to the constitution of the new nurse and more to the power of professional enculturation or our general need as human beings to belong. Being on the periphery, or 'marginalized' as a new professional is fundamentally inconsistent with the developmental need to be accepted as a new professional. *Enculturation* is defined as the process by which a person learns the requirements of the culture into which they seek acceptance. It is the process by which they come to understand and ultimately choose to adopt, challenge or reject the values and behaviors considered integral to that culture. Successful enculturation results in the inductee becoming 'competent' in the language, values and rituals of the dominant culture.

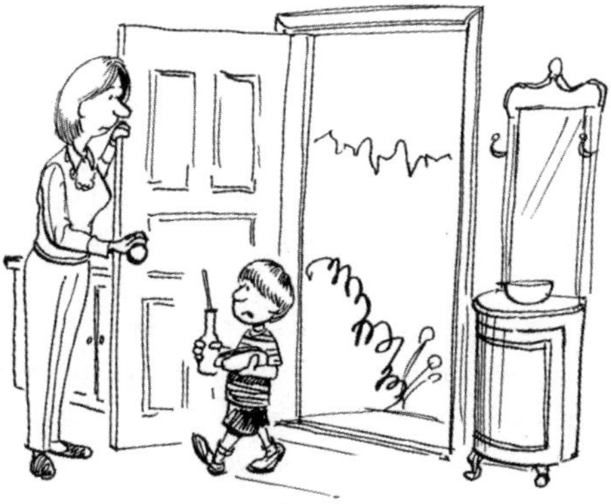

"The guy at the convenience store is the only one who understands me."

Becoming part of any cultural group involves **socialization**; the gradual but deliberate shaping of an individual over time by exposing them to cultural norms, customs, values, traditions, social roles, symbols and languages. There is an inherent assumption in socialization that the inductee will share the values of the dominant cultural group. While there are many traditional values of the nursing profession that the majority of nurses would likely agree are worthy of preserving, there are certain social customs, roles or ways of relating within the profession that could use 'a hot bath and a clean shave' ☺. Just because we've always done something a certain way doesn't make it the 'best' way or even the 'right' way. But tradition is steeped in a long history of 'doing it this way' and not likely to change easily or quickly. A few questions for anyone engaging in debate or critique are:

1) Do I have enough information about why this particular situation is the way it is currently to even critique it? Is there more than one way to approach this?
   <u>*Note to self:*</u> **There's ALWAYS more than one way to approach ANYTHING. GET MORE INFORMATION FROM ALL THE PEOPLE INVOLVED.**
2) What is my plan of challenge/critique?
   <u>*Note to self:*</u> **YOU CATCH MORE FLIES WITH HONEY THAN YOU DO WITH VINEGAR – people respond better when you can appeal to what works for them and not just what works for you.**
   <u>*Appended note to self:*</u> **THIS IS THE WAY IT IS FOR A REASON—DO I KNOW THE REASON?**
   <u>*Final note to self:*</u> **THERE IS ALWAYS A PROCESS TO FOLLOW IF YOU WANT TO BE HEARD—WHAT IS THAT PROCESS IN THIS SITUATION?**
3) Does my plan consider the other person(s) involved?
   <u>*Note to self:*</u> **It might sound cliché, but usually the BEST solution to any problem or issue is not YOURS or THEIRS, but OURS.**

Knowledge. It really is one thing to 'know' something as a student and then to 'know' that SAME THING as a fully accountable and responsible professional.

> *"I think so because, I mean, your ideals are what you hope for, you know, you're thinking of how great it's going to be and stuff and that's always good to try and achieve those goals and things. But…it's really tough when you think nursing is going to be one way and it ends up another so, in a way, yeah, what we learned in nursing wasn't necessarily applicable to what we really have to do. Cause it's not, even in terms of the big huge care plans we have to do in fourth year. Like I, I realize in first, second, and third year we have to do those big care plans to really learn and figure out, you know understand practice and organization and stuff but in your fourth year you do these huge care plans and you know everything about your patient and you have a really good idea of what you're suppose to do the next day after you go in. And then, when you're a nurse, you have sixteen patients, you know the top layer and you have to learn to nurse off of that. You have to learn your priorities by reading two sentences on their diagnosis and what operation they had and that's it. And you have to learn how to make judgments and how to organize your care in a split second and that's something that we weren't taught in nursing. That is something we had to learn in the real world and that was really tough. Cause you really have to learn how to prioritize your care and who you're going to look at first and who's the most important—in minutes."*

It is as if at times the knowledge that you had developed a relative comfort with as a student is unavailable when you most need it (which is usually in circumstances where you are under pressure, exhausted and distracted by your transition experience!!!). I want to be clear that this intellectual 'black hole' into which your mind seems to have fallen as a new graduate is often not about 'forgetting' what you knew, and it doesn't necessarily mean that you are incapable or incompetent. I would suggest that what you knew 'before' your mind, body and soul were consumed with transitioning into the roles and responsibilities of a professional practitioner has receded into the less accessible areas of your cognitive control and requires more energy and intent to bring it back to the FRONT of your thoughts—often having to make its way through the rather gooey mixture that represents the OTHER thoughts that are monopolizing your mind (if you still don't 'get' that, you need to re-read the initial 40 pages of this book.... ☺).

This is why I believe it is important to limit the level of EXPECTATION related to critical practice judgments and decisions that you are required to make and focus more on:

- taking in knowledge about your work environment and workplace routines (learning how to work nights for instance);
- familiarizing yourself with the common clinical presentations of your patient population or the situated concerns of the communities for whom you are responsible;
- getting to know who your colleagues are and how they work so that you can work more easily WITH them;
- experiencing what it is like to have a patient rapidly decompensate or even die on your shift; AND
- learning what you need to do in those uncomfortable patient situations that you didn't learn in school, like having to inform the spouse of a 56 year old man that you diagnosed with a sexually transmitted infection that she needs to be tested for genital herpes!

Much of this knowledge will be NEW to you! While you undoubtedly have a strong base of science and theory from which your colleagues and patients/clients will surely benefit, it is in the application of theory to countless combinations of variables that makes nursing practice so consistently complex, often unpredictable and always dynamic. As the saying goes: 'there's nothing like experience'.....

As has been outlined for you in the previous pages, knowledge of nursing theory and science related to normal and abnormal processes (biophysical, psychosocial, cultural or sociopolitical) is **ESSENTIAL** to practicing as a nurse. But, as a professional, there is knowledge related to workplace dynamics, professional roles and responsibilities, performance expectations and inter-professionalism that exceeds what you can be afforded in the relatively 'sheltered' experience of your education. There are few (if ANY) professionals, regardless of discipline, who 'waltz' into their new practice environments. It simply is not possible to prepare you for all the computations of issues, clinical presentations or dynamics that play out in real life in the few short years that represent your education. Even if we COULD prepare you, do you REALLY want to spend 10 more years in school????

"And you know all the senior nurses after that happened...said, 'oh, yeah when you have an abdominal pain in a male you always rule out a Triple A [abdominal aortic aneurysm] and then you go with whatever'. Not once have I heard that before. Not once....And that's the first thing that the paramedics teach...treat everyone with abdominal pain as a triple A. Not once in my whole entire stint of being in the ER have I heard that out of anybody's mouth."

I would like you to consider 'reprogramming' your idea of the contemporary nursing workplace; it is really the NEXT level of your education and builds upon the foundational knowledge you have acquired in your 'basic' program. To think otherwise is to misrepresent the dynamic and fluid nature of the human experience of health and illness and to under-appreciate the all encompassing essence of the nursing discipline: *interactions with human beings from all walks of life, throughout the lifespan and in all situations and dimensions of their health or illness experience.* Further, to think about your educational program as your time of 'learning' and professional practice employment as 'working' is unfair to YOU as well as to your practice. It sets up a polarizing experience when you get into practice and you see how much you have yet to learn. There is the potential, if you think of your educational program as completely responsible to prepare you for EVERYTHING that might happen in practice, to **blame** your education for the discrepancies between what you were taught WOULD happen and what you find IS happening for you as a new practitioner. Though I don't know too many nursing programs that would claim they have the 'perfect' approach to comprehensively preparing their graduates, I also don't know ANY workplaces that can lay claim to the perfect orientation or transition program for the new nursing professional. What we need to recognize is that both education and the healthcare sector have room to grow so that the 'gap' between them is lessened over time. While I recommend you wait until you have been in practice for a year (to gain a balanced perspective on your situation), be sure to provide both your educational program and your workplace with formal feedback on what might enhance a smoother transition to practice for the new graduate of nursing in your region.

Try as hard as we may for perfection, the net result of our labors is an amazing variety of imperfectness. We are surprised at our own versatility in being able to fail in so many different ways.

-Samuel McCord Crothers

"It seems like it's flown by but I'm at like such a different place than I was a year ago when I look back and like I still feel kind of anxious looking back you know. I just feel like I was kind of thrown in there and flying by the seat of my pants and all of a sudden you're responsible and it's just huge, huge, huge stress—huge, huge pressure and it's...like it feels like it wasn't that long ago but at the same time it does. Like I think the changes have been pretty subtle along the way but still a year's made a big difference. I hear that some places do a years worth of kind of orientation and buddying and that kind of thing and like when I did my buddy shifts—I did about a months worth full-time buddy shifts and at the time it was like, OK, I just want to be on my own but now I think 'If it was maybe more of a gradual time it would have been better.'"

NEED TO KNOW

- **Transition shock** occurs within the initial weeks to months of entering professional practice and results from an 'alarming' realization that the roles, responsibilities, knowledge and relationships you are engaging in as a new nurse are more challenging, dynamic and intense than you had expected;
- While you may be optimally **prepared** to practice as a new nurse by your educational program (you know what it means to 'do' nursing), it is likely not possible to be entirely ready to face the challenges of 'being' a fully responsible and accountable practitioner until faced with situations that demand these;
- Transition shock is not only **intellectual** (knowing something 'theoretically' is different than applying that theory in the 'real world'), but it is **cultural** (understanding what nursing is in relation to other professional roles in practice), **social** (there are certain 'unwritten' rules related to the relationships between nurses and between nurses and other professionals that can't be 'taught'), **physical** (plain and simply: nursing is HARD WORK most days as it includes a lot of physical effort—lifting, moving, walking, bending), **emotional** (we often deal with individuals and communities at the intersections of 'health' and 'illness', during times of vulnerability and in situations of despair or desolation and that takes its toll on practitioners. emotions), and **spiritual** (it is not uncommon for nurses to face demanding dilemmas that profoundly challenge their professional and personal ethics and make them question their own, others, or the healthcare system's moral underpinnings, resulting in disconnections or disharmony between the nurse's sense of 'self' and 'other');
- New graduates need to surround themselves with people and situations that are 1) **consistent**, 2) **predictable**, 3) **stable**, 4) **familiar**, and that support 5) **success;**
- IT TAKES at least 6 months to find your sea legs as a new nurse!!!
- Initial integration into practice TAKES practice—find a **SAFE ENVIRONMENT** to practice your fundamentals so that within the first few months you can 'lift your gaze' beyond **WHAT** you are doing to explaining **WHY** you are doing it—***<u>don't expect yourself to be thinking too much about WHY you are doing what you are doing for at least the first 4 months</u>***, particularly if there are many new situations to which you are exposed. Your primary goal will be to figure out what is expected of you and to learn to fulfill your roles and responsibilities 'without killing someone'. ☺

NEED TO THINK ABOUT

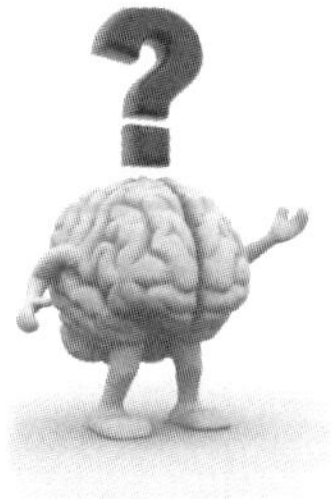

- Where is the **SAFEST** place for you to make the transition to professional practice (ask the following questions related to your plans)?
  - o Did you have experience in this area during a capstone practicum?
  - o Is there an adequate orientation?
  - o Will they assign you a mentor?
  - o Can you work days for the first month after orientation?[10]
  - o What kind of support[11] is offered to you as a new graduate?
    - Orientation and specialty certification;
    - Preceptorship;
    - Mentorship;
    - Supernumerary work;
    - Residency/Internship; AND
    - Transition Facilitation Coordinator
- Does the place where you are thinking about initially working provide:
  - o **Consistency**—are you going to be working with similar staff, consistent patient presentations/diagnoses?
  - o **Predictability**—do you know when, where and with whom you will be working, or can you predict with some certainty the kinds of patients you will be seeing?
  - o **Familiarity**—do you know where to find what you need when you need it, have you been with these staff before, have you worked with these particular routines before, and is there another new grad you can team up with to transition with you? AND
  - o **Stability**—how stable is your life? Do you have a consistent shift that you can predict and therefore plan around, are your patients at high risk of decompensating on a regular basis, is the staff turning over a lot, and is there a strong sense of support on the unit you are going to?

---

[10]This may not be required for all graduates but many new nurses struggle with the circadian rhythm challenges of working nights which can further exhaust you. As well, nights are notoriously 'short staffed' (there are no physicians making rounds, no diagnostic testing outside of emergent issues, etc.) and patients are encouraged to sleep, which makes caring for them less demanding but also reduces the availability of assistance from colleagues.

[11]All of the programs identified here vary in structure and format but all have the intent of supporting the new nursing graduate to gain experience with the routines and responsibilities of their new role, gain some familiarity with the staff they will be working with, progress SLOWLY in accepting greater breadth and scope of responsibility as a professional, and feel supported to grow at their own pace.

- Are you likely to be **successful** as a new nurse in this unit/center or are there situations (clinical or relational) of **high risk** that make your success less likely?
- What strategies have you used to **successfully manage stress** in the past? (i.e. exercise, journaling, socializing with friends, going for coffee with a good buddy)?
- What **negative outcomes of stress** have you experienced in the past? (i.e. irritable bowel syndrome, increased drinking, drug abuse, difficulty with anger)?
- What is going on in your **LIFE** that might influence your work transition?
    - o How can you stabilize the relationships in your life?
    - o What major financial decisions (moving, buying a home or car) can you delay for 6 months?
    - o What can you do to balance the intensity of the initial few months of transition (physical exercise, social activities, relaxation strategies)?
    - o How will you **PLAN** for this balance ahead of time?
    - o What do your friends, spouse, parents, children **NEED TO KNOW** about this phase of your career that will make it easier on you and them?
    - o Who are the individuals to whom you go to for support? Will they be available to you?
    - o What nursing peers can you routinely network with for support? When and where will you meet?

NEED TO DO

1. **Understand transition shock**;
2. **Know the limits of your practice** capability during this period of transition;
3. Remember that you need **CONSISTENCY, PREDICTABILITY, STABILITY** and **FAMILIARITY** to be **SUCCESSFUL**;
4. **Find a unit/center/community that will support you** to progress slowly into your roles and responsibilities as a newly graduated nurse (i.e. **SHOP AROUND!!!!**);
5. Determine what **level of patient is appropriate for you to care for** during your initial transition (**REMEMBER**: *stable, consistent, predictable, familiar*);
6. **Know your BOUNDARIES** (i.e. if someone asks you to care for a patient, or go to a unit that you feel is beyond your knowledge or experiential comfort level, **JUST SAY NO!!!!!** If you feel 'reduced', 'belittled' or 'coerced' by a colleague's response, **SAY "I sense that you don't agree with my decision, but I know this is in the best interests of the patient/the workplace/my coworkers"** and approach your mentor, educator or manager at the next most appropriate time—that might be at the end of the shift—to discuss your concerns);

7. **Meet with your manager, educator and mentor**[12] **EVERY SHIFT** for the first two weeks **POST-ORIENTATION** and then **EVERY SET OF SHIFTS** for a month after that:
   a. discuss how the shift went;
   b. outline what went WELL and what CHALLENGED you and why;
   c. formulate a plan together to deal with the challenges next time; AND
   d. modify the transition support as your needs change or are revealed.
8. Inform colleagues, family, friends, children, spouses and parents of the **POTENTIAL challenges** you will be dealing with during the initial couple of months after you begin working as a new nurse (AFTER orientation):
   a. **exhaustion** (sleep a lot but don't feel rested—sleep is consumed with dreaming about work);
   b. **fear of failure** (more defensive than usual or sensitive to critique/comments, tendency to ask questions repeatedly);
   c. **performance anxiety** (avoiding particularly difficult/new skills, avoiding patients who are ill and/or experiencing physical symptoms of anxiety such as sweating, racing heart, shortness of breath or inability to think/concentrate before or during a task);
   d. **labile emotions** (laughing one minute, crying the next—easy to provoke to tears or anger at work OR at home); AND
   e. **low self-confidence** (seem to react rather than respond to comments and many comments taken 'personally'; may need unusual levels of affirmation or reassurance).
9. **Be AWARE of how you COPE with stress**—prepare for stress during these initial months by PLANNING activities that relieve stress OR/AND avoid, delay, or resolve whatever stressors you can (i.e. if money worries stress you, try to put off major purchases until you have the energy to cope); AND
10. **Plan to get as much sleep as you can**—IF you choose to take sleeping aides, first talk with a Nurse Practitioner or Physician. While the 'odd' Gravol ™ or glass of wine might seem like a benign strategy to help you get through those nasty 'all night self-debrief sessions' that seem to haunt you after a shift, this kind of coping behavior on an ongoing basis should trigger an alarm for you. The line between healthy and dysfunctional coping is sometimes about the length of time you remain in 'coping' mode and whether or not that coping strategy starts to adversely affect other aspects of your life. YOU'RE A NURSE—you'd think you would know when you have crossed that line. But BEWARE—it CAN sneak up on you so if you feel yourself

[12]If you do not have a formal 'mentor' assigned to you, take an experienced nurse with whom you have a good working relationship into the meeting with you and debrief with them after the meeting to determine if you understood what was said the way they understood what was said.

sliding down the 'other' side of that slippery slope (i.e. someone comments about your unusual behavior or expresses concern about what they think are unhealthy habits you have adopted), reach out to another grad or trusted friend for support, or visit your primary care practitioner or even the occupational health nurse in your workplace. Any issues you share related to your health will be held in CONFIDENCE—these supportive health professionals are there to help you manage your stress appropriately and help you get back on track!

Stage 1
Professional Role Transition

DOING

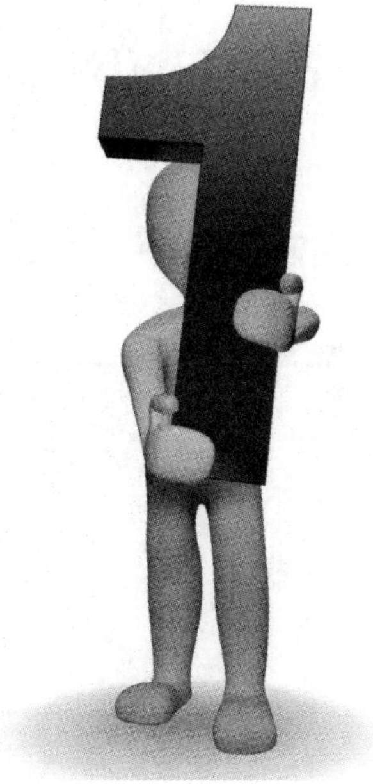

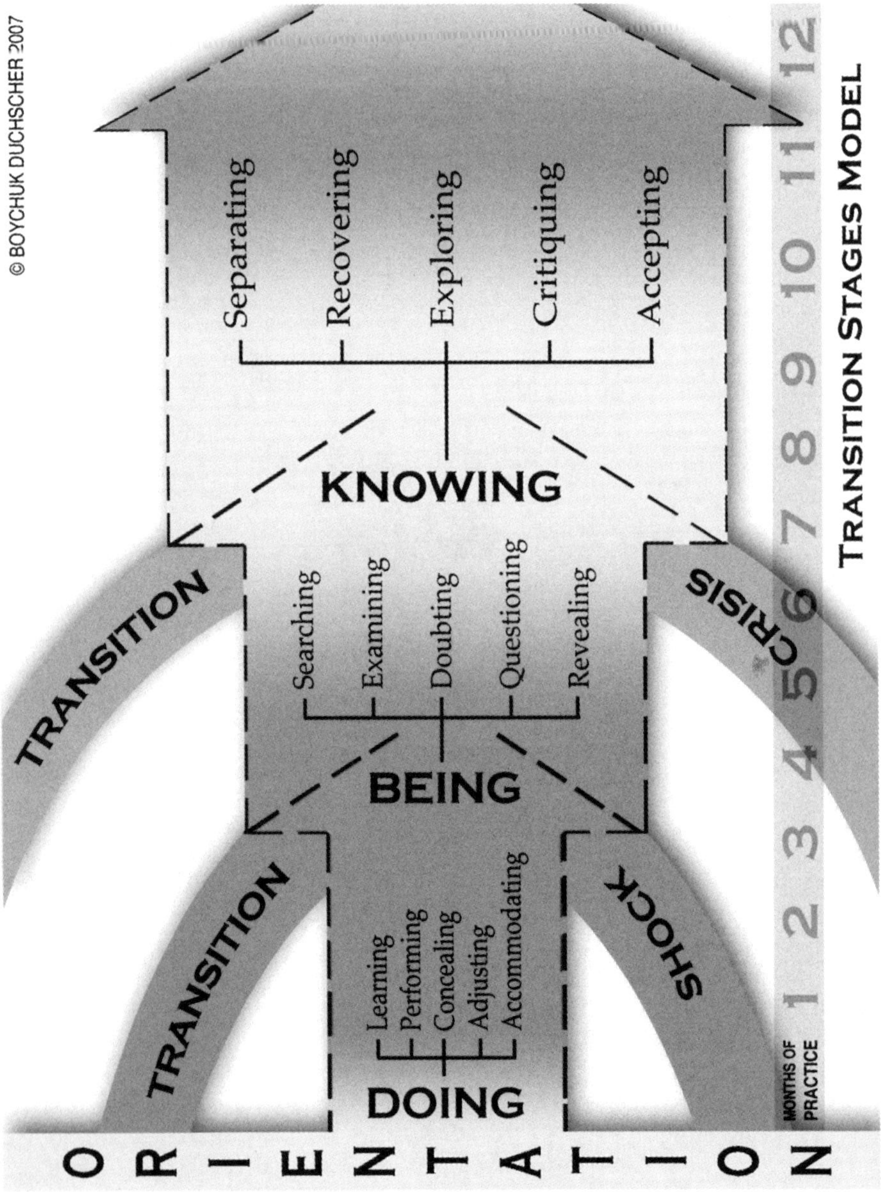
© BOYCHUK DUCHSCHER 2007
TRANSITION STAGES MODEL
ORIENTATION
TRANSITION
SHOCK
DOING
Learning
Performing
Concealing
Adjusting
Accommodating
TRANSITION
CRISIS
BEING
Searching
Examining
Doubting
Questioning
Revealing
KNOWING
Separating
Recovering
Exploring
Critiquing
Accepting
MONTHS OF PRACTICE
1
2
3
4
5
6
7
8
9
10
11
12

Some Things Come in Waves (like nausea ☺) . . . Transition Comes in STAGES

The transition into practice for the first 12 months after nursing school is a **process** of *becoming* a professionally practicing nurse. As with most journeys, it isn't a straight line from novice to expert, but more of a winding road, full of twists and turns, detours, and the occasional pothole☺. To be clear, this critical life experience will be very unique to every individual so I cannot tell you **exactly** what your transition will look like. I can, however, give you a sense of the experiences that the many new graduates have had[1] so that you can:

1) **begin to prepare** for your own transition by putting checks and balances in place for the possible challenges ahead, and
2) **know that you are NOT ALONE**—or in technical terms, 'normalize' your experience so that you do not get stuck thinking *'Am I the only one who is struggling?'*.

Trust me.....we ALL struggle with major transitions in our lives.
At this point, I believe it is prudent to remind you about the importance of **FAMILIARITY,**

> ***It is my daily mood that makes the weather. I possess tremendous power to make life miserable or joyous. I can be a tool of torture or an instrument of inspiration, I can humiliate or humor, hurt or heal. In all situations, it is my response that decides whether a crisis is escalated or de-escalated, and a person is humanized or de-humanized. If we treat people as they are, we make them worse. If we treat people as they ought to be, we help them become what they are capable of becoming.***
>
> ***- J. W. Goethe***

CONSISTENCY, PREDICTABILITY and **STABILITY** in your personal AND professional life during the next 6 months. As Michael Moncur's saying goes, *'life is what happens to you while you are making other plans'*. The message is that while we strive to plan, organize and direct our lives (which is not such a bad idea as ideas go), by doing so we often fail to leave enough 'space' for:

1) new events (moving, getting married or divorced, buying a car or a house, or ***starting a job as a new nurse***);
2) complicated relationships (conflicts in the workplace with co-workers, starting or ending personal friendships or intimate relationships); and

> ***Pain is inevitable; suffering is optional.***
>
> ***- Unknown***

[1]For an overall perspective on the Stages of Transition journey of the new nurse, please see the *Conceptual Model of Transition Support* in the Appendix of this book.

3) unfamiliar or complex practice situations or contexts (going to work as a professional nurse in an area that you never had the opportunity to experience as a student).

These interruptions can significantly disrupt the flow of things and may cause your transition to look different from what you had envisioned, or to be more challenging than you had anticipated.

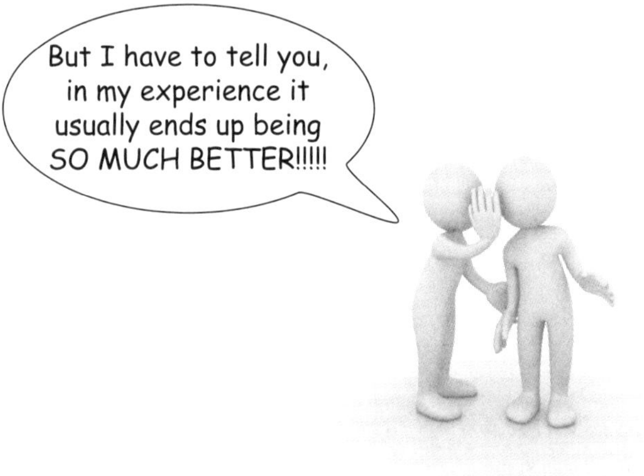

Well, welcome to the 'real' world!! Everyone at this point in their lives has likely come to realize that NOTHING turns out EXACTLY as you planned, dreamed, imagined or expected...... Ok, so let's talk about Stage ONE.....

Here you are! You have worked for years to achieve this goal and you can't WAIT to actually start applying the knowledge and skills that you sacrificed all that time and money to perfect!!!! It is SO exciting!

> *"It's all happening so fast! But it's exciting at the same time. Just knowing that you've come this far and you're going to go that much further. Every month I put $200.00 away for a trip to Australia and now that I've got some kind of security and I think, 'this really is going to happen. You're going to get to do these things and you can do them cause you've worked hard'. I didn't think I'd ever finish nursing, but here I am!"*

Now, I do **NOT** want to *rain on your parade*, but upon entering the practice environment as a new nurse, you may quickly come to realize that although you have been well PREPARED to assume the roles of a nurse (your educational program held you up to those high standards for a reason ☺), you may not feel READY to carry the full weight of responsibility expected of you, nor prepared to manage the significantly increased workload that comes with your new role.

"I've been experiencing numerous or various mixed emotions actually. At first it was nervousness and excitement and now it's more 'Wow, this is actually for real and now I'm feeling overwhelmed, stressed, still excited, but also wondering if this is the profession for me'. I've actually had that thought. It runs across my mind a couple of times. I'm not really sure and I've been told that that's a normal feeling. It's just all happening really fast for me I guess. I didn't really have a whole lot of time to let it all sink in I guess before actually starting."

"It's strange. I don't really feel like I am finished school. Like I walked to work one morning and as I was walking, I was thinking, 'I'm getting paid to do this,' because it's like I was still in school. And then, within my orientation week I was told that the staff had just run off this nurse who wasn't doing very well. They told me that they had made it so miserable for her that she would leave . . . and I think they were proud of it—that they had gotten rid of her. I think it's maybe to maintain quality control, but it's definitely one of my fears that I won't be accepted. That if I am failing, they won't come alongside me, but will show me the door."

This is NOT because you are not a capable, competent and highly intelligent graduate. It is just that learning how to manage dynamic, complex situations that are as variable as the people IN those situations, takes time and experience; that's why they call it a CAREER!

Reality is the leading cause of stress amongst those in touch with it.

- Jane Wagner

"I think part of the pressure for me is that I got the silver medal, and I think 'Well, OK, so if I had the highest marks in the whole province for my year and I'm floundering...was I marked accurately? Do I really have the potential to be as good a nurse as my professors all thought?'"

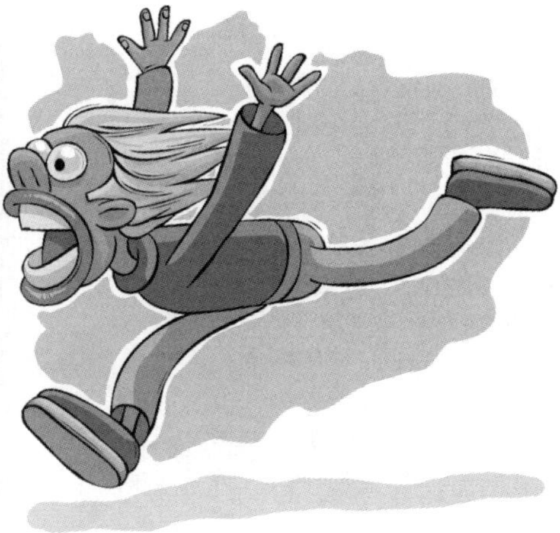

Many newly graduated nurses enter their professional transition with expectations and anticipations that are more idealistic than they are realistic. Seriously though, if pending graduates of ANY discipline knew EVERYTHING that goes on in the 'real world', they might stop, turn and run as fast and as far as they can in the other direction ☺! The trick is to strike an appropriate and realistic balance.

Leaders in EVERY profession, discipline and workplace fall a bit short in their attempts to create the right set of circumstances for their employees to reach the pinnacle of their potential. That's life. New nurses tend to blame a lack of educational preparation for the differences between what they had anticipated regarding their roles as professionals and what they are expected to do when they actually begin working in practice. When asked, none of the participants in any of my research over the years even considered the culpability of their workplaces in failing to adequately (in other words, gradually and strategically) introduce them to the roles and responsibilities of a fully practicing nurse. As a nurse educator I can appreciate that striking a balance between what we WANT to create as contemporary nursing practice and what we are ACTUALLY seeing in practice is difficult at the best of times. Having said that, I think that while nursing education programs have a responsibility to prepare students for the realities of the workplace, the healthcare sector has a responsibility to integrate new nurses into work roles for which they cannot be fully prepared during their education.

> *"I have a big problem with my final practicum because you go to school for years and you put in a lot of work and a lot of time. You finish school and you start your job and I feel that we shouldn't have the feeling of anxiety or the feeling that we aren't ready or aren't prepared. In school we didn't get our hands or noses into things enough. It's in the back of our head but maybe we weren't taught how to use our hands or wrap our head around those things but the knowledge is in there. They kept telling us to apply our knowledge but they needed to help us to do that more. But it's hard to take information from this class and this class and this class and put it all together. We maybe needed more clinical experience."*

Attempting to lay blame for what we are all clearly responsible is a waste of precious time and energy. Instead, I suggest educators and employers work closely together to identify and then seek to resolve the issues that prevent new nurses from experiencing a healthy integration into professional practice.

The fact that new nurses are surprised by the workload intensity and level of responsibility afforded them once they become 'practicing' nurses (particularly those working within an acute-care setting) is similar to what many non-nursing professionals experience when they first start their careers. Nurses who experience significant discrepancies in their practice environment relative to what they have come to expect during their educational preparation can feel disappointed by their work; some may even feel a sense of betrayal.

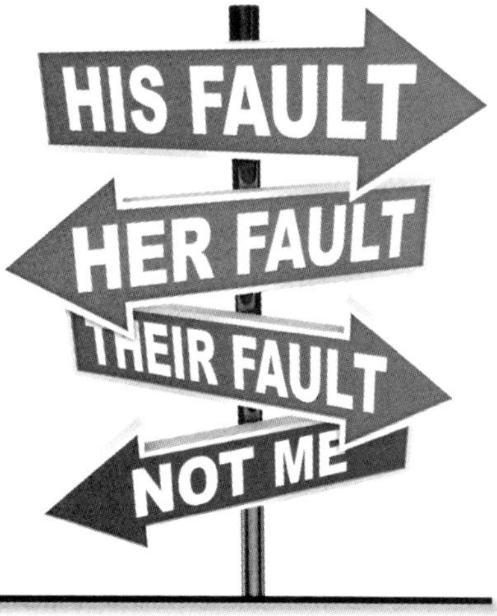

> *"I was scared. Very scared. I guess about a week in we had a buddy shift and then a week off and they were starting to call us. They needed staff and they started to call us to work on our own. I just said 'no' because I was too scared to start yet even though I only had two buddy shifts left. I just wanted to get those done first 'cause I was so scared to start on my own. Then I'm like, 'OK, I'm ready to start now', but you're completely on your own. Your preceptors are not there to double check your meds with you or ask questions...."*

These feelings can escalate over time, particularly if the new nurse is unable to reconcile the discrepancies, if they witness or experience further disempowerment, or if they feel personally or professionally devalued within their new workplace.

> *"It's gotten to the point where I don't even know if I like nursing anymore. When I was at that fair I had a ticket and I got to spin the wheel and I...put my ticket into this draw and I got to spin the wheel and you could win various prizes like T-shirts and buttons and mugs and it stopped and I won a button and I looked at it and it said, 'I love nursing' and I said, 'I don't want it'. I don't really like nursing anymore."*

The 1st stage of entry into professional practice is marked by tremendous intensity and a fluctuation of emotions as you work through the processes of *learning, performing, concealing, adjusting, and accommodating.*

> *"Like some days it's perfect—I had this day and I remember driving home thinking, 'I had a good night' and I was like 'I'm so glad I'm a nurse. I love this and I love working'. And then the next day I had a bad experience and was like in tears on my way home and it's just like it's one extreme to the next."*

The Process of Transitioning

> ***If the facts don't fit the theory, change the facts.***
> ***- Albert Einstein***

Progress through the stages of transition will vary according to the level of pre-graduate knowledge about professional role transition, the length and quality of your orientation, the transition and integration programs you are enrolled in upon hiring and the level of support you feel (or don't feel) from the experienced colleagues you are working with. Within the transition theory described here, stage one begins AFTER your initial orientation or introduction into the workplace[2]; the start of

[2] Note that ***Transition Shock***© has been identified as a 'separate' experience but is encompassed WITHIN the 1st stage of transition. The model of transition shock described in Chapter 2 serves as a foundational framework for the overall transition experience. The four intersecting elements (roles, responsibilities, relationships and knowledge) explicated in the transition shock model continue to act as the reference point for understanding the origins of both challenge and growth for new graduates throughout the initial year of professional practice.

this stage correlates with your first shift 'on your own' where, for the first time since graduating you feel the weight of a full clinical workload. IF you are fortunate enough to have an extended support period, you may experience a more 'muted' intensity and duration of this stage, although my research tells me that new nurses WILL experience each of these processes (*learning, performing, concealing, adjusting and accommodating*) to some degree within the first several months of practice.

Learning

Learning that all is not as you might have come to expect it would be in the professional practice setting can be disconcerting. Having said that, it is unreasonable to expect that your educational program would be able to afford you insight into every possible clinical situation, have you perform every possible skill required of you as a professional, or expose you to the range of relational dynamics that you might face working within a team of professionals under the kind of pressure that is now commonplace for the contemporary healthcare workplace. As a result, life as a newly graduated nurse often becomes a flurry of *learning and performing.*

> *"They're not my arms because, although it's my practice and I'm doing it, I still feel a bit like I need so much help from other people that my actions are not my own and I'm doing them but they're being orchestrated by other people. I still need so much help and I'm asking so many questions that I might be making the decision and I am talking it through with someone, but they're making it with me so they're not completely my arms yet cause they're not my decisions completely yet."*

At this stage of your transition you are likely discovering 'what you don't know'; which makes it easy to get trapped into thinking you don't know *anything*! It can be humbling, and even daunting, to realize how much MORE there is to learn after you graduate! But I encourage you to take comfort in the skills you come with—they will ground you, reassure you and save you so much time.

> ***All truths are easy to understand once they are discovered; the point is to discover them.***
>
> ***- Galileo Galilei***

A note here about WHERE you work during the early months of your transition. If you recall my comment earlier, the importance of consistency, predictability, familiarity and stability for a new nurse cannot be overstated. Remember to consider these elements in the whole context of 1) the patient/client population, 2) the staff, and 3) your personal life. IF you believe that the workplace to which you are going can provide these, PACK YOUR BAGS AND GET ON THAT BUS!!

BUT.....even if you are being encouraged, enticed or otherwise 'courted' to take employment in a workplace that in YOUR estimation cannot provide these fundamental elements of success, please reconsider.

> *"I think we're just trying to put everything together of what you learned in school and trying to think back on things and... you go though a lot of, 'should I do this, should I not be doing this, should I go back to school'...I found I was very hard on myself. Very critical of what I was doing and wanted to quit a few times. I think it really makes a difference on where you start and how what your experience is at that time. It changes your opinion of nursing."*

You have a lifetime to secure employment in a variety of nursing contexts so what's the rush??? I would suggest that it is wise to spend the first 12 months gaining a secure sense of yourself professionally, developing a strong set of basic competencies, understanding workplace 'culture' and what it means to navigate professional dynamics, and **<u>HAVING A LITTLE FUN</u>** while you're still young enough (I am speaking to the 2nd degree/accelerated track graduates ☺)!

> *"I'm on my 2nd of three nights here on [unit]. What a TREAT! I love the work here. Sure it's heavy, but it is mentally heavy, challenging my knowledge and skills, and at the end of the day allows me to be proud of myself for knowing what to do or how to react. I honestly can see that my confidence is increasing. I guess that is what working on the same unit for three days in a row will do. As compared to my wishy washy schedule where I am tossed between two units and never have time to really grasp what's going on. I have applied for a temporary at [hospital] so that I can find a little more <u>consistency</u> (participant emphasis). I don't feel that float position allows for adequate learning. It seemed like such a good idea at the beginning, but now I am really finding the downfalls."*

Performing and Concealing

Part of what makes this stage such a 'flurry' of activity is that while you acquired a base of knowledge and skill during your education, the variety of situations within which you are being asked to PERFORM those skills and apply that knowledge are as limitless as the human beings you are caring for. Learning what is expected of you, performing your various roles safely, taking responsibility for the professional decisions and judgments that are now yours to make, **and** completing all of this "*on time and without killing someone*" may well be your primary objective at this stage. Uncertain of who you can trust (this will depend on your prior exposure to the transition setting), and driven by a strong developmental need

> ***Never promise more than you can perform.***
>
> ***- Publilius Syrus***

to 'fit in' or 'belong' to your professional group, you may go to great lengths to *conceal* anxieties[3] you are feeling from your colleagues.

For graduates who have had experience working as professionals prior to entering their nursing education program (LPN/RPNs or Enrolled nurses moving into RN roles or individuals with prior non-nursing degrees who are variably referred to as '*accelerated degree*', '*2nd degree*', or '*Post- RN*' graduates), or for LPN/RPNs with extensive experience in nursing practice but now assuming RN roles, the need to conceal may be less of an issue, though it is normal in any 'new' situation to disguise feelings of inadequacy. This cautiousness, however expected, can isolate you from those around you as you 'appear' to others to be coping well with the changes, while inside you are screaming: "HELP!!! I am terrified and feel like I don't know what I'm doing!!!!" This contradiction between how you FEEL and how you APPEAR TO OTHERS can contribute to the loneliness you may feel as a result of being a new nurse in a busy and seemingly unforgiving workplace.

> *"Before shifts I have a hard time falling asleep 'cause all those thoughts run through your mind and anxiety and the feeling in the pit of your stomach before you're going to bed....Just mentally exhausted at the end of the day. Not so much physically but the mind never stops. It's hard getting it to relax when you're lying in bed and you find yourself tossing and turning and the next thing you know it's one in the morning and you think 'Oh my God. I need to be up at six and I only have this much sleep' and then you start getting worked up that you're going to sleep and then it's hard to get to sleep....I still dream about work quite frequently but it's not waking me up every two hours in a panic like it did during the first month. I dream that I didn't do something or that something's wrong and I don't know what to do about it....I dream about starting IVs, I dream about handing out pills, I dream about machines beeping, I dream about everything."*

Because so much of what you are experiencing is new to you, the learning curve that dominates this stage can feel steep. The solid professional identity you may have developed by the end of your education may fracture under the weight of your current performance anxiety and self-doubt. It may seem difficult to discern the exact origin of your anxiety as new graduates often feel stressed "*about absolutely everything.*" Your entry-level skill and knowledge may be

[3]While concealing anxieties related to one's LACK of knowledge or experience from others is a natural phenomenon in any new situation, it is equally important to understand that new grads coming with prior nursing, healthcare or even life experiences may seek to conceal what they DO know from those around them. This tendency is driven by fears of being thought pretentious by the very colleagues from whom they seek acceptance, having to deal with unrealistic expectations in the workplace, or being asked to perform roles or take responsibilities with which they are not yet comfortable.

challenged by the unfamiliar and sometimes unanticipated clinical presentations of patients that contribute to a wavering level of practice confidence. The relentless requests that come your way to assist with or perform procedures for which you have little or no reference can cause significant levels of anxiety. These situations pose a high level of risk to graduates who perceive such requests as having the potential to expose them as 'incompetent', subsequently reducing their credibility in the eyes of their colleagues; this perception of incompetence, alongside the potential for causing harm to patients, is the most significant fear of the new nurse.

> ***Life has no rehearsals, only performances.***
> ***- Unknown***

> *"A new graduate nurse....it almost feels like in the eyes of your co-workers you're seen as a completely different person. It's kind of hard to explain actually. At the same time you do get a little bit of, well not pity but they seem to be like 'Oh she's a new grad....she won't know anything' and it's almost like they look at you like they don't necessarily trust your care. I don't mind being looked at like that in some ways because I don't know everything and it's almost like they give you a little bit of leeway and I think for now that is a good thing. There's a little bit more understanding from the physician and some of the older more experienced nurses that yes I am going to be asking questions."*

> *"I asked my preceptor how much KCL should be mixed in how much NS since I had never mixed KCL in NS before. She said, 'What? I can't believe that, it makes me scared to think of what you yet do not know and lack experience in'. I felt ashamed for never doing this before and I felt stupid for opening my mouth and asking. Asking questions is how I learn and it prevents mistakes. While she was scared about my lack of experience, I was scared that this awful experience would stop me from asking questions."*

It is worth noting here that anyone who tells you that asking questions is not acceptable....IS DEMONSTRATING UNSAFE BEHAVIOR. That doesn't mean we ask the SAME questions for 2 years (that is another issue altogether...), but it does mean that by asking for information or clarification, we are practicing HUMILITY as professionals. It tells others that we recognize our limitations and we understand that we CAN'T know everything, no matter how long we have been a nurse.

When I was practicing as a critical care nurse (not a bad one if I do say so myself ☺) I recall one night when we were over staffed (yes, there IS such a thing....), so I was 'floated' to help out on an obstetrical unit. SERIOUSLY??? I have never even HAD a baby, so knowledge related to this area of practice is not 'common' to me. I was looking after a new mom who was experiencing post-partum urinary retention. There was an order for a straight catheterization (or as we called it, an 'in and out cath'), should this complication arise. So I catheterized this patient. Well, if she didn't have A LOT of retention—she poured out 2 liters of urine in about 10 minutes......which I thought would be a GOOD thing. That's when it happened—her bladder and uterus went into spasm from emptying too quickly (MY FAULT) and that woman screamed like I was killing her! Now, for those of you out there who think new nurses are the only ones that want to hide when they have made a mistake in their care, you are WRONG! But it was hard for me to hide from THAT situation!!! Anyway, I learned a BIG lesson and, accompanied by numerous other humbling practice situations over the course of my career, I have learned to ask a lot of questions.....things happen and we need to learn what we can from them and move on.

Graduates who are assigned the same workload as tenured co-workers within the first weeks of employment but who are NOT given access to expert counsel or practice support may feel as though they have landed on MARS! Being a new nurse in today's acute-care practice environment, where the clear majority of graduates make their initial transition, has been described by many as an *"obstacle course"*.

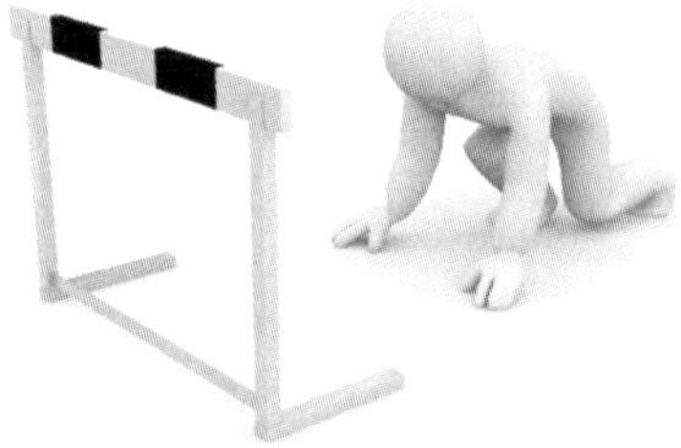

New professionals describe feeling overwhelmed by the weight of responsibility for new roles, responsibilities, relationships and expectations of knowledge application not previously experienced as a student.

> *"I'm so easily distracted and I don't know how to limit my visits to short ones so I can get back to doing whatever I was doing. I get very much tied into the patient so that's something I really need to work on. But watching the senior nurses, they can just walk in there in a few minutes and get all the information where maybe it would take me 15 -20 minutes to get what they did."*

> *"We haven't had a CODE while I've been up there working but you know housekeeping pulled the cord from the wall once and it goes off and all of a sudden people are running. I was like 'What's going on?' and someone said 'That's the CODE button!' and I was like, 'Oh I didn't know'. I was so busy I didn't even recognize what was going on, so I hope that changes. Because yeah the first few times it was like 'Oh my god what if I don't hear it?' What if something is going on down the hall and I don't hear it....I just don't necessarily pick up on those things right now."*

Adjusting

We cannot direct the wind, but we can adjust our sails.

- Bertha Calloway

The challenges of *adjusting* to the expectations of professional practice become particularly evident when the novice is expected to manage patients who are clinically unstable or if they are required to multitask (i.e. answering phones, speaking with physicians, processing orders, or dealing with multiple patient and family issues while performing difficult tasks such as starting an intravenous, giving medications, or doing a dressing change).

> *"I come in at 7:30 and I check in on everybody and I get my vitals done, get all my meds given and I sit there for a minute and I go, 'Okay, you have a minute to breathe'. Then I think maybe I should chart and then all of a sudden, BANG, call bells are ringing and doctors are writing orders and blah, blah, blah, and the next thing you know it's 10:00 and you have to do the next set of meds and 'Oh, I didn't get any of that charting done yet', and 'Oh, I haven't listened to so and so's lungs yet' and you know.....We got this admission that came in and it was through the pediatric transport team, so it was a kid that came in with meningitis and I was left alone and in charge on the unit and then we got this admission and I mean, he was sick. Like his oxygen was cranked up and everything you know, not alert—not stable really, and he ended up in PICU later. And so here I was all alone in the unit having to take this admission. I mean, I didn't even know where to start. I didn't know what to do or anything and I thought that that wasn't very right of them to send that other nurse home for those last four hours and then leave me all alone there. I mean I was still a grad nurse and hadn't been there for very long I felt that I wasn't very helpful because I didn't really know what to do or where I should start or anything. I was stressed out then you know? At the end of the shift, I hadn't finished all my work, we hadn't counted or anything yet so I was just kind of upset."*

It is not uncommon for graduates to have an intense focus on trying to remember or recall all the 'details' of the task that is *in front of* them. This often renders them unaware of what is happening **around** them. As a result, they worry about 'missing something' or inadvertently and unintentionally bringing harm to someone under their care because of their ignorance or inexperience. That is normal!

> *"But that night, both triage and charge saw that person and they're both very senior nurses. We saw him, the paramedics saw him, and he even said to me, 'he doesn't look good' and I'm like, 'I know, he's all pasty' like you could tell his color was terrible but he...didn't seem to be having lots of pain...I don't know what else we could have done. I didn't even ask for help so I feel bad, I do. When I look back*

on it, there were signs…I didn't know what it was but I just had this feeling that something wasn't right but I didn't question anything…cause I'd never been in that situation before and I didn't know any better."

The indispensable first step to getting the things you want out of life is this: decide what you want.
- Ben Stein

New nurses, like most professionals starting out in practice, have a relatively linear, theoretical 'keep my head down and get the work done' approach to practice. As a novice practitioner, you will tend to 'default' to what you learned in school; often this knowledge is based more in 'theory' than in experience.

"There's something to be said about experience. Like many of these experienced doctors and nurses get kind of a gut feeling about patients or a feeling…like they've experienced them before, they've seen them before. Say you have no clue what croup is…people come in and just cough a little bit, just a little like hardly don't make any…and there are nurse that say, 'Oh yeah, that's croup for sure'. The first time I was like, 'how did they know that?' It's like asking a person who's never seen a cat before to pick out a cat. So you trust people with the experience and the gut feeling. There have been times when I wish I had that feeling about a patient."

I remember one new nurse suggesting that the early application of her knowledge was like *"being in a private little bubble and things are going on all around me and I cannot hear them, I cannot see them."* The limits to your problem solving and clinical judgment are NOT surprising because you may have no actual experience with many of the scenarios to which you are now being exposed. While straightforward, stable and predictable clinical situations can be navigated with relative ease, the same is not true for *complex* clinical scenarios. This is generally because much of your energy and 'mind work' is consumed with an overwhelming amount of NEW information coming at you at the same time.

"Some things go so fast though I can't even process them….Like it's so fast that I can't even process some stuff and it takes like 5 or 6 times to catch it all. It's just going so fast."

The key to addressing this issue is to be cognizant of the clinical environment in which you experience your initial transition, and the workload afforded you during the very crucial first 4 months of practice. Those graduates transitioning into a moderate to high acuity practice context (active medical surgical, specialty, observation, emergency or critical care units) need to be cautious about the patient workload (both level of care required and quantity of patients) they are assigned and try to 'gradually' increase workload intensity and complexity.

Start with fewer patients and those who are ready for transfer (more chronic), have been on the unit for a period of time and whose issues are known, those who are waiting for placement in a long-term or convalescent unit, or those whose clinical situation is relatively stable. The process of 'admitting' patients to these units should be first done WITH an experienced practitioner and, when comfortable, then alone. You should always have access to a senior nurse with experience on the unit and advanced clinical knowledge of the patient demographic common to that practice area.

> *"This one particular day where I came home and that was it I thought. I quit. I hate this. Um it was just really rough on the ward. Everything seemed to be happening all at the same time....and so fast. I can't think like that....Like when I give my meds I'm so cautious and it just seems to take me longer than the other nurses at this point and I either don't recognize or I'm not 100% on so I'm always checking them. Always double-checking. Even triple-checking."*

Starting out your professional practice in community or public health, or in long-term care, is a good idea. The challenge is that these positions are often 'sought after' and many new graduates are not hired into these areas (outside of 'casual' work) initially. While the challenges related to professional role transition remain, these environments tend to be more *forgiving* (the practice error outcome risk is not as high) and the roles and responsibilities of this work are easier for new nurses to adjust to.

As a rule, new nurses tend to focus on completing their work (roles, responsibilities, skills) and applying existing institutional protocols within the prescribed time frames without thinking much about "why" they are doing something. While these protocol-oriented boundaries may feel like they distract you from providing quality care (doing baths at certain times in the evening because of staff availability and not because of patient preference; rigidly imposing 'visiting hour' protocols), you may find it equally difficult to face the consequences of NOT complying with existing workplace routines. The 'attention' that can come from 'standing out' amongst your colleagues is in fundamental opposition to the new professional's desire to fit in to the workplace and is often the cause of dissonance within the new nurse.

> ***If you chase two rabbits, both will escape.***
> ***- Unknown***

> *"You're just so busy doing other things. More of the organizational things. Trying to get things all set up and done, but I feel like I've lost that patient relationship. When you're a student and you have two patients, you can really get to know them and now I know what the nurses meant when they said 'Oh you know these students......' cause as a student it's great, like you know so much about your patients. Cause you do; you just have the time to sit there and talk with them—that's what you do. You have maybe three or four patients and that gives you lots of time to really spend time with them so I feel like I've lost that part of it right now. I think that I need to learn how to make that happen a little faster."*

Accommodating

As a result of the pressures to meet deadlines constructed by the unit or institution within which you are working, you may feel the need to *accommodate* practices you see in more experienced staff without necessarily critiquing those practices for their soundness. Sometimes this happens without you even realizing it (I mean REALLY—you are BUSY TRANSITIONING!!!!), but then again, sometimes you may find yourself accommodating substandard practice because to NOT do so might be perceived as an indirect challenge or *criticism* of your colleagues. Although new nurses understandably feel an immediate need to adjust their practice to what may be accepted unit practices, many later identify discrepancies in standards of practice as primary factors contributing to their lack of professional fulfillment in their nursing role.

> *"I was so focused on knowing the routine, knowing what I'm doing, getting things done, knowing the way different nurses like things done, knowing where I fit in, what I'm supposed to be doing, when I'm supposed to be doing it. I had total tunnel vision. I was just focused on getting the job done and getting out of there on time. Then I would go home and I would feel guilty for not being more."*

> *"I've never had anyone's blood sugar who was critically low before so I asked one of the more experienced nurses, 'Okay, what's the next step—like who do I call and what do I get ready and what will they probably order?' I would say I was slow—slower than them."*

> *"Blood—well I've given it a few times but I had to give a chemo drug for the first time and so I was thinking back to my orientation in the classroom: 'Okay, what do I need to do? What do I need to check?' So yeah it just took me 5-10 minutes to review everything, get things ready and go over in my head what I'm going to do and then going in and doing it."*

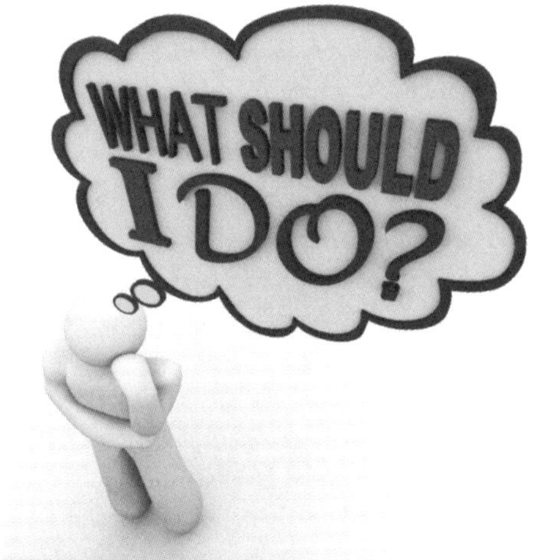

In part, this accommodation may be warranted as nurses with years of experience performing particular skills or making certain decisions and judgments repeatedly acquire 'tacit' knowledge; a deep sense of 'know how' that comes through repeated success in dealing with varied clinical situations. Such expert knowers not only 'see' what others do not (relying on a deep knowledge that comes from a subconscious synergy of the senses), but 'know' intuitively WHAT to do, WHEN and HOW to do it, and WHY they are doing it. Invariably, the new nurse watches the application of this knowledge with awe wondering, *"How did he know that?"* or *"Will I ever be able to practice like that?"* Indeed you will, but that kind of knowledge development takes time, practice experience and circumstance. You cannot even **buy** that kind of experience.....

> ***If you can't live through adversity, you'll never be good at what you do. You have to live through the unfair things, and you have to develop the hide to not let it bother you and keep your eyes focused on what you have to do.***
>
> ***- Maurice "Hank" Greenberg***

> *"For me, this is what made my first few months BLOW SO SOOOO much…if you have really good role models in your workplace, you still sort of feel like a bag of dirt. But you really feel like a big bag of dirt when these nurses act like they came out of nursing school this way! It's just nice to know that these role models once felt like I do now…."*

I would be remiss if I did not speak to the frustration and disappointment some new nurses describe when they see what they believe to be archaic ways of thinking about, or practicing nursing by their experienced colleagues. This includes the rigid allocation of 'tasks' that may be arguably outside of the job description of a professional nurse (i.e. emptying dirty linen bags or cleaning patient rooms after discharge). Notwithstanding the need to perform whatever tasks ensure the health and care of patients/clients (i.e. sterilizing a vaginal speculum at 0200 hours on a weekend when central supply is not in the hospital because you are admitting a rape victim OR cleaning an observation room after you have urgently transferred a more stable patient to accommodate a transfer from critical care), it IS important that we ensure full application of ***each team member's*** skills, knowledge level and practice capacity.

As a nursing graduate, you may struggle with the expectation that you assign or delegate[4] tasks and responsibilities to other licensed and non-licensed personnel, many of whom may be older and have more clinical experience or work seniority than you.

> *"What overwhelms me the most? Definitely being incompetent. Feeling like I'm not prepared to handle the patient load and delegating when I don't even know what*

[4]It is important to understand the distinctions between **'assigning'** and **'delegating'. Assigning** care implies that you are collaborating with another healthcare professional who is licensed and works within a scope of practice for which they can be held accountable. IF, in this case, you are 'assigning' care, it is assumed that you are transferring responsibility for that care to the individual to whom you are assigning the task (in other words, they are responsible). Conversely, **delegation** encompasses requests for the performance of a task for which the individual to whom the skill or task is being delegated is NOT licensed and therefore is NOT able to be held ultimately responsible for the performance of that skill within their professional scope. In this case, YOU (the delegator) retain responsibility for the performance of that skill or task.

to delegate cause I don't know what should be done. Where I work we have really delineated roles but sometimes I find it hard to give other people direction. Sometimes it's hard for me....Especially if they've been there longer than I have, it's kind of tricky because we were expected to do all of the care for our patients as students so when we take on the RN role we do everything for the patients that we have been assigned."

> ***Pride is concerned with who is right. Humility is concerned with what is right.***
>
> ***- Ezra Taft Benson***

While it may be initially difficult to consider having to 'tell' someone what needs to be done, it is often more a matter of APPROACH than substance (you know what they say: *it isn't WHAT you say but HOW you say it that matters*.....or put another way, *people may not always remember what you did or even what you said, but they will always remember how you made them **feel**....*). I have provided some ideas in the Appendix on how to approach these sensitive situations, but here is a summary:

1) **Use 'I' more than 'YOU'** – *I was hoping I might get some assistance to bathe this individual this morning – would you have time?* OR *I am new to collaborating on workload – how would YOU recommend we work with this group of patients/clients?* OR *I have never partnered with a practical nurse except when I was a student – can you help me understand how our roles work together on this unit?*
2) **Listen CAREFULLY** to the other person – understanding is crucial – *My first thought is that we should do ____ - what do YOU think we should do in this situation?* OR *Have you seen this happen before? What would you do in this situation?* OR *How would you approach this?*
3) **Avoid judgmental statements** – *You didn't ask me* OR *I wouldn't have pulled that dressing off the way you did* OR *You were so unsupportive to me in that situation.* Instead, **stay with YOURSELF**, and offer insight into how it felt or what you are thinking: *When you didn't ask me for my opinion, I felt invisible* OR *I wondered why you removed that dressing when you did – I know you had your reasons and I want to understand so that I can learn* OR *When we were in the room with that patient, you seemed impatient with the way I was taking out those staples – it didn't feel very supportive.*
4) **Use QUESTIONING with HUMILITY whenever possible! I call this *'The Columbo Approach'*** (OK, that might be 'dating' me but *Columbo*™ was a popular television drama from the 1970s whose main character was a private detective. For more insight into his approach to inquiry, go to http://johncaswell.posterous.com/columbo-questions-and-the-semantic-answering). In approaching ANY situation, if you can change a 'statement' into a 'question' that implies a level of humility in your own understanding, it can smooth the edge off statements that might be perceived, however unintentional, as judgmental, accusatory or even confrontational. Try this instead: "*I noticed when we were in that situation that you didn't ask me what I thought – would you mind if I shared that with you now?*" OR "*I noticed that you removed that dressing without gloves and I am not accustomed to that – can you tell me why you would*

do that so I can learn?" OR *"When I was removing those staples, I felt you being a bit impatient with me. Was I doing it incorrectly or is there a way you would have done it differently?"*

5) **UNDERSTAND** what the roles and responsibilities are of the 'other' nursing and allied health personnel you are working with. Ask THEM what the relationships are in the workplace, look at any role descriptions the manager or educator might have, or spend time BUDDYING with each of those individuals so you get a sense of what their days consist of.

During this first stage of transition, your overall energy is usually divided between demanding professional adjustments as discussed above, the broader issues related to the 'culture' within your workplace (working with people who have individual ways of thinking, behaving and relating with others) and changes in your own personal life.

Your life, and reactions TO your life, may be labile and 'extreme', so be aware that your response to situations in MANY facets of your life may have as much to do with the stage of transition you are in as the situation itself!

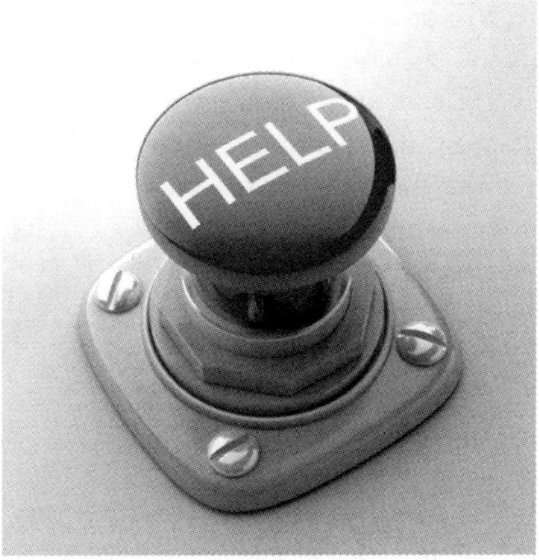

"It's up and down depending on the day. Some days I'm fine and it's like 'This is great!', and other days it's like 'Wow, I've got to look for another job' or 'Maybe this isn't for me'. I just thought this is where I want to be and I was so excited when I got hired and I was like 'YES, this is where I'm going to be!' Then it was like 'Well maybe this isn't where I want to be and if it's not, then where do I want to be....like where do I belong? Where should I go?' Like if I thought this was where I wanted to be and it's not working, then now what do I do now? So I don't know. It's kind of confusing at times, but overall I am enjoying it—it just has hard moments."

"I try to remember that it's just a job. It's not my life and it shouldn't be my life but I don't know. It's hard. It is. Yeah. Yeah but it's only been a month and I just hope it's going to get easier. I hope it doesn't get any worse....To tell you the truth I really expected it to be easier and when it was hard, I was surprised when I found it difficult. I mean it's so naïve of me."

"Work is very, very stressful right now. It's been causing me so much grief. We're really busy and we have some really sad, sad cases right now that I'm having a hard time dealing with it....I'm having a hard time separating myself from it, so like I can't sleep. I'm dreaming. And then outside of work I've been really busy too so I just feel like my head's been spinning. It's still good days bad days so it just sort of depends on what is going on in the unit that day. Some days, I just come home saying, 'I have to find a new job because if it's causing this much, like leakage into my personal life, then I'm going to burn out in no time, or else I have to learn how to separate myself better.' So...it's been tough."

You may have just moved out 'on your own', decided to end an intimate relationship (they often say that one major change begets another), or START one (getting married is a common experience for young graduates). Now that you are making all this money ☺ you may decide this is a good time to purchase that new car or home you have always wanted (really, that makes sense now that you are a working professional!!!). Stress comes in a variety of forms, but remember that even 'good' stress is still STRESS!

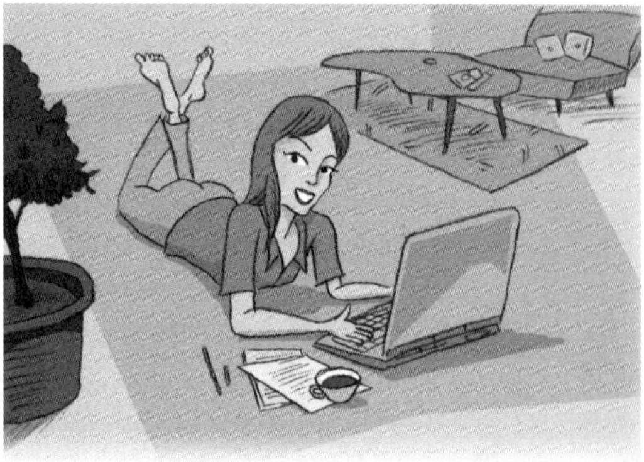

"It looks like dinner, sleep and sanity are not to be."

"I feel it's harder to get things done just because I want to escape from work and get out of the city and see things but then I feel so disorganized in my life when it comes to things like laundry and dishes and all that stuff that builds up when I'm at work and I don't want to spend my day off doing that stuff. When I'm not at work, I really need that escape. I feel I need that but at the same time I think that may be contributing to the overwhelming feelings cause my personal life is so disorganized."

If you are a 'mature' student, perhaps completing nursing subsequent to working within another field or line of work, you have likely sacrificed family time or suspended what might have been a stable income, to move in this professional direction.

"You know, it is a lot of work just trying to remember everything and I have kids at home. This is just one part of my life but it's consuming right now and I find it hard to balance everything. I don't have the time I thought I was going to have and the kids want me, and there are meals to get ready and I can't always ask [husband] to step in for me—I think he is tired of that actually. It's not that I stress totally about work, it's just that it's EVERYTHING—all together, that seems a bit much right now."

Further to this, individuals who have chosen nursing as a second career may have to balance child-care and family responsibilities within an often condensed and intense period of study. While graduation can be a welcome relief from the burdens of balancing multiple roles and pressures, returning to such a 'full' life (children awaiting your attention now that you are 'free' and spouses expecting you to resume prior roles within the family) while navigating the stresses of transition can be daunting.

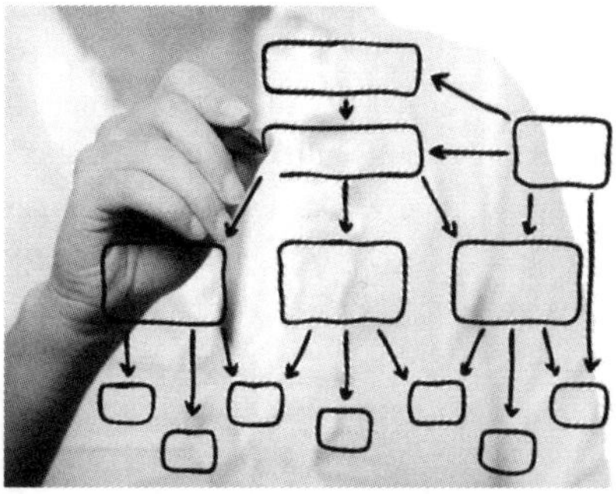

The changes that come with completing your education and moving into professional practice can be as stressful as they are exciting! Particularly when, at the same time, you are: adjusting to intimidating levels of professional responsibility, trying to get a sense of what it is like to work with other professionals on a team, struggling with what appear to be changing relationships with individuals you knew 'as a student', and seeking acceptance into a tradition-bound and somewhat *hierarchical* nursing culture.

> *"I know I could ask someone else to do it. That's one problem I have though. I have a hard time delegating things especially to senior nurses because I feel this is my job. I should do it. But I need to ask someone else to do it and I'm a little hesitant because I guess I feel a little bit inferior. I know I shouldn't but I do because I'm new and they know what they're doing and they would have had it done and I don't."*

> *"When I was a [senior student] we got along great. She orientated me. She was great. And now that I'm an RN I have a hard time saying, 'Can you do this' cause I feel like she's looking at me like 'Oh you think you're so high and mighty' and I'm not trying to act like that and I hope I'm not acting like that but you just really think in the back of your head that they're thinking that—I've never heard anyone say that but I'm just always behind and I don't like asking people to do things. I don't know why. I'd just rather get it done myself."*

Then there are the physical demands of adjusting to intense, alternating, and sometimes unpredictable or inflexible day or night shift schedules without the advantage of 'breaks' that used to come in the form of pre and post conferencing with your instructor!

> *"Oh there's definitely no routine. Not with shift work. It seems like I have complete opposite schedules to friends that are up here and that when you do want to go for coffee or you do want to go out that it just seems like you never have the same day off.*

Yeah it definitely takes the routine out for sure. And maybe that's why it makes it a little bit harder to adapt to. I don't think I always deal with change very well."

NOW you realize for the first time what it means to work THROUGH a complete shift and the energy it consumes can take you by surprise. When you think about taking responsibility for significant clinical judgments and practice decisions when so much else is going on, you are feeling the full weight of Stage One transition. I encourage you to go a bit easy on yourself. It has been my experience that, despite the fact that many of the responsibilities you are charged with as a new nurse, as well as some of the new clinical situations in which you may find yourself in, may be beyond your intellectual or practical familiarity (and maybe even capability), that you tend to blame YOURSELF for 'missing' something or failing to identify or appropriately intervene in a changing clinical situation.

> ***All blame is a waste of time. No matter how much fault you find with another, and regardless of how much you blame him, it will not change you.***
>
> ***- Wayne Dyer***

"It's just still like the uncertainty and the second guessing and then the wanting or needing or reassurance that sometimes I feel like I can't just go and do something. I always want to make sure that I've checked or that I am doing the right thing. That I am making the right decisions for this patient. And I wonder 'Is there something more that I should be doing?'"

"I still kind of worry about missing something....being detrimental to my patient. I don't know how to keep all that stuff in my head and how to pass everything on. I can't remember everything and, you know, I try to keep notes for the day but there's always something....not knowing the answers and maybe I'll do something wrong or forget to do something and cause a patient harm."

Seriously, the workload of a nurse challenges even the most experienced practitioners, ***so go easy on yourself....***

NEED TO KNOW

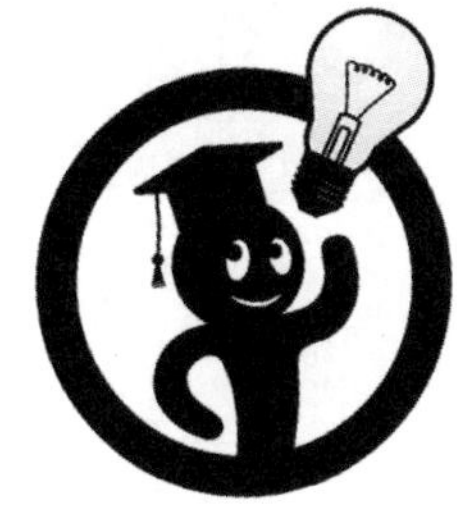

- This stage is all about **CHANGE**—if you are familiar with the workplace to which you will be transitioning (i.e. you have worked there before when you were a student or you completed a final practicum there), the intensity and duration of this stage **may** be reduced.
- During the course of the initial 3-4 months of practice, you will be:

1) **Adjusting** to new roles, responsibilities, relationships (both personally and professionally); you are also adjusting to expectations that you will apply the knowledge you have come to know theoretically from your formal education at the same time as you are learning the NEW knowledge that comes with working as a professional nurse in practice. Adjusting takes time!
2) **Accommodating** new routines for practice that may be embedded in prescribed timelines and strict policy guidelines and are different from what you knew as a student (BID medications may be given at 1000/1600 instead of 0800/1400 ***OR*** all patients being seen in clinic for a suspected STD must be seen by a Nurse Practitioner for sexual counseling ***OR*** female nurses are NOT to do perineal care on incarcerated male patients). While you may have options or choices related to the practices you adopt as your own, and while some established ways of practicing can be challenged using current evidence or your prior experience, there will be certain policies and procedures that you will simply have to accept as 'the way we do things here'. In fact, you may find yourself in situations where you will see practices that you DO NOT feel able to accept (i.e. substandard, unethical or illegal) but that are being adopted by those around you—maintaining or adhering to a professional standard of practice is always a decision!
3) **Learning** new skills, roles, responsibilities and clinical knowledge that relates to a specific area of practice. It can feel like EVERYTHING is new when you start out in professional practice; even OLD feels NEW when you have to take responsibility for it!!
4) **Performing** skills, tasks and procedures can feel daunting; even those you have expertly performed before can take on a different level of complexity when the context within which you are performing is intense, dynamic and unfamiliar. Knowing that YOU are responsible and accountable now for your actions (or inactions) can be intimidating. For instance, being charged with the decision about WHAT and HOW MUCH narcotic to give your methadone patient WITHOUT 'consulting with your instructor' can feel overwhelming the first few times. Don't forget that there is ALWAYS another nurse you can check with—even

if you have to page a supervisor, text a peer or call a friend or another nurse at home from your workplace!

5) **Concealing** your level of insecurity, your fears of inadequacy or your feelings of anxiety from the experienced colleagues around you is normal; after all, you want to FIT IN and be accepted by them as a practicing colleague! Depending on the support you have received from your manager, educator, preceptor or mentor, and depending on the availability of open and accepting co-workers, you may feel more or less comfortable asking questions, thinking 'out loud', or sharing your concerns, ideas, practice decisions and clinical judgments as a new nurse. Remember, it is ALWAYS better to be CAUTIOUS and prevent an error than be OVER CONFIDENT and have to correct your mistake! If you feel unable to ask questions when you need to, or if you do not have access to an experienced colleague for consultation as a new nurse—you are in an UNSAFE WORKPLACE and should be addressing this with management as soon as possible. While it is normal to find yourself in the rare position of having to respond to a situation for which you are ill prepared or inexperienced, being PLACED in these situations consistently (i.e. frequently feeling 'over your head') is **NOT ACCEPTABLE**. If your manager or clinical educator are unable to reconcile this situation to your satisfaction, and if you do not have access to, or perhaps do not feel comfortable approaching a workplace union/labour representative[5], you should seriously consider alternate employment. In such circumstances YOU and those under your care are in danger.....

- This stage is **EXHAUSTING**—physically, emotionally, intellectually and spiritually—and may leave you terminally tired by the end of the 4 months. Initially you will be sustained on the pure, raw excitement of graduating and the 'nervous' energy of being a new professional. Over time though (usually as you approach the 2nd stage of transition), you may find yourself demonstrating signs of energy depletion that include:
  - o feeling tired despite prolonged sleeping periods;
  - o poor quality sleep due to dreaming about work;
  - o disengaging with friends and family;

[5]For graduates working in 'unionized' professional environments, it is important to appreciate the distinctions and differences between unions and professional regulatory organizations. **Unions** function to advocate for the socioeconomic interests of their members, lobbying on behalf of nurses with regard to their salaries, conditions of work including professional practice environments, and safety in the workplace. **Professional regulatory organizations** are primarily focused on the protection of the public by setting requirements to enter the profession and establishing and enforcing standards of practice. There are situations in which these separate organization overlap in the mutual interests of patient safety, quality work environments and promoting excellence in nursing practice.

- o forgetting appointments or commitments;
- o losing interest in social activities;
- o gaining or losing weight (too tired to exercise or eat);
- o feeling depressed, short tempered, unusually anxious, angry or detached; AND
- o experiencing a sense of grief.

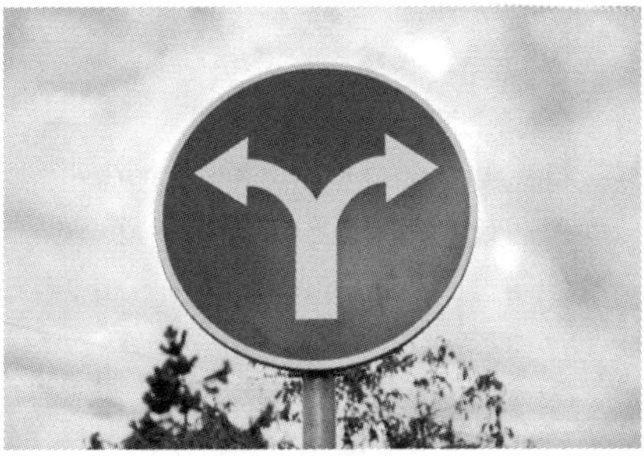

- You may experience **dichotomies** (things that go *"WHAAAAAT???"*) in your practice:

1) **caring dichotomy**—you find yourself caring for patients efficiently (with a focus on the workplace) rather than effectively (which would be a focus on the patient's *needs)* as you had come to expect during your education;
2) **quality dichotomy**—instead of witnessing, or personally providing compassionately competent care that speaks to the needs of patients and their families (again, something you were taught you would be doing), you find yourself and your colleagues maintaining and supporting the powerful structures, hierarchies and ordered routines of the institution where you are working;
3) **dependency dichotomy**—while wanting to be perceived as an independent, capable practitioner by your colleagues (isn't that the goal of every new professional?), you frequently need to reach out to others for assistance, exposing your 'newness' and perhaps even your lack of knowledge and skill;
4) **practice dichotomy**—you begin to see the differences between what you were taught in school and what is actually practiced in the clinical setting; this results in confusion, frustration and sometimes a need to determine who or what 'failed' to prepare you for these discrepancies;
5) **focus dichotomy**—you feel guilty about the fact that your focus is often about how a situation will impact YOU (how you will be perceived or judged in that situation) instead of only how it impacts on your patients and their families (that isn't 'selfish' in a new professional, it's normal);
6) **experiential dichotomy**—while you understand that experience is key to your progress as a professional (and the means by which you acquire the respect, mutual recognition, acceptance and independence all professionals desire), you have little control over how you get that experience.

THESE are the things that keep you up at night, with your mind racing as it tries to 'understand' how things that don't GO together, ARE together….

NEED TO THINK ABOUT

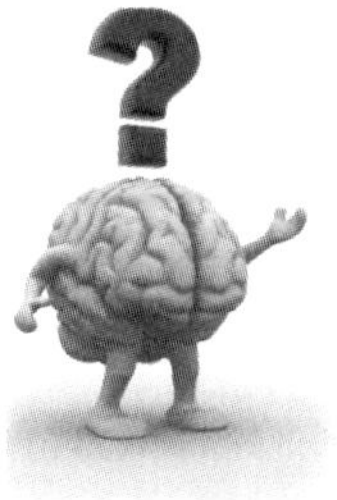

- How can you plan for **familiarity, consistency, predictability and stability** in your personal life and professional workplace during this first 4 months?
- What **MAJOR decisions** can you **POSTPONE** until the 2nd stage?
- How do you normally **cope with stress?**
- Are you at risk for **substance abuse**—if so, how can you prepare for/manage this risk?
- How can you **relieve your stress**—can you plan ahead of time to take several mini-vacations or ask for 3 spa treatments as a graduation present and book them for 1-2-3 months post orientation?
- How can you **plan** with parents, siblings, children, friends or spouses to do what needs to be DONE in your PERSONAL life while you experience this transition in your PROFESSIONAL life?

NEED TO DO

1. Ask to be assigned a **consistent preceptor during the initial 4 months of your employment** who has *volunteered* for this advanced teaching role and received SOME kind of preparation that includes knowledge of the stages of transition.
2. Find a **mentor** who can offer support and encouragement over the next couple of months. If you are NOT assigned a mentor, ask the manager or educator who might be a good 'match' for you ***OR*** make the effort to connect with a senior nurse in your workplace who gives you an indication of acceptance (i.e. perhaps they say 'Hi', or smile at you—ask them to go to coffee and talk to them—you will know whether or not they are interested in supporting you). **Keep searching** until you find someone to support you in the workplace (it DOESN'T have to be someone you WORK with, but it would help if they were a nurse). It is generally a good idea to find a mentor who shares your scope of practice; they are most likely to understand the challenges of your role. Having said that, I have had numerous professional mentors in my career! Sometimes all we need is a good listener, someone who is willing to support and encourage us or someone who can lift us to higher ground when we feel like we are drowning.
3. Request a **predictable schedule** or 'staffing line' so you can learn the practices and particularities of a consistent group of co-workers as well as experience the scope of clinical presentations related to the patient/client population you will be caring for in your work.
4. **Gradually and SLOWLY advance** your skills and ask your supervisors to limit the **level of complexity of patients** you are assigned for the first 4 months. GRADUALLY increase

the complexity of your patient load over the initial year of practice.

5. Give your close friends and family a **copy of your shift schedule** and try to plan time to socialize, time to be alone, and time to do personal errands.
6. Provide **guidelines** to family and friends regarding **WHEN** to call you, particularly if you are working nights (i.e. call NO EARLIER than 2 hours before the start of your shift and NO LATER than 1 hour after you arrive home from your shift).
7. Make your **meals the DAY BEFORE** your shift.
8. Arrange to **meet with your mentor/support person after EVERY set of shifts** for the first 2 months—then meet with them every month for several months—then as needed.
9. **DON'T WORK OVERTIME** or if you have to, **LIMIT** the overtime shifts.
10. Try to find consistent part-time or full-time work where you can work with the same colleagues and patient population. **Don't FLOAT** if you can avoid it—if you HAVE TO FLOAT, limit yourself to 2-3 units.
11. Negotiate your **orientation schedule** with your educator (see Appendix VI).
12. Organize **debriefing sessions** with a friend or peer after every set of shifts.
13. Don't plan any activities **the day AFTER a stretch of shifts**—sleep in, do your laundry, vacuuming and dishes, and CHILL!!!
14. Find a way to **work off your stress** (i.e. meditate, do yoga, exercise).
15. **Talk to other new graduates** who are going through the same thing you are!
16. **Keep a journal** of all the things that well went during each shift. Jot down positive feedback you receive from co-workers or patients. It is so easy to focus on what went wrong or how you have to improve that it can be easy to forget what you are excelling in. Staying positive and consistently focusing on what went well during these first few months will increase your confidence as a new practicing nurse.
17. **Get together with your nursing friends or other new graduated nurses!** Go for coffee and discuss or vent about your experiences as a new graduate nurse. You will be surprised that you are really NOT as alone as you might feel.

Stage 2
Professional Role Transition

BEING

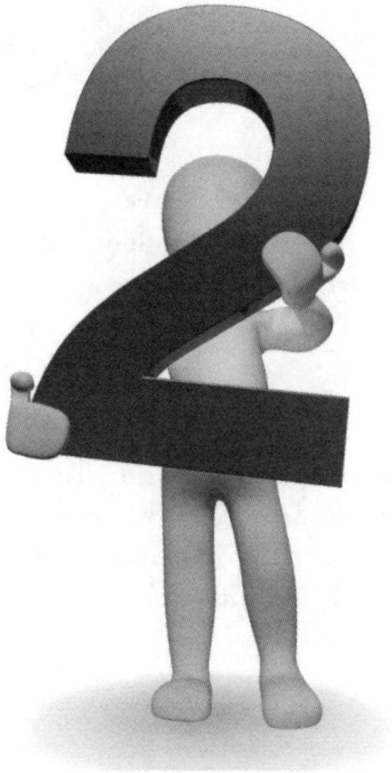

"I have thought of the many other things that have happened in my life but so far this has been the most difficult time in my life. Surviving the first six months. And I don't know if I really communicated to you how stressful it was. I like to think I did in my journals and in our interviews, but it was stressful on so many levels. On every level and like I said, it's stressful now, my career is stressful now but in a very different sense. In that I know that I'm going to survive the day, whereas before I literally didn't know if I was going to survive the day. I honestly wasn't sure."

Can you BELIEVE you made it through the 1st stage of transition....essentially unscathed! WOOHOO!!!!!!

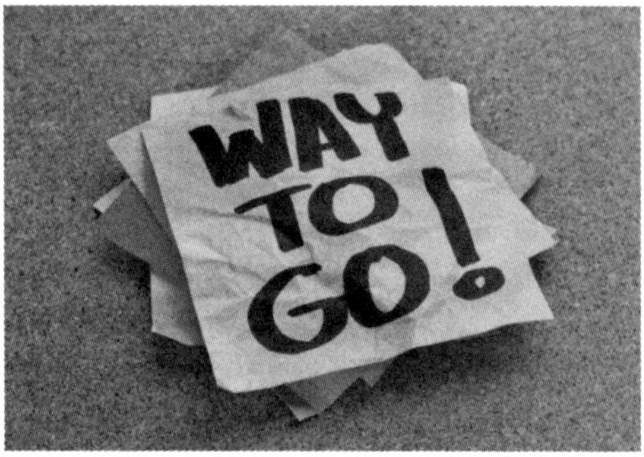

If you are simply 'reading ahead' in hopes of finding out what happens during the next stage, READ ON DUDE!!!! The good news is that you are moving from SURVIVAL mode to THRIVING mode as a new nursing professional!!

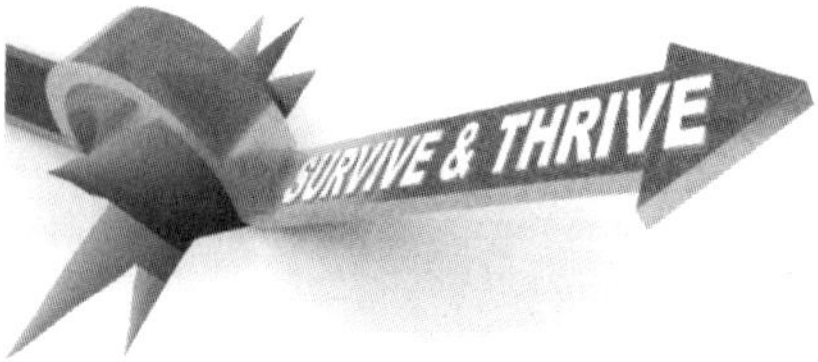

The next 4 to 5 months of your post-orientation transition experience will be marked by a consistent and rapid advancement in your thinking, knowledge level, skill competency and....BEST OF ALL, your confidence.

You gain strength, courage and confidence by every experience in which you really stop to look fear in the face. You are able to say to yourself, 'I have lived through this horror. I can take the next thing that comes along.' You must do the thing you think you cannot do.

-Eleanor Roosevelt

"And I've definitely learned a lot more about time management. Like if I need to give somebody this med and I need to flush their catheter I need to grab them a gown, so I'll do it all at once. Where as before I'd be in and out of the room four times to do all these things. But now, I can think better in my head and I'm like 'OK, I've got to do all this before I go in'."

"I'd probably say [the biggest change is] the confidence. Just being confident in my knowledge and what I know, and confident that I know where to get the answers

or who exactly to go to instead of going to ten different people. Just being more confident in myself and my knowledge so I know when I need to do something. I'm not always second guessing what I'm doing."

"Yeah, I think it's getting better. It feels better because I've had situations where I have picked things up and then I feel like, 'Yeah, I went to school to learn how to do this and I will recognize these things'."

Just a word of caution here—while the 2nd stage is not as 'daunting' as the 1st, this stage can spark disquieting doubt regarding your professional identity and purpose.

"The reason I'm finding this part of the transition to be the most difficult is because the excitement about being done and the shock that I was in has worn off. I feel as though I'm on a raft that is drifting farther and farther away from the shore (my safety net of being a student or a new grad). And I'm floating toward an island where the experienced nurses are, but I keep losing sight of them due to all the waves."

Perhaps it is all the '*waves*' that make the initial part of this stage so challenging. To date, the transition has been dominated by **physical** adjustments to the hours and demands of work (particularly if you are working shifts in a hospital environment); **emotional** ups and downs brought on by the anxieties of practicing 'on your own' or taking responsibility for practice (in particular, skills and decisions) that you had significant support for when you were a student; and **intellectual** strain from having to THINK ABOUT EVERYTHING with a level of intensity that can be more draining than invigorating.

"I was doubting myself. Everything was happening so fast....I felt like I was on the edge and was losing control. I thought maybe these feelings and these emotions were going to overcome me and I wouldn't be able to get out. It felt like I was drowning....It seems that there is always something new and it's always stressful to be doing things for the first time, figuring out the process, making sure I do it right. Do these feelings of anxiety every go away? When does this job get less trying? I guess some things are becoming repetitive, but it will feel a lot better when I can attack more things with confidence and not fear."

Now your energy is going more (or additionally) to the **social** (establishing relationships with colleagues, adjusting to individual personalities in the workplace and reconfiguring a personal life while being a working professional), **cultural** (understanding how 'power and influence' are exercised in your workplace and who the formal and informal leaders are) and **political** (determining what control you have over your practice and how to use that power to 'get' what you need for those under your care) aspects of your life as a nurse. These are elements of your day-to-day functioning as a professional that you might not have NOTICED before. Now that you are able to 'lift your gaze' from the more immediate *tasks* before you, you will start to notice what is going on AROUND you.

Take note that the need to coexist in all 6 of these spheres (physical, emotional, intellectual, social, cultural and political) at the SAME TIME accounts for the majority of energy consumption during this stage. As one new grad put it: "*This is why you are SO SO utterly bagged and tired in this stage*".

> *"I get the bigger picture a little bit more now. Not always, but I know where I want to be and I'm still not there yet but I feel like, 'OK, at least I know more how to get there.' Just even knowing and feeling more comfortable with other staff, like the physicians, and knowing them more…it's not so lonely."*

> *"Lately, patients have been driving me CRAZY (participant emphasis)!! Demanding, rude, ungrateful. Some days I come home and wonder what the common belief is as to the nurse's role. Because let me tell you I feel like a waitress not making tips. I need to start sticking up for myself a little more, but I am quite unfamiliar with how to be confrontational."*

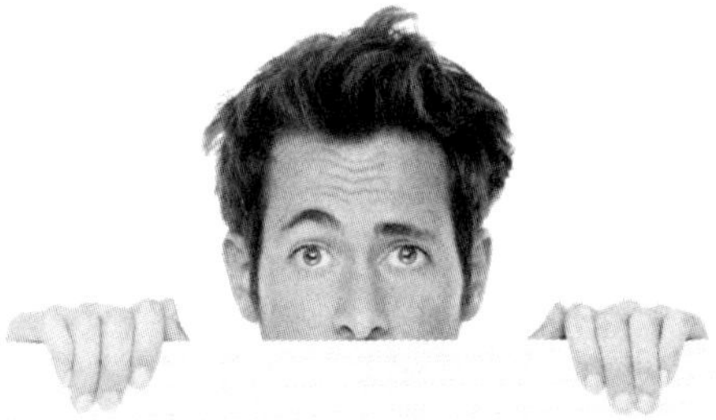

You may find yourself challenging pre-graduate notions of nursing and you might even notice inconsistencies and inadequacies in the health care system. This can be very disruptive to the impressions of nursing that you had come to believe when you were still a student. One of my research participants articulated it as follows:

> *"I like the nursing aspect of it, it's not stressing me out much anymore. It's other things now. It's the politics…everyone's burnt out. I'm not even focusing on myself and my skills anymore, it's my surroundings and just the atmosphere."*

This can be a stage of significant 'flux' for new nurses—a time of 'awakening' to all that IS and all that IS NOT. *Restoring a sense of equilibrium* is the name of the game in this stage, marked by: 1) *searching*, 2) *questioning*, 3) *doubting*, 4) *examining*, and 5) *revealing*.

> *"Like in the real world you are understaffed and you are working hard. It was a real eye opener to me. You know, the things that go on and the things that they let fly. Like do you know that now we have patients in the hallways on our units? I had a patient in the T.V. room the other day. Like this is the real world and welcome to it, you know? You're nursing someone in the T.V. room today! It's a bit bizarre. It's*

just we're full to the max mostly with medicine on a surgical unit and we have these surgeries that the surgeons don't want to cancel so we take our least sick patient and put them in, well we could put them in the equipment room or in this case the T.V. room, and you nurse them there and hope nothing goes bad 'cause you don't have any suction, you don't have any oxygen. So you put a note on the door saying 'Patient Room. Please don't enter.' I just think it's crazy. Like I just couldn't believe it when they were asking us to do this. I thought are you nuts? Like on a general day I take care of ten patients. I can't take care of twelve or thirteen patients! That's too many—there's a lot going on. And the other thing that happens is if we need a bed early in the morning, the patients that are being discharged later that day have to get out of that room and go sit in the T.V. room until someone can come pick them up. But they've just had surgery, they're in pain and maybe they would like to rest for another three hours until their husband can come pick them up, you know? But we need that bed, we need it cleaned, we have a fresh O.R. coming in so, 'Pack up your stuff cause you're in the T.V. room.' I feel like the hospital is being run a bit more like a business than a caring community. It's really business-like so whoever is making these decisions obviously has no idea what goes on in a nursing unit."

Searching

The confusion, doubt, frustration and anxiety that characterized the initial stage of your transition will continue at a slower, but seemingly relentless pace.

"I'm exhausted. You hear people say, 'Well I work a week of twelve hour shifts' but you could never do that in nursing. By the end of four [shifts] I'm either one of two ways: I feel like I could go on forever working those twelve hours because you're in that routine, you're totally switched around; or I could sleep for two days because I'm so exhausted....I think it's the mental part. The thinking—you're so busy doing stuff, trying to remember the numbers, trying to remember this, do that, did I do that? It's just more mental exhaustion is what it is."

Feelings of 'energy drain' are common during this period. Truth be told, it may be that you are just **noticing** your lack of energy now, but the 1st stage of transition was more likely where it was depleted. While it can be frustrating, I have come to believe that the exhaustion felt by new nurses at this stage is a normal and healthy part of the disengagement process. The exhaustion essentially FORCES you to make the separations necessary to gain back your equilibrium and in doing so, motivates the creation of a larger 'whole' that can encompass the multiple and complex dimensions of real life.

"I value my personal life over my work—that's changed. Sometimes I get frustrated because nursing should be my career and I like to believe that it is my career but sometimes it is just a job. Some days I go in and it is just a job—sometimes you're

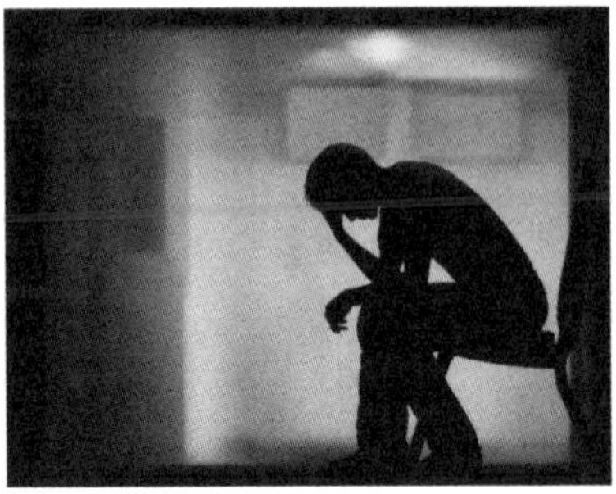

so drained and everyone's been working overtime and you go in and just do your job. It's unfortunate that my patients are on the other end of that because I'm not giving my 110% but sometimes I just do the tasks that I need to do to get through the day and then go home....I really am enjoying the fact that I've got a fulfilling career and I'm paying off my student loans and able to have a nice lifestyle for the first time. I'm developing a relationship with my husband and so I'm not prepared to give up the time...I like being with my husband and I like keeping my house in order. I go to work because I like being a nurse but I also know that there are other things that define me so when I'm not at work, I don't really think about it very much."

"Right now the issues turning me off of nursing are related to the shift work. I have a very active social life with friends all over the country and we are always coming and going. Unfortunately, my job interferes with my social life too often, when the majority of my close friends work business hours and we are trying to plan trips and events. Do I love nursing right now? No not today. What will I think tomorrow? Who knows?"

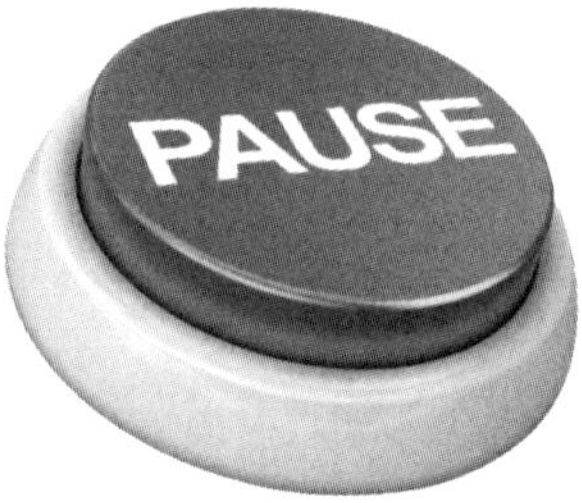

To cope with the drain on your energy you may seek refuge in your your personal life. This desire for distance from that which is stressing you (WORK!!!!) may express itself in a need for separation from your work environment (e.g. you may refuse overtime or you may call in sick to avoid having to face the workplace) or a need to put distance between you and your colleagues (i.e. choosing to forego staff functions or isolating yourself during breaks).

"I don't mind going to work but I think that sometimes maybe I'm taking too many shifts and it's starting to catch up with me. Once you're there, you're there and you just go and you work, but on my days off I think I can really feel it."

"After awhile, I wasn't interested in making friends at work. I just wanted to come, do my job, and leave....It was too much work to try and build new relationships with the strain I was under from being a new grad."

Realize that true happiness lies within you. Waste no time and effort searching for peace and contentment and joy in the world outside. Remember that there is no happiness in having or in getting, but only in giving. Reach out. Share. Smile. Hug. Happiness is a perfume you cannot pour on others without getting a few drops on yourself.

-Og Mandino

New nurses will need to make important adjustments in their social lives. There are times, particularly if you are working shifts, when your schedule will be opposite to those with whom you regularly interact, making getting together for support or just fun much more challenging. Having been accustomed to engaging with friends and family on weekends or statutory holidays as a student, the inability to do so with any regularity now can throw quite a wrench into your social life. Given that this is happening at a time when you MOST NEED that social support, it may add to the strain of your situation.

"Working nights and weekends when a lot of your friends are out having fun or going to bed for a good night's sleep when you are only going to work can leave you feeling sad and left out. There are times when it is hard to go to work because you are going to miss out on stuff you would really like to do. Simple things like going to the gym, grocery shopping, and even cleaning the house and getting errands done become more difficult. You struggle with finding a routine that works for you, IF (participant emphasis) you can even call it a routine, but you will learn to get organized in a hurry because when you work 3 or 4 shifts in a row, not much gets done."

During periods of relaxation after concentrated intellectual activity, the intuitive mind seems to take over and can produce the sudden clarifying insights which give so much joy and delight.

-Fritjof Capra

Now that we have the DOWN side out of the way, there are real advantages to working shift!! Once you get a relative rhythm down (see Appendix IX for more information on managing shift work), you can actually enjoy having time off when everyone else is working. Seriously, not too many people get to go to the gym at 10am or 2pm and (think of all the cardio equipment that will be YOURS for the taking!), and what about all those amazing shopping bargains—well, guess who will be FIRST IN LINE on Tuesday morning???? You got it—YOU will be!!!! Seriously, *shifting* can work, but it will take you some time to find your groove, and even more time if you don't have a shift schedule that is predictable. The sooner you can find that the better. Until then, you simply do the best you can and you learn to be ORGANIZED!

Fundamental to this stage is an increased awareness of yourself professionally—you may begin searching: 1) for more insight into the role of the nurse relative to other health care professionals and, 2) to understand the influence of the nurse within the larger 'system'.

"And even dealing with some of the senior staff. When I have a problem I can come to them with a little more information. I can think a little more critically, 'Well they're going to ask this question so I'll have that answer when I go to them'. Or when I go to them I say, 'Well this is my problem and this is good, and this is good and they're not doing anything wrong here. Is there anything I'm missing? What do you think?' And you get in to some good discussions."

"I spoke with my mentor and she completely agrees with me that being in charge of 12 patients on nights and assessing them all is too much. She spoke with our nurse manager regarding this but got no response. I thanked her for that but in the end there is no talk of anything being changed. It is as though everyone on this unit just accepts that this is how things work, that [unit] always does it this way, therefore that's the way it will be. It's as though we [the new grads] are fresh new eyes and minds and are able to see how things could be run differently. However no one cares or understands. I think I need to grow some [courage] and say something because my inexperience as a nurse shouldn't matter over my concerns for patient safety."

Equally fundamental to this stage is finding a balance between your personal and professional lives.

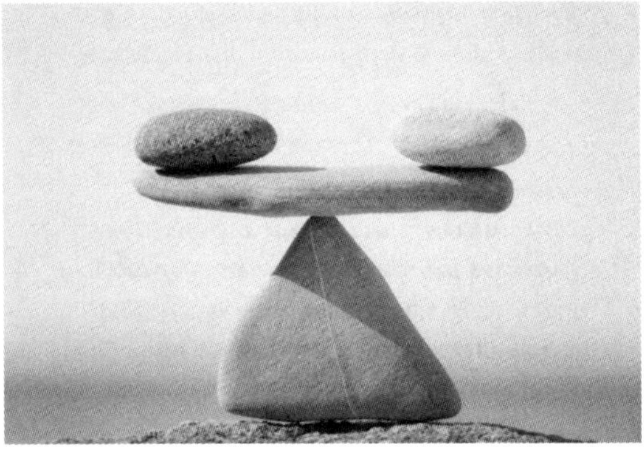

"It's stressful. Obviously, I still really enjoy it. I always have, but I don't think this is something I want to do forever—not ward nursing. I'm enjoying it. It's more comfortable. I like it. I see that I need this experience and you know, it's great experience but I just can't imagine myself when I think of the future, I don't see myself anywhere. I don't know exactly where I see myself and that's sort of another issue. Nursing's a hard job and a very different job. I was discussing with some friends about the differences even just between my fiance's job and my job and that he can go out for his lunch break and, you know, do a few errands or he can leave if he has to or if he sleeps in he can come in late and stay a bit longer. It's so much more flexible—like we can't go to work in our job and say 'I don't feel like working today.'"

During the initial half of this stage, you become increasingly comfortable with your roles and responsibilities as a nurse[1]. This comfort may permit you to begin an examination of the underlying rationale, appropriateness and effectiveness of what you are doing.

> *"It's having some experience I guess to draw from. You know, when you have nothing to draw from it's really hard but now it may be limited but at least I have something that I can remember. I remember doing this the last time we had this kind of case and I draw from that."*

> *"In terms of work it's really actually starting to get better as I hoped it would. I feel like things are starting to come together, like the whole picture you know, and I've noticed it because we have students. And for me it's sort of like, 'Wow, I do know something'. And I'm not saying that the students don't [know anything], but they ask me all these questions and I have answers for them whereas, I always thought I was the one asking all the questions and that I didn't know anything. I've been there six months but I still feel like I'm new and then all of a sudden these students come in. They've never even, I don't know, hooked up a tube feed and I'm thinking this is so, *snap fingers* you just do it now, bang, bang, bang, bang, bang and I mean I can relate to where they're coming from but at the same time I really feel like I've progressed. Even keeping track of the whole unit. You know, as a student you tend to get your one or two patients and that's where you're at, so that's sort of a new thing that I've had to deal with, having more patients. There's still bad days and there's still days where I'm just overwhelmed but for the most part it feels better."*

> ***They who lack talent expect things to happen without effort. They ascribe failure to a lack of inspiration or ability, or to misfortune, rather than to insufficient application. At the core of every true talent there is an awareness of the difficulties inherent in any achievement, and the confidence that by persistence and patience something worthwhile will be realized.***
>
> ***-Eric Hoffer***

[1]As noted in previous chapters, the relative presence of consistency, predictability, familiarity and stability in your work to this point will dictate how you 'recover' from the initial stage of transition. To minimize the delay in moving through the stages of transition, it is recommended that you seek a clinical environment that provides you with ***consistent*** colleagues and care demographics (the types of clinical situations you are exposed to, and the roles and responsibilities you are expected to perform), ***predictable*** work expectations (some control over the intensity, scope and conditions within which you work), some ***familiarity*** with the work expected of you (working with the same colleagues and seeing similar clinical situations repeatedly), and a ***stable*** practice context (there are not extreme ranges in the clinical situations presented to you and the risk of 'disaster' or 'crisis' is limited).

While this stage is initially about disengaging from the intensity of your workplace (pulling back), another intensity soon takes its place—that of questioning the motives and rationale behind your work, searching for meaning in what you do as a nurse, and trying to recover the physical, emotional, spiritual and intellectual strength that might have dissipated during the first stage. The goal of your 2nd stage is to come to terms with the many changes in your life and work, and to re-engage with your career; the difference this time is that it will be more on **your** terms.

> *"I really have tried to not let myself get so worked up before I go to work. I've just been able to put it aside and just deal with it as it comes that day. Like if I thought that I was going to be in the observation unit[2] one day I would be fretting about it all week or worrying about it and I wouldn't sleep the night before. Now I'm just like, 'Whatever, I'll deal with it tomorrow when it comes and we'll see' you know? Cause I've never had a day that's been as bad as I thought it was going to be. Even though there's days where situations might be hard, for the most part it's like, 'OK, I don't know why I was so worried about that.'"*

> *"Well I just…I don't want my job to ruin my life because my outside life's really important to me: my family, my friends, my boyfriend. They're all really important and I just don't want to become one of those nurses who are crabby and hate their job and don't like the work and complain everyday. I don't want to become that, I want to love my job and I want to work with people and enjoy it so if I find myself becoming one of those nurses then I'll have to make a change because I just don't want to become that. That's not who I am."*

Questioning

As one of my research participants suggested, the initial segment of this second stage feels like you are "*caught up in a turn.*"

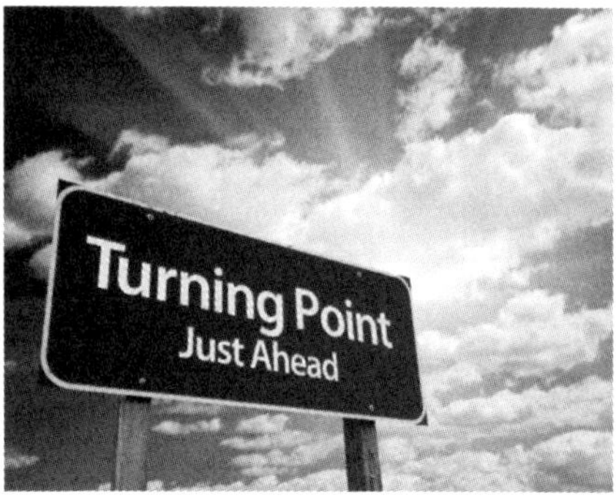

> *"I remember coming home and telling my husband I made my own decisions and acted on them without asking anybody and it was the right one and to me that was a turning point. I did it without asking anybody else and I had a favorable outcome so then it was, 'You know, it's OK to try again.'"*

[2]The term *observation unit (obs unit)* is used to reflect practice areas responsible for the higher acuity patient with complications or complexities that require more nursing care or vigilance, but whose conditions do NOT warrant placement in a Critical Care Unit. These units may also be referred to as *high dependency units.*

> *"Life's a dance you learn as you go.…that pretty much sums it up. I accepted the dance, am caught up in a turn at the moment, but as this crazy dance continues, I will learn the steps and be able to not feel so awkward…I HOPE!?%! If I sit down now and don't finish the dance, I fear I will never try it again. The question is, how long is the dance and when will I learn the steps?"*

You are aware that something is different, but it may still take several months for you to feel like a 'real' nurse. Because you have arrived at a greater level of overall comfort and familiarity with work and role expectations, some of you may find yourselves questioning why you left the comforts of your established school routine only to expose yourself to the daily onslaught of daunting responsibility that sometimes leaves you feeling incompetent, inadequate, exhausted, disappointed, devalued, frustrated and powerless.

> *"I don't know. When I talk to other new graduates, a lot of them seem to be thinking to the future right now, and I don't know, they're not happy where they are or with the job they're in. And so I'm thinking, 'OK…do I want to do this for the rest of my life? What am I going to do?"*

> *"This isn't acceptable—this is not who I am. I am not mean, short, [grumpy], so why can't I stop acting that way? Can you burn out after 8 months? I've certainly got the cynicism and attitude part down-pat! And what's that, 'Oh, because I look young and am a somewhat new face to you, you think that is a license to treat me like an insolent child?' And this perpetuates your cycle of being frustrated with new nurses all the time. But who is going to stay when you treat them like that? I wonder what would really happen if I treated people with the level of respect that they treat me with? I would really love to—it's not how my momma raised me, but it may be coming soon.…Wow, this is all really negative—but it is how I have been feeling. It's not the best place for me. I am starting to feel like my job is less an extension of myself and more just something I do. Something I am competent at but I know this can also make me cold toward people, patients and families."*

This can motivate a downward spiral, during which you may find yourself withdrawing from your surroundings in an attempt to protect your energy and focus on re-establishing a sense of control over your life. It is not uncommon for new grads at this stage to long for stable and familiar patient situations that require less thought and energy to care for (given that you HAVE less to give.…), and I have seen new grads seek casual employment at this time so they can choose the work hours they want. Most grads are simply *TIRED* of the constant 'newness' and are looking to escape the barrage of learning, growing and changing they have experienced to this point.

Now that you have the ability to 'lift your gaze' from what is directly in front of you, the NATURAL questions that allow you to '*let go and move on*' must be answered:

1. *Why did I go into nursing at all?*
    - It is normal to feel a lack of confidence in yourself. This is still a time of learning and you may not yet be sure of what you offer to this profession when compared to those you see around you—do not forget the unique gifts that YOU bring to your work that NO ONE else does and value them!
2. *Am I capable of reaching the level of expertise I see in my experienced colleagues and mentor(s)?*
    - Witnessing what may appear to be innate and seemingly 'effortless' abilities and skills in your experienced colleagues becomes the yardstick against which you measure your own, as yet unrefined, fluctuating and often tenuous abilities—this can undermine your confidence and is not a realistic comparison.
    - You may draw relationships between your 'confidence' and your 'competence', thinking that because you do not feel CONFIDENT you are not COMPETENT—remember that these are NOT always directly linked and that it takes time for you to build both competence and confidence.
    - Frequent debriefing with your mentor, an experienced colleague or just someone you TRUST who understands your experience is essential to cultivating a 'truthful' perspective about nursing work.
3. *Will I ever experience the professional respect that I feel I deserve?*
    - Claiming your 'rightful place' on the healthcare professional continuum is an ongoing process. This struggle may be particularly evident:
        a. within institutions or unit cultures that are more hierarchical;
        b. where nurses of varying levels of responsibility do not act collegially or collaboratively;
        c. when nurses and physicians do not work together as a collaborative professional team;
        d. if nurses are not valued for their knowledge, practice skill, clinical judgment and decision making.
    - Everyone deserves to be respected by others for the unique knowledge, skill and character that they bring to the care of their patients/clients but oftentimes the respect we REALLY want and need is from ourselves—this is where you should focus your attention.

> ***Believe those who are seeking the truth; doubt those who find it.***
>
> ***-Andre Gide***

4. *Will my life ever be well balanced?*
    - You may well be exceptionally tired at this stage and this exhaustion can feed your doubt. Be sure to 'ground' the questions and doubts you might have during this stage in the knowledge that things always look different when you have had a good sleep (or perhaps several weeks of good sleeps in your case).
    - You WILL achieve the balance your experienced colleagues seem to have and some day, you too will be able to come to work and banter about how your

weekend went without even THINKING about all the work that lies ahead until you have to do it ☺.

5. *Who am I as a nurse?*
    - It is normal to compare yourself to other nurses within and outside of your own scope of practice—we often 'measure' ourselves against others like us, particularly when we are new.
    - At this point in your transition, you have seen enough to come to some conclusions about what you DO and DO NOT want to see in YOUR practice; you are starting to crystallize your own professional identity.
    - It is in this 2nd stage that you make decisions about 'what does it mean to be a Registered Nurse, Licensed/Registered Practical Nurse, Enrolled Nurse or Registered Psychiatric Nurse' and how will I honor those credentials?

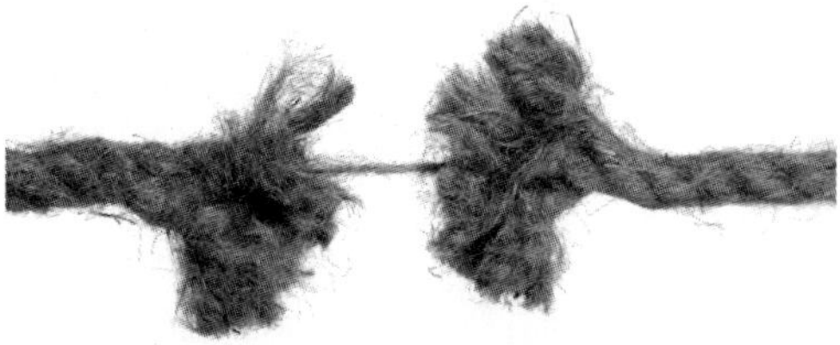

Doubting

You may find that your sense of self-trust is fragile during the initial phase of this 2nd transition stage. It is common to seek validation for decision-making and clinical judgments from experienced coworkers whose level of practice you respect and admire.

> *"I think it's coming, but I don't feel like I have proven anything to anybody yet at work. I feel like they still look at me as the little grad nurse that asks so many questions and needs so much help. And I feel like even in the last month that I have learned a lot and changed a lot and I had a lot of light bulbs go on and I think I'm asking a lot less questions and requiring a lot less help. But I still feel like people…I don't know how to explain it and I can't really think of anything to prove it, but I don't think they respect me yet as a nurse."*

> *"I was asked by my mentor, 'Well why would you do it that way?' and I said, 'Well, ____ told me that this was the way we do it and I agree with her and I believe this is what we should do', and she was quite, well I mean it was a Monday morning after all, but she was quite short with me and I think it's because she doesn't trust me as a nurse. I'm just the silly young grad nurse that she doesn't trust and she didn't believe that I knew what I was talking about. Whereas I think if I was a senior nurse she wouldn't have questioned it. So it just made me feel like I was going backwards again and it was like, 'Oh you still don't respect me as a nurse. I still need to work on you.' *chuckles*"*

Unlike the 1st transition stage where you called upon your colleagues for more prescriptive directives about "*what should I do*" in particular clinical situations, you are now able to generate ideas or strategies for addressing clinical challenges you face and are looking more for clarification, confirmation or validation of YOUR thoughts and actions.

> *"I don't have to consciously think as much about doing some of the care. I can think beyond that. You've worked with enough of the nurses to get a feel of everybody's personality and what they do, and I'll ask some nurses, 'Why do YOU do this when this other nurse DOESN'T do this?'"*

> *"Yeah, before when I was asking questions, I didn't care. I was like 'I need to know this. I don't want to hurt my patients'. I just needed to get this done quickly because I had so much to do. Whereas I think I have a little bit more time now. Rather than running to someone and saying 'Give me a quick answer' I look it up and do it myself. I think I'll earn a little more respect doing that."*

Knowing you can make decisions and implement nursing actions that are not only safe and appropriate, but astute and thoughtful is important for your confidence. This is where the feedback from colleagues is particularly helpful so do not be afraid to ask for it!! For instance, you might ask your preceptor/mentor, "*I wondered what your impressions were of my decision in this case. Is this a decision you would have made?*" OR "*What did you think about how I approached that situation? Were my nursing actions the best in that case or would you have done something different? Can you explain the thinking behind your own decision in that situation?*"

> *"I think I'm much more thorough and also more focused on what's important. Also just understanding—you know you sort of get the routine down so you know what to expect and then that helps you in your preparation and then you start thinking, 'OK, what are the usual orders for that? Well these orders aren't really fitting so maybe I should call the doctor and make sure that they don't want antibiotics or want the morphine or whatever'. I think I analyze more and the whole critical thinking you know, like what am I prioritizing, instead of just starting at room number one and working down to room number ten, it's 'OK, who do I need to see first? How can I organize my morning? Who has 08:00 meds'? Or you know, 'This person didn't have a very good night' or 'This person might need something for pain so I'll go see them first'. I think I have gotten a lot quicker at things like processing orders. Like we do all of our own orders so trying to find things in the computer before it was like, I don't even know where to look. Whereas now it's like I know I've entered it before. I know I can be a little bit faster—I mean I'm still slow compared to most of the nurses but I'm faster than I was. It sounds silly but at the time when you're doing it for the first time, you forget all these little tiny things whereas now it's just like *finger snap* 'OK, we should just do it'. It's being comfortable I guess *laughs*, you know?"*

It is important to note that during the initial several months of this 2nd stage, it may be tempting to accept leadership positions. For example, managers and educators who witness the increased level of comfort and confidence that accompanies this next stage may take this as a cue that you are 'ready' to be put in charge of units or students, or made responsible for orienting new staff. A consistent but disturbing finding in my research was the frequency with which new grads were placed in clinical situations beyond their clinical competence, cognitive or experiential comfort levels.

> *"I'm scared of the same things I've always been scared of. I'm always scared that I will miss something or something will happen and I won't pick up on it. Or that I'll get in over my head and not recognize it."*

A significant percentage of participants in my research have claimed that prior to five months of experience, they were either requested to go to, or were assigned shifts in an *observation unit.* This caused significant discomfort but these new grads: 1) felt too 'new' to make demands about where they were being asked to work, 2) did not want to disappoint the manager, educator, or senior colleague making the request, or 3) interpreted the appeals for advanced responsibility as a statement of confidence in their abilities. All of these situations made it difficult for them to refuse the requests.

> *"Well, here I am in obs [observation unit] AGAIN! I don't really feel I should be in here seeing as I have never been orientated to obs. This is the second time they've put me in here but the first time there was much confusion and they shipped me to [somewhere else] after report. I mentioned that I thought I should get some training but that sort of seemed to fall on deaf ears....I don't understand how they can justify an unsafe situation by saying 'Oh you're only the 2nd nurse so you won't have to give meds'. HELLO, people are not put in obs because of the meds they're on, it's because of their increased acuity. Something I don't feel I am qualified at doing with my present level of experience!"*

While it may be hard to say 'no' to such an offer as it may represent positive affirmation of your growth, it is essential that you CAREFULLY weigh this decision against the risk accepting this opportunity may hold for you and those under your care. Remember what I said before—it takes a CAREER to make an expert nurse!!!

> *"I feel like the staff have accepted me, which is great, but with that I feel as though they forget that I am still a new grad. There are many things which I have still not done and many others that I have very limited experience with."*

The key to realizing a dream is to focus not on success but significance - and then even the small steps and little victories along your path will take on greater meaning.

-Oprah Winfrey

While it is obvious relatively early in this stage that you are 'on your way' (WOOHOO!!!!), it can also be a vulnerable period in your professional role transition. Though there is a relative comfort and familiarity that comes with working in one place consistently for the initial 6 months, think carefully about moving on too quickly. You will continue to develop your fundamental professional skills for at least the first 12 months of practice, and making a change prematurely can set you back.

> *"Oh, I feel like I'm back to the beginning right now. I left a job where I knew for the most part what I was doing, I knew what to expect, I knew how the ward worked and now I'm kind of back to square one and it's frustrating. I really feel that I don't know what I'm doing. You know, I have some general experience with surgeries so I don't feel like I'm that far behind but in terms of routines on this ward and the nurses here are very strict with how things are done and what's done. So being new again is really hard. I feel like I'm back to square one. I feel like I'm a new grad again, and I've been out six months, you know? Like it's tough. And then you feel incompetent like I'm getting all those feelings again."*

It is my sense that the experience of stability, consistency, familiarity and predictability may be as important in this stage as they were in the prior months of your transition—but for different reasons. In the early months of transition, you are sustained by the excitement of graduating; you can deal with almost ANYTHING!!! That may not be the case after several months of learning new roles and responsibilities, dealing with inconsistent, unpredictable and sometimes unstable situations, and working hard to establish that all-important, but usually hard-earned professional credibility. I liken this stage of your transition to how it feels AFTER a CODE (forgive me here, but I AM a cardiovascular critical care nurse so my experiences reflect this), where the adrenaline that got you THROUGH the experience (a.k.a. Stage 1 transition) is still running through your veins causing a sense of hyper-vigilance and an accelerated level of energy. Eventually that adrenaline level DROPS (a.k.a. Stage 2 transition) and you feel shaky and drained. This 'shakiness' is another reason why you need consistent and predictable assignments with an 'appropriate' level of challenge. Depending on how smooth your journey was through Stage 1 and transition shock[3], you may feel more or less depleted at this point. Remember that the only solution for depletion is **<u>regeneration</u>**—give yourself permission to COAST!

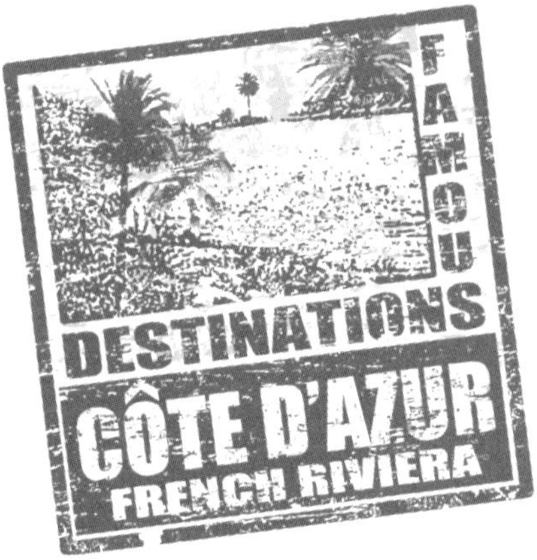

[3]As previously identified, ***Transition Shock©*** is a component of the 1st stage of transition—to review, re-read Chapter 2 or review the ***Stages of Transition Model©*** in Chapter 3.

"Comfort, confidence, level of responsibility and just, I think the personal and professional growth that you go through. You do a lot of changing. Things are a lot different. You're not living that student lifestyle anymore. You're not always worried quite as much about money and you can spend it on that or you can do this. And you have to be more responsible. I think there are definitely changes. It's a lot different having days off or having a week off. You can do a lot more things. And I think I'm still searching for some stuff to do constructively in my time off."

The period of 4-8 months post-orientation is a delicate balance of wanting to ***hold on*** to what 'was' because it seems safe and comforting (mostly because it is recognizable), while being equally aware that in order to move beyond who you ARE to who you could BECOME, you need to ***let go*** and trust in the process of development. At this point you need to be willing to keep walking even though you might be unsure of what is ahead.

"I just loved it. Every day I enjoyed going. If I had to work four nights in a row, I wasn't worried about it, you know, I just really liked the work. But now it's a different story. I just don't know. And partially it's because it's new and I just don't feel as confident. But nursing in general, I mean, I still do love nursing, I just don't love my job right now."

"It was a bit scary for me to admit that I was so uncertain about my career choice. It feels so silly to go to school for so long, and then once being finished, saying 'I don't know if this is for me'. It's like I should have thought of that before it started....I'm so uncertain as to what I think about nursing and where I'm at right now, that I need to wait until I have some definitive thoughts and feelings before I make any decisions."

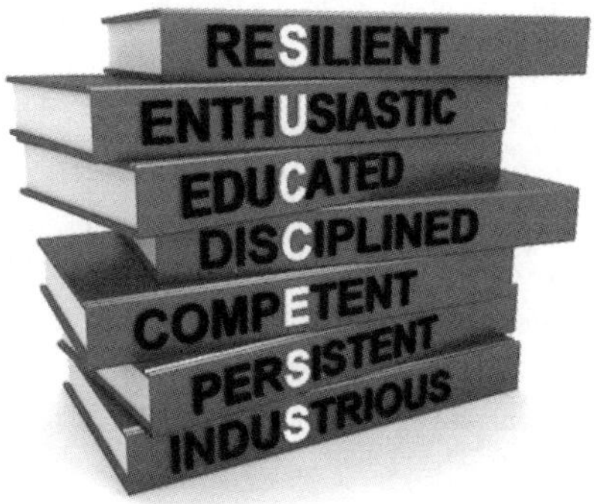

Unlike the initial months of transition where you felt reassured by the presence and oversight of your experienced colleagues, this stage of transition is about transferring your *dependence* on others to a *reliance* on yourself; you need to know you can trust your *own* abilities, skills, assessment capacity and practice competence. Therefore, overly attentive 'supervision' of your practice by well-meaning mentors or supervisors may now be interpreted as a display of doubt in your abilities. The peak of this struggle usually occurs around 6-8 months when a crisis of confidence[4] results from the intersection of your remaining insecurities about your practice competency, the need to become more independent, and fears you might have of failing your patients, colleagues and yourself if you are unable to meet expectations (your own AND others).

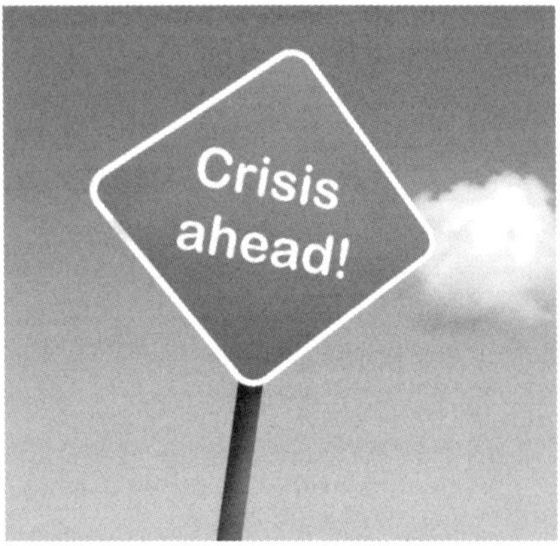

"It's odd how I work a 3 day stretch and however those days went often reflects my attitude on my days off. If work is going good, I am in a good mood to experience the rest of my life. If work didn't go well, it affects my social life, my relationships with family and friends. It is the difference between me achieving productivity in my personal time or wasting it laying on the couch hung-over and dreading the next stretch of work. It shouldn't have this much control over my life. Work is supposed to be a significant portion of my life, but the key word is 'portion'. I am feeling the same way I felt when I started; unable to keep up with everything occurring around me, patients unsatisfied with their care, families asking me questions I can't answer, coworkers having to take the brunt of the extra work needing to be completed and physicians intimidating me more than ever. It is not that I never began feeling comfortable in my work. There were a couple of amazing months where I felt comfortable in my position, confident in my problem solving skills, aware of my new time management skills, and proud of my assessment skills and detective work when issues came up. Now I feel I am back to square one wondering where those months of experience disappeared to. Questioning if that comfortable feeling was a figment of my imagination."

"I remember that I was emotional because nursing wasn't how I wanted it. You know, like I had this dream of like the perfect house and all this money—that was the thing, money. I always was excited about that and being able to take trips, you know, plan a family and stuff and then of course the first six months you have so many other things you have to do and so what you think as soon as you start nursing is, 'I'm going to be out there and, yada, yada, yada', but it doesn't happen and it was hard fitting into 'the circle' at work for the first little bit so that was difficult. And then being new I didn't know my rights as an employee. I wanted to quit after like the first six months 'cause I just thought, 'This isn't what I wanted'. But my mom made me stay. And I'm glad she made me stay. I went to go see a counselor and she

[4]See ***Stages of Transition Model***© in Chapter 3.

> *said, 'You know, like you're only in the first six months' so my mom made me stay and I thank her for making me stay. But I would also say if you ever came in contact with someone that wanted to be a nurse, to encourage them to really meditate and think on if that's what they really wanted and if they can come across experiences to make that decision 'cause it's a long road to walk down and then find out that it's not right for you."*

This is a relatively precarious time in your growth; you can feel impatient with your colleagues' 'watchfulness' while at other times you feel like you have been abandoned if they leave you alone in unfamiliar, unexpected or unstable situations. It is difficult to prescribe a workable solution to this predicament because it is one of those '*darned if you do and darned if you don't*' situations. I have always believed that respectful honesty and dignified transparency are the best approaches so I would suggest you sit down with your preceptor/mentor and let them know EXACTLY what we talked about above. Thank them for their vigilance and let them know it is not about THEM but about YOU—that in order for you to move forward, they need to let go of you a bit. If you are NOT comfortable saying this, approach your educator or manager for confidential advice on how to handle the situation. Finally, if your preceptor/ mentor IS that watchful, you may want to start the conversation with, "*I have noticed that you are still very watchful of my practice and I wonder if perhaps you have concerns about what I'm doing or the way I'm doing it? I have SO appreciated your support and guidance, but thought I would ask if you think I am ready to do more on my own?*"

> *"I had a senior nurse helping me with some work today—she watched over my shoulder constantly and made me nervous. I know that I take longer at doing everything—a few minutes longer at drawing up a medication, a few minutes longer to chart, etc. She was always one step ahead of me, pointing out what I needed to do before I could do it myself—that just made me fumble a little more!"*

Examining

Somewhere around 6-8 months something changes and the remainder of this stage is about finding some 'middle ground' between your past experience as a student, with the primary goal of learning about nursing, and your current experience as a professional *applying* what you have learned to your practice.

> *"For the most part I think that's been really a conscious decision especially about the anxiety. It's just like 'that's enough'. You know what I mean? I'm usually OK now with just leaving it or I'll just, you know, tell [my boyfriend] 'this happened and it was really hard' but then that's it and I go to sleep. It's not looming over my head or anything, like 'did I make any mistakes'? I don't usually think that so much anymore. It's sort of just like, 'OK, I did my best that day or I made sure everything was done and what didn't get done well...I'll just have to let that go because there's nothing I can do about it now.'"*

Growing into your new identity as a nurse may well depend on your ability to engage in a critical but fair examination of your experience to date. There will come a time (likely during this stage) when you become acutely aware of the differences in what you are actually doing as a nurse relative to what you were educated or prepared to do. **That's a big one**....

> *"It's definitely not what I thought it would be. I mean by the time I was done school I thought I knew what it was going to be, but when I started, I have no idea what I thought nursing was.....I can remember learning the principles of sterile technique in school. Now I'm standing here watching an experienced nurse pull off a dressing with no gloves, and slap another dressing back on the incision without even cleaning it, and I don't say anything."*

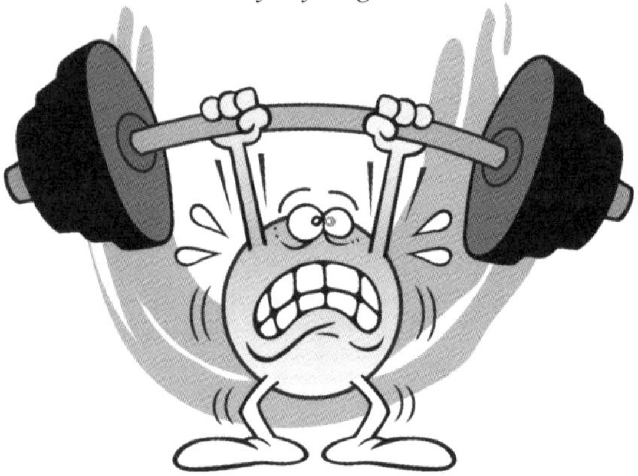

It is advisable that you consult with 'wise elders' who themselves have wrestled with issues like this over the course of their career (and EVERYONE has). As I said earlier, a defining moment in any professional's life is when they come to realize that THERE IS NO NIRVANA.....that reality is NEVER ideal, but that we are all obligated to get as close to it as we can. You may struggle with 'what to do' when witnessing substandard practice in a colleague—what you choose to do is a critical decision in your developing professional identity—choose carefully.

It is very strange that the years teach us patience—that the shorter our time, the greater our capacity for waiting.
-Elizabeth Taylor

> *"I basically told myself that it was OK if I didn't meet all of those standards. There is just so much to learn that it's impossible...to do it all as well as you would like to. I don't know if that's really good, but that's where it is. There's definitely the temptation to become complacent when you say, 'Well, I've been managing OK.'"*

Professionals working on the edge of people's lives the way that nurses do quickly learn that there are 'lines' we must NOT cross when things get hairy (and believe me, things will get hairy). The lines that distinguish *good* practice from *bad* practice cannot be **BOLDED** and *ITALICIZED* for emphasis like I have done here! The knowledge of which I speak (the real life application of theory and knowledge that we call *tacit knowledge*) is subtle and more grey than it is **black and white**. Much of what we learn as nurses is accomplished through thinking-in-action[5] (a.k.a. thinking DURING practice) through a critically reflective debriefing process AFTER practice.

> *"Yeah, I think a little more about it [things I'm doing], like 'I don't think that's a good way to start an IV [intravenous]'. You know, once you watch those really skilled nurses put some of these IVs in, you're like, 'Yeah, that's a lot different than the way this other person does it', and that must be working because people seem to come to her for IVs. So yeah, you can judge a little more."*

Everything that we do as nurses can likely be done better, and each day is a new day that holds possibility for progress and advancement. The new graduate needs to understand that while no practice is perfect, we continuously STRIVE to optimize our care, clinical decisions and judgments; this implies an ongoing intentional synergy between what we THINK and what we DO.

> *"I really think it all goes back to the workload. You become exhausted…even myself, I never wanted to start doing this 'cutting corners' thing. You find yourself doing that and that's not nursing. …You've been running around all day, your back is sore, you're exhausted. This patient is a sit-down lift…it is a good idea to get her up into the chair at least once during the day but you don't. That's cutting corners."*

> *"I feel I have really grown in my skills, knowledge and confidence as a nurse, but there is always so much more to know and do to gain comfort as you become a competent nurse. Getting over that hump of being terrified each time you set foot on the ward for a new shift has allowed me to feel comfortable in what I am doing and to ask questions when I am not sure. I think the old saying 'practice makes perfect' does not apply to the career I have chosen, because there are so many ways to do things and so many practices that change with time, you really never become the perfect nurse. I have given up on that goal. I think it is safer to say 'practice makes you more efficient.'"*

Find someone (or MORE THAN ONE because different mentors connect with you on different issues) you can trust to help you negotiate the minefield that comprises the daily issues and clinical situations about which we make nursing judgments and decisions. This stage is about struggling with self-doubt and "*its like night and day walking onto a shift knowing I can completely trust the nurses I am working with and go to them for help.*"

THOUGHTS become ACTIONS that can have life altering consequences for those under our care. Nobody can nurse well in isolation.

---

[5]Schon, D.A. (1983). *The reflective practitioner: How professionals think in action.* Cambridge, MA: Basic Books, Inc.

"Some affirmation would have been nice. That's something that I've noticed we don't do well. I don't know if it's nurses in general but on our unit they don't compliment each other very well. Like sitting you down and saying, 'You know you did a very good job'. I haven't had that. I mean they do write people up, when someone isn't doing well, and I don't think it's necessary. I would like to see them make an effort when a new grad makes a good decision to say, 'You know, that was the right thing to do', because you need it. You can't always rely on your self-talk to pull you through."

Revealing

As you progress toward the latter part of the 2nd stage of transition, all that has been revealed to you over the past 6-8 months stimulates an increasingly moderate perspective on your professional experiences; there will be *fewer* HIGHS and LOWS and *more* 'neutral' days (seriously, who can sustain those kinds of highs and lows!!!!). Having been previously frustrated by your perceived lack of progress, you might find yourself relaxing into a more comfortable space that permits the mild angst that comes with revelations about what you DO NOT KNOW to co-exist with the growing confidence in what YOU DO KNOW. You begin to gain trust in yourself.

"I think relying on yourself and trusting yourself go hand in hand because if you don't trust yourself, if I don't trust my own judgment, I'm never going to be able to say, 'Oh that's the right choice'. I'll always be like, 'Oh I better ask somebody else'. So I think it's very important. And I think in order to move on I need to trust myself, or I don't think I would ever move on. Even if it's that I'm going to screw up and it's going to be OK."

You might feel a bit detached from your surroundings (friends, colleagues or even yourself) as you find your way through this stage. This is a normal response as you locate that middle ground we spoke about earlier.

"I can just prioritize what I need to do. It doesn't bother me as much and I just do what I need to do or what I have to do and then delegate what I need to delegate and get everything done. Then hopefully by the end of the day everything is done, and I can go home. Life used to revolve around work so much and I felt almost depressed in those first few months. [My husband] was gone and I was starting this new job and it felt like that was all I did—I went to work and came home and prepared to go back to work again. But I was switching over and having trouble sleeping and dreaming about work and just everything revolved around work. But it doesn't anymore. I still don't sleep wonderful the night before but I can sleep OK between shifts and I don't lose sleep afterwards thinking 'Oh what did I miss? What did I do wrong? What should I have done differently?' I can go out and have a life and not worry about work."

An essential element in your recovery during the latter part of this stage and into the final stage of transition consists of reacquainting yourself with personal goals and aspirations that you had put aside in order to experience professional growth. Less cognitive, physical and emotional energy is needed to manage your now familiar nursing roles and responsibilities and less anxiety is generated in dealing with clinical situations. You may find that you require less energy to debrief about work, your dreams are less disturbing and that you spend less time before work thinking about what might happen or after work debriefing about what did happen. This extra energy affords you more time to adjust to and accept the changes in your personal and work life schedule; you might even spend your days off relaxing and enjoying your new-found liberation!!!

> *"I feel like a hermit some days and I know a lot of [my friends] that I went to school with that I still am in contact with, they're doing the same thing. Not wanting to go out. Not wanting to deal with all the people at the pub. I just want to stay on my couch and watch my TV."*

By about 8 months post-orientation, you should see a rejuvenated spirit reawakening in yourself; one that might even inspire you to seek out new challenges to your thinking and more complex situations in your practice. WHO you are as a nurse is being revealed, and that self-knowledge releases you from the constant doubting and questioning that was necessary to arrive at this new place.

> *"I finally feel that I am moving into a different stage. I don't feel new anymore, and I catch myself saying 'this is new to me' a little less often. I feel a lot more comfortable. I feel a lot more confident in some of the skills that I was anxious about when I first started....I even notice that my assessment skills are getting a lot better, and I know they will only improve because the more you do something, the better you get."*

> *"I'm happy where I am now and I think I just want to leave it that I'm happy and not have to think about the future too much. When it gets here it will get here."*

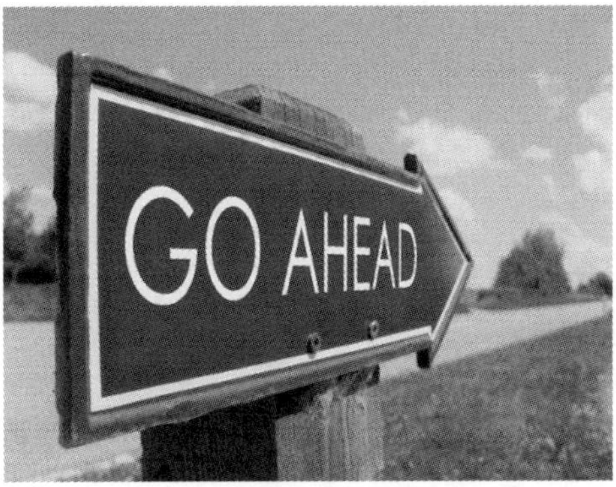

NEED TO KNOW

- This stage is about **FINDING BALANCE** it is a time when you become acutely aware of what has just happened and you are trying to find your equilibrium amid the chaos of your professional integration—I am not suggesting that the chaos you are experiencing is unnatural, abnormal or even negative—it just IS. Figuratively speaking, *transition* is a time of *disorder and confusion.*
- During the 4th to 8th month period of your initial year of transition, you will be primarily:

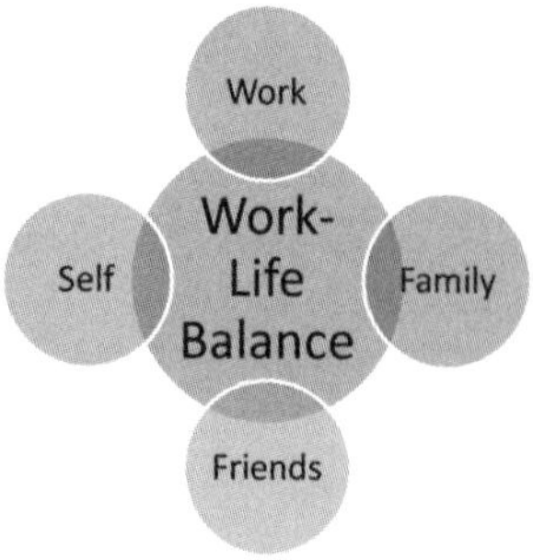

1) **Searching** for a sense of balance in a life that feels out of control! This search may lead you AWAY from the intensity, if only to get perspective and 'protect' yourself from further energy depletion. You will begin a concerted exploration of yourself professionally AND personally (something like doing an inventory of your clothes closet in the spring – guys do that too ☺), trying to understand what to let go of and what to keep. You are looking for MEANING in this transition experience, in your work and in your larger life (the saying "*there's got to be more than THIS*" applies here). Much of what you had put on hold personally in the 1st stage (that might be your kids, your spouse or your friends) starts to look appealing. This is a chance for you to re-engage in those hobbies you enjoyed BEFORE school started to consume every waking moment of your life!!
2) **Questioning** why you left your life behind to study all these years, only to discover that nursing, like every OTHER profession in the world, is about '*working for a living*'! While nursing is often gut wrenching, soul moving, heart warming and life transforming, it is also work. You are expected to be there for a full day, you must DO certain things and WORK WITH certain people that you may not have chosen. But outside of changing jobs (where you will likely face the same challenges), the reality is that nursing is a job. You just want to do it WELL....and enjoy it most days, right? Now we're talking...this can be a difficult period in transition because the exhaustion that feeds this questioning sometimes skews the results, or your perception of the

results. Hang in there, question what you must, and know that all is unfolding as it should.

3) **Doubting** whether you have made the right choice in nursing, or whether this particular workplace is right for you is NORMAL!! Even doubting your decisions and judgments is expected as you move from being more 'dependent' to being more 'independent'. In fact, like most things, we go from one end to the other before we find our way to the middle; INTERDEPENDENCE is the ultimate goal but often comes last. The interesting thing about doubt in this stage is whereas in earlier months you doubted EVERYTHING (your thinking AND your actions), now the doubt is expressed primarily as ***caution*** related to implementation. You usually arrive at a request for consultation with your colleagues after having thought significantly about the challenge you are facing, and often have several ideas and strategies to address the challenge that require clarification, validation or confirmation. The trust you have in yourself is growing but it is a big step!
4) **Examining** the differences between what you came to know about nursing as a student, and what you are learning about what truly exists in the world of professional practice can be disconcerting! I have come to believe that it is not feasible, nor even desirable, for students to be made completely aware of what lies ahead for them as fully accountable and responsible professional nurses. So much of any professional role cannot be realized until it is EXPERIENCED! This is NOT to say that we cannot or should not be constantly examining our educational approaches as well as our workplace structures of support for transitioning professionals. But no matter how much time, content or support one receives, the move from student to practitioner is a distinct process that challenges the best of us. **The key is in providing you with the space and resources to make that transition a healthy one.**
5) **Revealing** what you DO NOT KNOW as a new nurse should not make you feel incompetent and should not be accompanied by fears of being disciplined. It is as important to know our limitations as it is to appreciate our strengths, but as a new grad it can feel as though that is somewhat lopsided ☺. During this second stage, what you KNOW starts to be revealed as you experience clinical situations consistently and repeatedly and your role in responding to these situations takes on a certain familiarity. This gives you a sense of confidence and reduces the relative weight of what remains unknown to you. That's the good news…..but as you *lift your gaze* from the somewhat narrow vision you have had during the initial months of your transition, you begin to take notice of the larger picture. It may become evident that the system you are working in does not always work; it is not always constructed with the patient/client/family in mind and it does not always facilitate professional nursing practice opportunities nor produce optimal health outcomes.

NEED TO THINK ABOUT

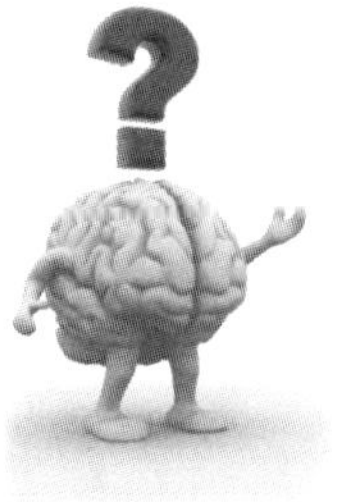

- What are you noticing about nursing and healthcare where you work?
- What are 3 things you are doing well in your practice?
- What makes you feel GOOD about coming to work? What frustrates you now about practicing nursing?
- Have you connected with your nursing manager and educator? What do you need from them and how can you get those needs met?
- What do you do on your days off? What hobbies did you enjoy before school consumed your life and which of those do you want to reconnect with?
- What practices have you seen around you that you can hold up as a model for your own? What practices have you seen that you do not want to adopt for yourself?
- Who are the individuals in your workplace that you most admire? How can you spend more time with them?
- When you look at your schedule, how balanced is the personal with the professional? How can you increase the balance between these?
- Are you being encouraged to take on leadership roles and responsibilities? How does this make you feel? Are you prepared to take on a charge nurse or preceptor role? What rights do you have to negotiate these requests in your workplace[6]?

NEED TO DO

1. **Limit overtime** work—you need to rest on your days off. While it will always be enticing to earn more money or gain more experience, this additional work exposes you to the very thing that you need LESS of right now—WORK and STRESS. And trust me….debt is inevitable and enduring ☺.
2. **IF you want to take on leadership roles (i.e. charge duty, preceptorship, or project development/management)**, ensure that you are given adequate opportunity for formal orientation. Most institutions have programs that train you to take advanced practice roles, so try not to get pulled into taking on a role because 'they need someone' and you happen to be available. Formal leadership is a professional decision and you have the final say.
3. **Join a club or pick up a hobby** that brings out a different side of you. Because you

[6]For individuals in unionized workplaces, your union representative might be a good person to talk with about your rights to refuse work that you believe is outside your experience, scope of practice, or professional readiness. For individuals working in '*negotiated contract*' contexts, find out who your labor relations advocate is and speak with them about how you negotiate advanced practice or leadership roles as a new nurse.

have expended so much of your time and energy working for the past number of months, you might begin to feel like a new mother who longs for the company of adults—remember that you are a complex and multifaceted human being who does best when exposed to a variety of stimuli. Challenge yourself in ways OTHER than work and you might find it easier to relocate your balance. For some people this requires a concerted effort that is akin to DRAGGING yourself away from what has become routine (work, work, work) in order to see how it has monopolized your life. But once you STOP the focus on work, you will begin the rejuvenation process and be able to return to work happier and healthier.

4. **Spend time with friends and family** who do NOT remind you of work. During the initial stages it might have been somewhat frustrating to spend time with family and friends, particularly those who could not appreciate the transition you were going through. At this point, however, it is refreshing to spend time with people who talk about something OTHER than nursing. And, it is amazing how putting yourself in situations that do not allow you to think about work actually give your active mind a reprieve from the constant barrage of pre-briefing and debriefing that is characteristic of the new grad transition process. As the adage goes, '*a change is as good as a rest*'!
5. Find a **mentor** from your workplace or within the profession whose practice or attitude (preferably both) you admire and ask to spend time with them talking about nursing. This might be an educator from your nursing program with whom you had a particularly strong connection or someone you met during the initial months of your transition. Engage them in an informal discussion (over lunch or even a dinner out together) and direct these questions to your mentor to get the dialogue started:
   a. What do you love most about nursing?
   b. What has changed for you over the years about your work?
   c. Have you ever felt frustrated by what you see going on in the workplace? If you have, what frustrated you and how did you cope with it?
   d. How did you come to this place in your career? Why do you work where you do?
   e. If you could 'do it again', what might you change in the way you have lived your professional life?
   f. How do you deal with negative people at work?
   g. Have you ever had to approach a colleague about their breach in practice standards? Can you share how you approached that situation?
   h. How do you balance work with the rest of your life?
6. **Find a buddy with whom you can debrief after each shift**—maybe you could drive to work together and debrief on your way home—by the time you get home you might be more likely to settle into the 'personal' side of your life. This approach might not always be feasible because that is part of the problem—you aren't working similar shifts to your buddies. But IF you are, EUREKA! The alternative is to get together after every SET of

shifts with a trusted peer and talk about how things went. Be cautious that this debrief doesn't become JUST a venting session—venting IS important as it allows you to release the emotion connected with the experience, but then you have to move BEYOND the emotion to the FACTS. Focus on WHAT happened, WHY it happened, WHAT you might do differently, and HOW you can learn from the situation. NO situation is a BAD situation—it simply IS what it IS. Learn everything you can from it and move on.

7. Consider **connecting with other new nurses** who understand your experience. Discuss your desire for peer mentors with your nursing manager or educator; they may be able to find a way for recent new grads to come together to discuss their experiences confidentially. Alternatively, contact Nursing The Future at newgraduates@nursingthefuture.ca where we ALWAYS have someone who can speak with you about your transition!
8. **Journal/blog** about your thoughts and feelings related to nursing and work—write down one POSITIVE story about an interaction you had at work after every shift. Remember that journaling or blogging doesn't have to feel like it did in school (NO APA or CHICAGO STYLE here)! You could get an inexpensive coil-ring book from the store and draw pictures, write poems, inspirational quotes or just the thoughts that come to you over the course of a day that express how you are feeling. Date them and then you can see patterns in what you are thinking and feeling that can mark or guide your growth. You don't need to SHOW this to ANYONE[7] and you AREN'T being graded on it!
9. **STAY IN THIS JOB** for the first year if you can. Outside of an abusive work situation (see Appendices on *Conflict Management in the Workplace* and *Dealing with a Bully*), it is recommended that you 'stay the course' for the initial 12 months of your professional practice experience. It is enticing to think about switching your place of work for one that seems more open to new nurses or where the care population is more 'interesting', more challenging, or represents the practice context you always wanted to be in. It becomes even more appealing if you believe that changing workplaces will ease the struggles you

[7]A NOTE ABOUT SOCIAL MEDIA: Be attentive to the vehicle you choose when 'venting' about your transition journey or work experiences in general. Twitter™, Facebook™ and other social networks are GREAT avenues of support, and certainly allow you to talk to, and be supported by peers and colleagues around a host of issues. Just keep in mind that these are essentially public (a.k.a. NOT confidential) modes of dialogue; be respectful of the topics and be wary of posting content. Also, be aware that the use of social media has become a relatively contentious issue in most workplaces around the world! Speak with your nursing manager and educator about existing institutional/health region policies regarding the use of social media and be sure you abide by these. As well, when you are using a hand held electronic device to access healthcare or nursing practice information, just let your colleagues and patients/clients know what you are doing. Just being transparent goes a long way in dispelling concerns about how you are 'spending your time'. Remember, this isn't necessarily about YOU—it is about the varying generations of people AROUND you. When we are ALL respectful of the 'other' (that includes people respecting your mode of communication!), and willing to talk about and try to understand our differences, things usually work out!

are having as a new nurse. While I would NEVER recommend remaining in a work environment that is unsafe or unsupportive, issues that new grads face during transition usually transcend practice areas and people (there are good/nice/happy/supportive and not so good/mean/unhappy/unsupportive people everywhere). If you can '*stick it out*', you are more likely to develop the essential skills required to deal with challenges like conflict, change, frustration, disappointment, clinical decision making and judgment and workplace collaboration; challenges that exist in every country, city, workplace and job! If you are NOT working in the practice area that you want to be in, focus on what you ARE learning or CAN learn rather than what you AREN'T learning or CAN'T experience; eventually you WILL practice in your dream specialty!

Please remember that there may be other workplaces and specialties that you have never considered, so learn ALL you can from the areas of practice you find yourself in! You might even have difficulty FINDING a job (see the Appendix VII for more tips on this) so take the work that is AVAILABLE and learn SOMETHING about nursing from it (oh, and you CAN—tell me anything you would do that you couldn't learn something about nursing from and I'll buy you something really expensive). I can't tell you the number of times I struggled to find work and ended up practicing in areas or roles I would not necessarily have chosen. For instance:

1) Early in my career I worked in several remote northern communities (not that I was prepared for this level of practice, but they were desperate for relief nurses and I needed the work) where I performed a nasal scope on a child to retrieve an embedded pea from his nose that had been there for 2 weeks (seriously, the smell was overwhelming), removed a fish hook from a man's hand (just thought my way through that one because I was alone and 'on call'), sutured an intoxicated man's head (at least he wasn't belligerent), scaled down a roadside ravine to retrieve a car accident victim, prescribed antibiotics for a multitude of upper respiratory ailments, delivered a stillborn child (gave last rites and helped the family bury their child), and treated venereal disease (including having to call 'unsuspecting' spouses to inform them of their risk);
2) After having returned to Canada after years studying and working in the US, I was unable to find work in my specialty (or anywhere for that matter—I had entered a unionized environment and I had NO seniority) but needed work and money (I see a pattern developing…). I happened to meet up with a wonderful woman who owned a private homecare business. In the months that followed I performed personal care for a quadriplegic social worker who had installed an ELEVATOR in his home so he could be more independent, and I assisted with the daily mobility of a 22 year old man valiantly enduring multiple sclerosis (and I learned some great tricks for reducing the odor in chronic urinary catheter leg bags!);

3) Once back in Canada (see above), I applied for many nursing positions but was 'bumped' out of most of them. In the unionized environment where I worked, nurses with more seniority were offered positions BEFORE those with less seniority, allowing them to 'bump' the incumbent out of their position (and yes, then THAT person bumped ANOTHER person out and so on and so on and so on....). As a result of being bumped out of several positions, I ended up assuming the role of Nutrition Nurse in a large urban hospital. My mandate was to prevent and, if necessary recommend treatment for, parenteral and central line infections secondary to intravenous nutrition delivery. I remember one case (a case that made me question my suitability for this role ☺), I squeezed 2 tablespoons of PUS out of a man's forearm after I removed his septic parenteral access site (by the way, the charting indicated that the site was 'healthy'....hhmmm what do you think I learned from that situation?);
4) I was asked to be on the medical team of the 1988 New York Marathon (and OF COURSE I ACCEPTED—I was desperate for work remember?) and during that time, I witnessed true love, endurance, resilience and persistence, all in a 72 year old woman who was 'running' (actually she was walking by the time she got to me on the 25 mile mark) for her husband who had died of leukemia the year before. It was a gorgeous fall day in Central Park and I had on my sweats, a pullover that said 'MICHIGAN' on it, and leg warmers. Our job at this particular station was to do 'whatever' the runner needed to assist them to the finish line, or convince them to pull out of the race. So when I asked this petite and clearly laboring woman what she needed, she said "*walk beside me and talk to me. I MUST get over the finish line*". So that's what I did. I walked beside her and we talked. Within 500 feet, you could hear and then see the crowds—they had gathered in the stands that lined the final ¼ mile of the marathon route. As we approached the finish line, all I could hear was 'GO MICHIGAN'!!!!! Yes, and that is the closest I have ever been to finishing a marathon. This courageous woman crossed the line (well, fell over it after which we carried her to the med tent), and I kept walking. Unfortunately I got lost and after about an hour the sun was beginning to set and I was alone in Central Park (apparently, NOT recommended even by New Yorkers), scoping out the wooded areas that I felt might be safe to spend the night in....until I heard a familiar voice, "*Judy!!! Where have you been? We've been searching EVERYWHERE for you and we were scared to death!*" (YOU were scared to death????). I was reunited with my team and we left the park to enjoy an amazing dinner and make even more memories....I can't even begin to tell you what I learned as a nurse THAT day;
5) I was taking another specialty nursing education program in a city where I didn't know anyone and, as usual, I was desperate for work and money ☺. I opened my door one day to an amazing, brilliant and caring woman who also happened to be a Jehovah's Witness. She was canvassing my dormitory and I invited her in to talk about some of the JW cases I had worked on. I was struggling with how some of their

religious doctrine had influenced and impacted on the care of some of my patients and I was looking for answers (I was young and thought I had something to say about something I knew very little about). Over several visits, she graciously taught me about JW, and in the process we became friends. She also happened to own a personal care business and offered me casual/relief hours as a care aide anytime I wanted so I took her up on it (I have noticed that opportunity knocks often....but you have to answer)! Oh, and she dropped off a box of food with hams, canned food and lots of cookies ☺ on my doorstep, knowing I was a student and........YUP, desperate!! Then, on my graduation day from this critical care specialty course, she sent me roses.....and THAT, my friends, is what opening your door (and mind) to a stranger can do.

These are just a few examples of opportunism at work. If you want to work, do what is *possible* and *available*, secure in the knowledge that what you WANT will come eventually. Hey, you never know, what you 'want' might even change.....

Speak to your educator/mentor/coordinator about any concerns you might have about any practice situations you find yourself in because this will help you to move forward. Strategize with people you trust (there will be more about career planning in Chapter 5!!) and begin to identify ways of working towards your career goals AFTER your transition year.

Stage 3
Professional Role Transition

KNOWING

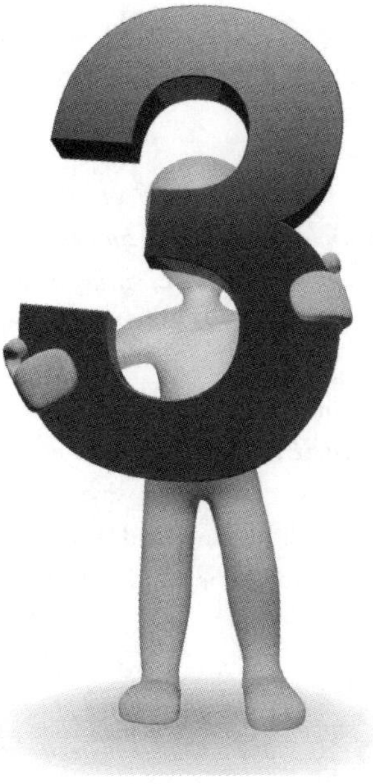

NOW THIS IS MORE LIKE IT……

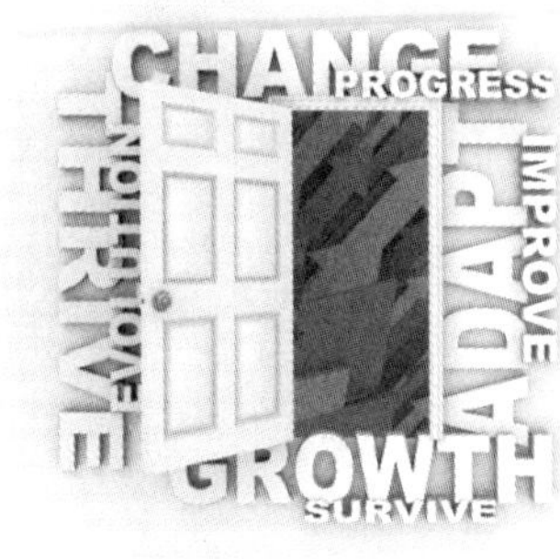

Having survived the physically, emotionally, intellectually and spiritually exhausting period that encompasses the first several months of transition, and having hopefully found a restorative balance during the subsequent 'mid-year' transition stage (2nd stage), I anticipate that you have *arrived* at the final leg of your initial professional role transition journey.

> *"There's not as much worry or fear really. Like in the beginning there was a lot of fear of the responsibility I had, of the decisions I had to make, of what was riding on me I guess. Just like all of a sudden having, you know, the full patient load and all these things and you know, parents asking questions. Just everything. It was like, 'I'm not going to be able to keep up' or 'I'm going to miss something important'. Whereas now, I can plan better and look ahead and sort of, 'OK, what can I do to help the night staff out today?'"*

> *"It's weird, like it just was, it was, it was, you know, just kind of rolling along thinking it is, it is, it is and then, all of a sudden I realized 'Hey, it's not so bad anymore.' I don't even remember the month it would've been. And in some ways it almost feels like it's just been getting better for a long time."*

When I say 'final leg', I do so with the full knowledge that the socialization to professional practice as a nurse is called a ***CAREER*** and it happens over a lifetime. I have been nursing for 32 years and something new is always coming my way; most times that is because I invite it in. On occasion, however, it creeps in like a dense and strange smelling fog (like out of a Stephen King movie), finding its way under my door despite strict instructions to **STAY AWAY** ☺.

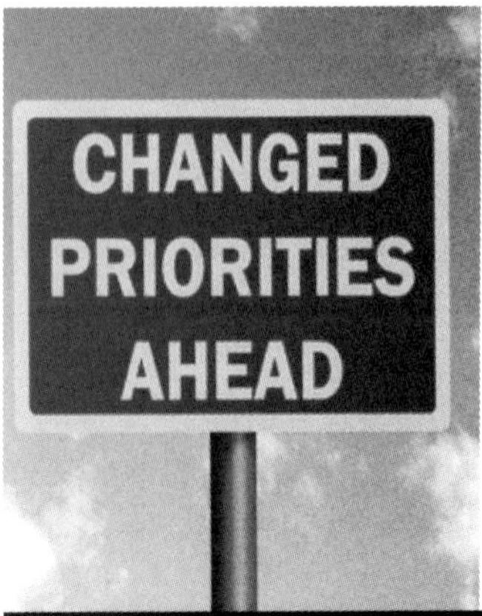

> *"It still comes and goes too and like I've said before, I'll have a day that's bad and you feel like 'Oh, I haven't even made any progress'. I'm giving report and they'll ask me a question and it's, 'Of course, why didn't I think of that?'"*

Whether it is viewing our profession with a different lens, or simply watching the discipline grow as the world changes, being a professional is *a work in progress.*

Your role as a new nurse, developmentally speaking, is to achieve a relative uniqueness that both distinguishes you from the established practitioners around you, and allows you to work interdependently amongst them within a community or on a team of professionals. It is normal to harbor some apprehension about moving out of the learner role and into a role that holds greater expectations for performance and a narrower margin for error.

> *"How I define good days has changed. A good day before was surviving to the end, feeling that everything was done. I knew what tasks I needed to do and I had the list in my head so I could check another thing off this list and so I wouldn't get caught not doing something. Now I don't even look at time…as long as I can get done what I need to get done I'm ok."*

> *"That first period, the first three months were a time for debating whether or not this is the profession for me. I was doubting myself; I was doubting my skills; I was doubting everything that I had learned in nursing. It started to progress a little bit, but then I had a little stint again at about the 6 month mark where again, the stress, the overwhelmed feelings, like just everything seemed to be piling up and it felt again like 'I don't know about this'. But now I would say probably within the last month it's been feeling really good. I actually don't dread going to work and I don't lose sleep over it."*

> *"A friend of mine bought me a name tag and it says 'Jenn, RN' and once I actually felt comfortable in that role, I started wearing it but I didn't start wearing it until about probably a month ago. Ever since I've been wearing that name tag I've had, and again it might just all be in my head, but their respect level and the physicians approaching me have been a lot more respectful. I don't know if it's just because of the RN behind my name. Because I know before with my other nametag, they would actually ask 'Who's the RN down here'. But now they look at my name tag some of them even call me by my first name and, oh yeah, it's been very different."*

During this final stage of your initial transition to professional practice, you will continue the recovery you started during the 2nd stage, but this time you will be engaging with a more future-oriented set of priorities.

> ***The future, according to some scientists, will be exactly like the past, only far more expensive.***
>
> ***-John Sladek***

> *"Like I said from the beginning, things are so much better. I know I'll never forget how hard it was because I still bring it up and even some of the girls that I'm friends with now were the ones that were kind of rough on me in the beginning and I still*

bug them about it because I don't want them to forget. I want them to realize that they need to accept new students and new nurses, and that people who are new to the unit need to be welcomed and accepted."

This stage is about settling into a deeper understanding of what nursing IS and who you ARE as a practitioner within the larger discipline. It is a time of 1) *exploring*, 2) *separating*, 3) *critiquing*, 4) *recovering*, and 5) *accepting*.

Exploring

The detachment from work (and sometimes from life around you) that may have settled in during the latter part of the 2nd stage continues through the early months of this 3rd stage. You may simply want to "*get up, go to work and come home to my life...eyes and ears open, but mouth closed*".

Laughter and tears are both responses to frustration and exhaustion. I myself prefer to laugh, since there is less cleaning up to do afterward.
-Kurt Vonnegut

"I guess I thought it was going to be the big defining career. My kids would be like, 'My mom is a nurse'. But that's not how they introduce me, because it's not how people see you. You know, people see you as [given name] you know? I wrote a letter to my Mom awhile back because I was frustrated—for a couple of weeks it had become just a job and I think it was mostly because of the people I worked with, 'cause to them sometimes it IS just a job and so you fall into the same rut as them. So I was frustrated and my Mom said 'Well you just have to stick it out. You know, you just need to stick it out and maybe this isn't where you're going to be for the rest of your life and that's OK because nursing is so diverse'. I know I won't be here [name of workplace] forever because I enjoy it but it doesn't energize me all the time to go to work. I don't get all excited. I want to be in a job or a career where I do the foot-work but I also want to be part of a committee to make the unit better."

As is alluded to in this narrative, more time may now be spent exploring and critiquing your new professional landscape and taking stock of the more disquieting aspects of your socio-professional, cultural and political work environments.

"I think…it's a little bit of everything and I think I need a break. Badly. Like I think I need to just get away and not worry about it and not have staffing call four times a day for overtime. Like I said, I used to see my job as an extension of myself and now it's just something I do and that I'm competent at it. And I know that

Reality is a crutch for people who can't cope with drugs.
-Lily Tomlin

makes me probably not as caring as I'd like to be but I guess that's just how I've dealt with the fact that I don't want to be there. Right now I don't see a lot of other options for myself. Like I use to think that…it was like I would do this for a while and then I would try this, and this, and this, and this and now I'm just like, I don't know. It was suggested that maybe trying a different hospital might be better because I guess things are different at [this other hospital] and there's a lot of the crap going on at [this hospital] that doesn't happen there and that might be worth a try. I don't know. I just feel like, it's only been 8 months and I'm kind of stuck between a rock and a hard place—what do you do really?"

What we need to do is learn to work in the system, by which I mean that everybody, every team, every platform, every division, every component is there not for individual competitive profit or recognition, but for contribution to the system as a whole on a win-win basis.

-W. Edwards Deming

Your level of stress during this stage can vary considerably, but the factors contributing to your stress have likely changed from a focus on your *individual* capacity to cope with new roles and responsibilities, to feelings of frustration in dealing with the *system* at large (i.e. the workplace, institution or healthcare in general). An overwhelming majority of participants in my studies over the past 12 years took note at this stage of their position of power and authority relative to others, with many identifying nurses as "*being at the bottom of the pile*". Some were understandably disturbed by this perception.

"I wish I could say that work is going great. I wish I could say that nursing is everything I ever thought it would be and more. But I can't. Sometimes it takes an army of courage to drag myself from my oh so comfortable bed to that stressful place. I feel like I am back at square one wondering where those nine months of experience have gone. I was feeling so good a couple of months ago and it's like I don't even remember that feeling. I wonder, 'Could I be experiencing burnout?'"

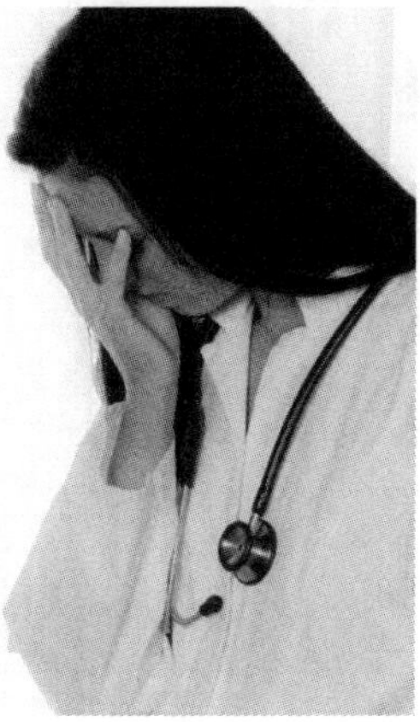

Growing discontent with what you might perceive as professional devaluing can motivate another, albeit less dramatic reduction in your momentum. In my research, for those making their transition in a hospital environment, this peak (really the peak of a chronic level of discontent) ultimately served as a tipping point that started them searching for professional fulfillment beyond the role of an acute-care bedside nurse.

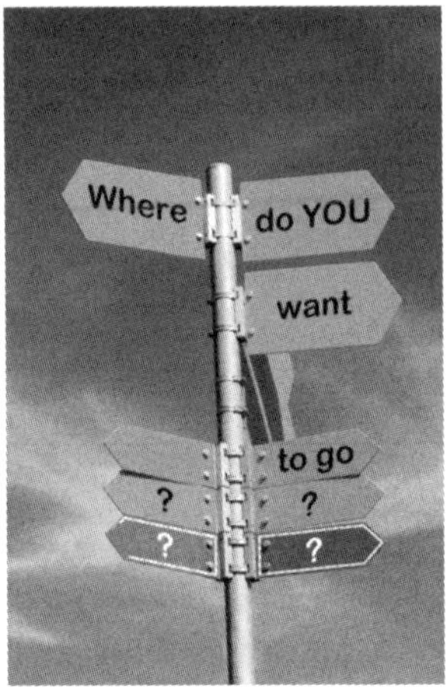

At this point in your professional journey, you can expect a change to occur in your primary support relationships. Prior to graduating, you most likely relied on non-nursing friends, pre-graduate student peers and family members for support. Now, you may see your support relationships shifting to current coworkers and experienced nursing colleagues. It is important to recognize that any change brings about both gains and losses; you must be willing to shed the 'old' in order to make room for the 'new'.

"I think one thing that has really helped me is having a sounding board with my colleagues who can say, 'That's normal'. It's having great relationships with all the staff members, and going out together and socializing; it's like a family you know? We get along and we really try to help each other out, work as a team, back each other up. I've gotten to know some of them a lot better too and they genuinely care about their co-workers. So some of us are friends outside of work so I think it's good."

This does not mean that ALL past relationships will go by the wayside, but that your relationships may be altered somewhat in form and purpose. You may start to notice that your new *multidimensional* life (personal and professional) has relative components (for instance there may be your '*professional nursing*' life, your '*creative photography*' life, your '*family*' life, your '*social*' life) into which some relationships fit while others do not. Many new nurses, particularly younger graduates, may make crystallizing commitments with partners at this stage such as getting engaged, getting married or taking steps to cohabitate if they haven't done so earlier in their transition process. For grads of 2nd degree programs or for those with established families of their own, this stage creates space (time and energy) for reinvesting in family connections or time honored traditions, engaging in a partner's career or a child's activities, or thinking about where your personal and professional lives are going or what they might '*look like*' in the future.

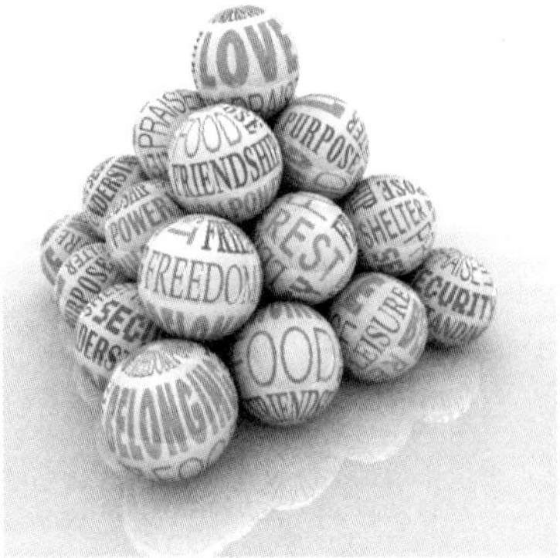

"I find it very stressful at times and there's a lot of things that bother me about it like not being able to complete my work and be satisfied with my job all the time. But I don't think I'll ever do anything else and if I do, it would just be temporarily. Like I might take some time off to have children some day but I'd always go back. Even

if I got some other type of job for a short period of time, I would always, always go back to nursing."

"I just, I have a really good feeling that this is going to get better. And I just know myself from having past jobs and just everything I've ever done in my life, I'm always kind of a little bit behind the rest of the crowd. It always seems to take me a little longer, to catch on to stuff but once I catch on to it, I'm really good at it. Yeah, I just know that I can be an expert in nursing and I will be one day, but for now I just need to focus and hold with it and it will happen. I know it will."

Separating

I can say with relative assurance that by the 12-month mark most of you will reach a stable level of comfort and confidence with your roles, responsibilities, knowledge and professional relationships[1].

"I just definitely cannot look into my future at all. I'm so happy where I am right now that I just want to stay here right now. Some of my friends are going to California for three months and working there and they asked me to come along. I know I could do work over there but I'm not ready to leave yet. Like I know it would only be a temporary thing but even for myself, like I don't think I'm ready skill wise and confidence wise either. I'm just not really forcing myself to look in the future because I'm happy where I am now. Sometimes I think that I'm going to be a lifer on [this unit] but I don't know."

"As far as being neutral about the profession, I don't think that's necessarily a bad thing at this point or that it means anything. It just takes awhile to get to that place

[1]At the risk of sounding like a broken record, I find it is necessary to qualify my comments on the NGs level of comfort at 12 months by reinforcing the pivotal influence of ***stability, consistency, familiarity*** and ***predictability*** in the evolving development of a new nurse. The healthiest transition experiences for NGs will be facilitated when they:
1) have personal and professional lives characterized by **stable and supportive relationships**;
2) receive **consistent workplace support** and **constructive feedback**;
3) are able to safely deliver nursing care and perform skills appropriate to their scope of practice,
4) have opportunities to consult and collaborate with experienced nurses about increasingly complex clinical decisions and judgments;
5) are **repeatedly successful** in responding accurately and appropriately to practice scenarios;
6) are provided with **positive reinforcement and reassurance** as to their progress over time that is evidenced by a strengthening of their knowledge base and positive care outcomes; and
7) are supported within their workplaces to **deliver quality care** and influence policy related to care and practice standards.

> *where you identify yourself with the bigger things. It's less about me and how scared I am and how I feel and it's more about the patient and the family. Less about the little things, the minute things that don't actually matter but it takes awhile to figure out what's important."*

It is natural at this stage to compare your practical skill level and cognitive prowess with that of the newest graduates entering your clinical environment, or with students that you are asked to preceptor.

> *"Once fall hit and we started having students and I started working a lot again that seemed to make a difference. In talking with my friends, it seems like most kind of went through the same things. Like it was really hard and they were really terrified and they worked their way through it and I think for the most part people are comfortable. And I remember having the discussion with them and they said the exact same thing, 'Holy smokes! We had students the other day, and I didn't realize how much I'd learned until I saw how much they didn't know."*

> *"It seemed crazy. It just seemed like you're running, running, running and now everything seems slower. I think it's 'cause we have a bunch of fourth year nursing students and new grads starting and I was trying to picture myself being them right now and it's just weird because they looked so scared. They're just always asking lots of questions, which is what I was like too. Unsure about yourself, you're doing your best but your best is still fairly little. And you're just starting to deal with shift work. Not having much time for yourself because you're always thinking about your work or being stressed out or wondering what's going to happen next shift. I guess you're just starting in a new area so you don't know the people as well and that's always a challenge to get to know people, get to know who all the doctors are, who everyone is that you collaborate with like social work, PT [physiotherapy], OT [occupational therapy], homecare, everybody...so you don't know any faces and you don't know who you should be talking to or where to go. I don't know, it just seems like, 'What if so many things got missed when I didn't know about all this stuff?' I think of causing harm to somebody, of not knowing what the [heck] I was doing, feeling stupid every day and not knowing any answers. It was just overwhelming and a large amount of responsibility for which I didn't feel prepared. I mean, all of a sudden you're a professional nurse—well what the [heck] does that mean? I don't know. All of a sudden everybody's coming to you, you're the one with the answers but when you don't have them, it's not much fun."*

Your objective here is to establish a 'new' identity that moves you beyond both *nursing student* and *graduate nurse* labels.

"Perhaps I noticed such a difference because I reported off to a new grad. And the contrast between our reactions is what made me realize I have changed. I watched as her eyes became bigger and bigger as I gave report. She almost started panicking before I was even done and stated she felt really overwhelmed. I remember exactly how she felt, but I was surprised (and relieved) that I no longer felt this way about work."

"I've come home increasingly thankful for my life. That's one thing about nursing, it really keeps me grounded in the sense that I don't really take things for granted and it's a constant reminder of…you know, very easily that could be me and my family member, anybody in that bed, and you should really be thankful for what you've got. Families? Yeah, they've been causing me stress. I guess that I don't brush them aside anymore or I'll sit there and I'll talk to them because sometimes it's just so hard. Just families having a really hard time with death and letting go and wanting to do everything for their mother when the mother is telling me that she wants to die. The two daughters came up to me and one was really level headed and had faced the fact that her mother was probably in her last week/months of life and wasn't doing well. But the one daughter came up to me and was just in a frantic panic and said, 'Her legs are about three times as swollen as they were yesterday and what can we do about this' and 'What can we do about the swelling in her legs. We need to fix that. It's a sign of heart failure isn't it? My mom's going to die of heart failure isn't she?' I had to sit there and listen and try to be calm and it was really good that her sister said 'Yes, she is going to die, this is going to happen.' Instead of being task focused, running around trying to get everything done, instead in my head I'm trying to think of what I can do to help them deal with their fears of losing their Mom."

> ***The path to our destination is not always a straight one. We go down the wrong road, we get lost, we turn back. Maybe it doesn't matter which road we embark on. Maybe what matters is that we embark.***
>
> ***-Barbara Hall***

Being able to answer the questions instead of always asking them, and finding the time and energy to assist others with their workloads instead of being consumed solely with your own, are signs of your progress.

These changes are a culmination of advancements in your ability to organize and prioritize, the experience of managing increasingly complex clinical and relational situations, and a growing confidence in the performance of nursing skills and competencies. While all of this has been an evolving and progressive process of growth, you may find that "*all of a sudden, you look back and it's like, 'How did I get from there to here', because it's gradual and it happens without your realizing it.*" In fact, some graduates have claimed that "*it could be exactly the same scenarios, but my ability to cope has changed.*"

> *"I remember in first year nursing school we needed to 'find ourselves'. We needed to 'self disclose'. Hated that class. Absolutely hated it because I've always been a concrete thinker. It had to be black and white with me. But now I'm seeing the gray areas of myself and I've learned a lot not only about nursing but about myself and I finally 'get' that class *chuckle*. I feel like I'm on the mend and finding out who I am, where I need to be, where's my place in this world. Just overall, the confidence has changed drastically since I started in May, [when I was] so nervous that I would lose sleep about it and now it's just another day."*

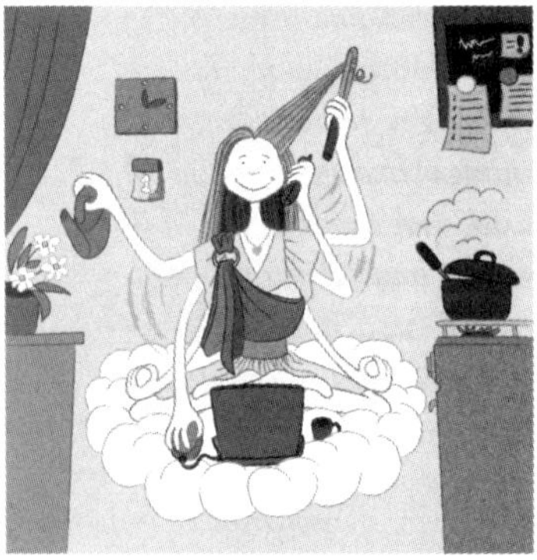

You will likely be seeking opportunities for a more advanced and independent level of practice. These opportunities can come in the form of enhanced clinical complexity in the patient/client demographic for which you are caring, preparation for and assumption of charge nurse duties (if those are within the scope of your nursing role), preceptoring of new staff or students, or the addition of more in-depth client care program development responsibilities.

> *"I don't know what happened in the past few months, but I really love my job! If I've ever doubted in the past, I don't anymore. I've noticed myself looking forward to challenges that I once dreaded and feared...I've also noticed a change in the way I deal with unstable patients or rapidly changing situations. One of our patients on the ward suddenly went unresponsive and we had to quickly move a patient out of the observation unit to accommodate the changing medical condition of this patient. I was able to stay calm and think about what needed to be done...That is not to say that I don't still have moments of anxiety or uncertainty when dealing with situations for the first time. But I think I approach them differently. I seem to have the ability now to see a situation more holistically, taking into account the family and the patient. As well, I break it down and deal with one thing at a time, making it much more manageable. I find I require much less reassurance and I deal with challenges or problems often without needing to consult others, which I think is a testament to my increasing confidence. I've developed good working relationships with the staff members. I've created my own routine and that seems to work for me. I've begun to learn from my own experience now as opposed to relying on others. I still ask questions and I take the opportunity to learn when I can. Though I have in the past regretted going into nursing, I certainly no longer feel that way. I couldn't be happier with the choice that I have made."*

To manage the advancing roles and responsibilities, you may require more give and take, negotiation, and collaboration in your professional relationships. In an attempt to take on more depth and scope in your roles and responsibilities, you may put some distance between yourself and your experienced nursing colleagues. This is natural!! If you can, share with your colleagues how you are feeling and how your needs are changing—negotiate a different way of relating, informing them that as you become more independent they will need to 'let go' of you a bit; be present for you, but not hovering as intently as they might have before.

A vision without action is called a daydream; but then again, an action without vision is called a nightmare.

-Jim Sorenson

Critiquing

In order to reconstruct your vision of nursing and understand how that vision fits with who you are now, you will likely engage in a certain level of critique.

> *"I'd say that's probably one of the most frustrating parts of the job. Just systems things like the other day I had to move two patients around so I could get this patient up and she didn't even have oxygen. I mean, she was a simple patient that didn't need it but we still had to do all these moves and stuff to bring her up. It's just political. Like that floor doesn't want that patient so we get them—it's expensive and it's a waste of nursing time. And things like entering orders into the computer—I don't think nurses go to school to be data entry clerks and I think it's a waste of nursing time when we could be doing other things instead of running around like crazy."*

Critique does not equate with *criticism*—while you may be critiquing individuals with whom you interact or the situations in which you find yourself, this does not mean you are *criticizing* those people or those structures (practice settings or institutions). But people may take your need to critique 'personally' so be careful about the way you approach these situations.

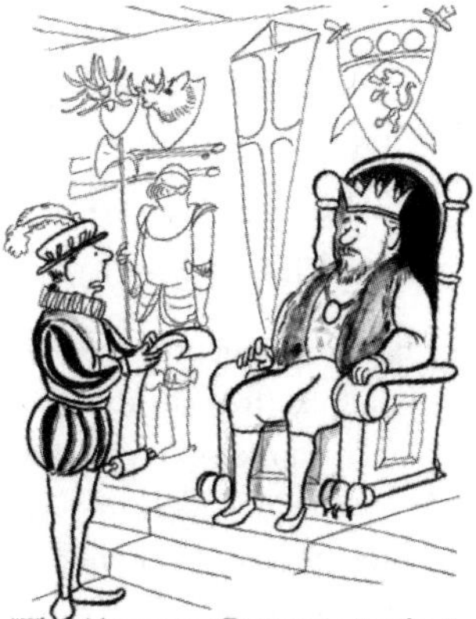

"The Humpty-Dumpty project is way over budget."

Try to stay with '*I*' as often as possible or begin your conversation with "*This is not about YOU personally*" **OR** "*I am not criticizing or even talking about what YOU personally have done, but....*" **OR** "*Please know that I have absolutely no desire to offend you when I say this, but I am wondering about...*".

What you NEED to do is deconstruct what exists in your professional world for the purpose of reconstructing it so that there is a better 'fit' between what you are experiencing, who you are becoming as a nurse, and your expectations and aspirations. This process might be easier for YOU than it is for those around you. You may need to help them understand WHY you are critiquing things and illustrate for them the ways they might assist you to move your concerns, questions, or practice issues forward. Do you recall the '*Columbo*' approach I talked about in the 1st stage? While I **fully endorse** this approach and continue to use it when the circumstances are right, this indirect, stumbling over yourself, '*excuse me but I don't know what I'm doing*' kind of style is intended to catch the unsuspecting off guard. You may be beyond that approach at this point because SERIOUSLY, you can't say you don't know anything anymore ☺ (YOU'RE A NEW GRADUATE, PROFESSIONAL ROCK STAR!!!!!!!). So, let's switch it up a bit and go with what is referred to as the '*Socratic*[2]' method (NOW my blood is pumping! If you are a previous student of mine, you will recognize this).

Quite simply, the Socratic method turns STATEMENTS into QUESTIONS for the purpose of challenging, clarifying, or even changing the way one thinks about an issue. The purpose of this method is really to facilitate, encourage, and provoke evidence-based discussion that assists all participants to discover the '*caves*[3]' (unexamined beliefs) in their thinking. **NOTE TO SELF**: *statements* CLOSE conversation while *questions* OPEN conversation. The Socratic process begins with deconstructing the issue to get UNDER or BEHIND what is really driving it. Then, those involved can reconstruct the issue so that it more accurately reflects what is really going on.

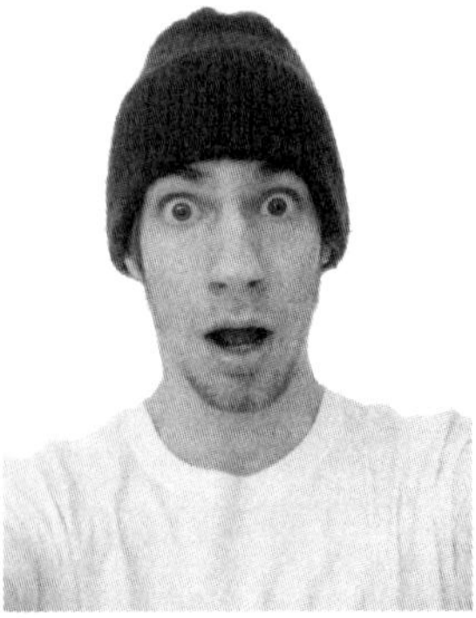

Finally, keep in mind that the more experienced colleagues you are working with might have *valuable experience or information* on how best to 'make change' that can help you succeed, particularly in the environment within which you are all working as they know the 'players'), so try to stay OPEN to their ideas! MANY heads are always better than ONE!

Recovering

WOW!!!!!!! What the heck happened there??????

You might be wondering what on earth happened to you over the past 8 months and now need time to recover from the draining experience of making your initial transition to professional practice. This process is related to separating in that the separation of your personal life from your professional work is important as you advance your identity WITHIN and AWAY from work. The dimensions of your life are now becoming distinct and it takes time to figure out how to manage them all.

[2]Gross, R. (2002). *Socrates' way: Seven master keys to using your mind to the utmost*. New York: Penguin Putnam Inc.
[3]Gross, pages 116-119

"I definitely feel more comfortable where I am now. I like what I'm doing, I like where I'm at. It's a nice privilege that they chose you to orientate new grads and take on heavier workloads because someone thinks you're competent at what you are doing and that you've been there long enough that you do know the routines…I was also saying that I kind of feel like I had a little plateau at work for the last month; like I am not as passionate about it as I once was. I think I was work, work, work for a straight year and it's all that I thought about and it was stressful at the beginning and I wasn't really doing much on my days off. I don't feel burned out, just not as excited about work as much."

You may want to spend more time with family and friends, in part because you feel as though you have neglected them for the past several months while absorbed in making this transition. You may also want to engage in personal activities (i.e., hobbies you want to reactivate) or you may simply need to spend time away from the work environment. It is very important that you be encouraged to pursue activities OUTSIDE of nursing (NOT spending all your unscheduled hours working overtime!!) that can give you a balanced sense of development, success and fulfillment.

"I definitely have more energy at work and at home. I think I just got to a point where I either had to do something or I was going to fall apart, you know, have to leave my job because I was feeling so stressed out and it wasn't going well for me so I think I just stepped back a bit, went on some holidays and I came back feeling better. I don't feel that attached to the nursing profession right now. Not that I don't enjoy being a nurse or anything, I just feel kind of neutral you know? I will be fine, I will just keep doing what I'm doing and I think right now that is all I need."

You may be making decisions at this point about the place of nursing in your life and about the meaning of your recent transition for your plans as a nurse. Depending on the degree of adjustment you have experienced (this is individual), your recovery will vary in intensity and duration.

"I just can't see myself doing anything else, and I think I said this before, that nursing's got that beautiful balance between the science and the caring and you have all of it. You can touch people's lives in a certain way and then you can run and look at their lab work and grab their meds and you can do all that fun stuff—all the science AND give them a backrub. It's just amazing…"

"Sometimes I feel like nursing isn't enough for me, or that where I am isn't enough for me. Like I need to go back to school or I need to do something else so I can't say that this is enough. I think it has more to do with me and my personality than anything about nursing. Like it's nothing to do with nursing; it's not the profession, it's just

who I am. I just need more than what I'm doing... To me the expectations just aren't high enough. Like I feel like I have a lot more knowledge than I get to apply but I don't know yet—that's the problem I guess. I just don't know where I want to go necessarily or what I want to do."

Accepting

Accepting is about distinguishing, during the course of your *critique*, what you can and cannot 'live with' about both the practice and professional relationships that surround you. This may mean that you have to reconfigure your expectations about some*thing* or some*one* (i.e. in navigating your daily workload, you may need to find a way to assess AND educate your patient/clients at the same time), or it may mean that you need to initiate a change (i.e. approach your manager to discuss practice issues, request targeted clinical experiences, or address a specific issue/conflict with someone in your work environment). Learning from a mentor how THEY coped with their initial practice adjustments and how they integrated THEIR nursing standards into the contemporary nursing context may assist you in generating your own creative ways of approaching your evolving practice. Remember that this mentor could be a nursing grad who has been out a few more years than you! It's about experience and a willingness to support you, it's not about age....

Acceptance is not a state of passivity or inaction. I am not saying you can't change the world, right wrongs, or replace evil with good. But acceptance is, in fact, the first step to action. If you don't fully accept a situation precisely the way it is, you will have difficulty changing it.

-Peter McWilliams

"I feel like they've accepted me and I feel good about being here. I guess I don't have to worry about that anymore. I mean when you work with great people you want to help them and you want to do good in your job so it's positive. It's something that feeds on itself once you get the momentum going. For instance, once whatever is necessary clicks into place, you feel more welcome which increases your sense of comfort in the area which increases your confidence, which then increases your tendency to reach out, which then increases your 'team'manship....it's sort of a cycle. Just being more comfortable and not having work hanging over you as such a stressor makes your life outside of work better too."

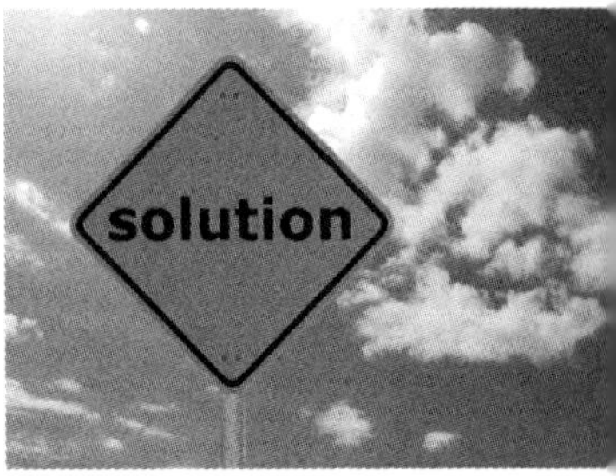

It must be acknowledged that untenable conflicts may occur for you as you work your way through the process of accepting, or NOT accepting what you find in the real world. It is important to ensure that both you and your mentor, nursing unit manager, educator or experienced colleagues try to steer away from perceiving all practice or work incompatibilities as a statement of failure. Your responsibility, in consultation with your support team, is to recognize IF an incompatibility exists, determine what steps can and need to be taken to understand the situation and then, if possible, resolve it (i.e. meet with your manager, educator, mentor or preferably ALL of the above to strategize on an approach).

Resolution may mean that the issue cannot be altered to your satisfaction and may require that you change your perception of the person or situation. Or it may mean that this is not the workplace for you. Again, just be OPEN to all possibilities!

NOTE OF CAUTION: I do not want to leave you with either an unreasonably optimistic or an unnecessarily pessimistic impression of what your arrival at the 12-month mark of professional nursing practice might look like.

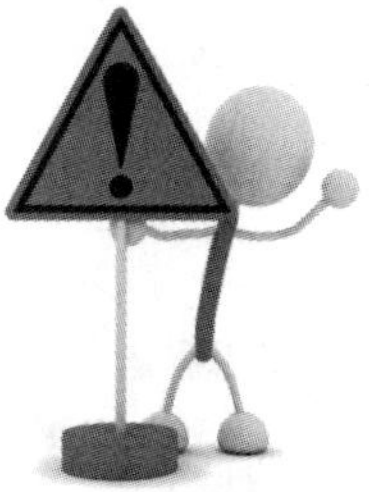

HOWEVER......

There is always the chance that your experiences to date have been NEITHER consistent nor stable, and that these experiences did NOT give you the sense of practice familiarity or predictability that you needed to feel successful as a new nurse. It is possible that your transition to professional practice has been fraught with overwhelming challenges and has left you with a residue of discouragement or disappointment from which you are struggling to recover. I have seen this and my heart aches at the thought of witnessing even one more lost nursing soul.

Emergencies have always been necessary to progress. It was darkness that produced the lamp; it was fog that produced the compass; it was hunger that drove us to exploration; and it took a depression to teach us the real value of a job.
-Victor Hugo

IF THIS IS YOU, please connect immediately with your regional/institutional occupational health nurse/office or the *Employee Assistance Program* where you work. These meetings are intended to be STRICTLY confidential so that you can openly discuss your feelings and experiences. If you are wary of your safety in this situation, make sure you ask for the sessions to be confidential at the outset—this is about being transparent so that you can be honest about your experiences. As well, *Nursing The Future* (www.nursingthefuture.ca OR newgraduates@nursingthefuture.ca) is always there for you—contact us so that we can talk together about how to move you from a place of disillusionment to one of hope and possibility—a place where you can *thrive* in a profession that both WANTS and NEEDS you.

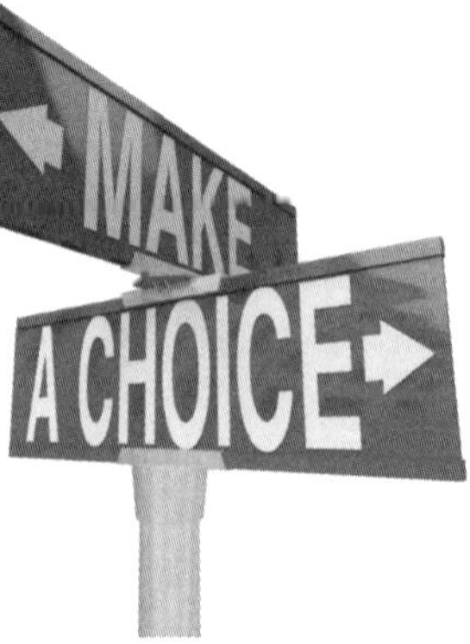

Make the choice to STAY! I know from my own, extremely diverse career, that there is NO OTHER profession in the world that can accommodate as many varying interests, unique styles or work preferences. This is a broad and deep profession and it has room for us all!

There ARE nurses out there who have successfully found their way BACK from career disappointment and could help you work through the challenges you are experiencing. There are also psychologists, counselors and social workers whose whole professional purpose it is to assist healthcare providers with traumas they have encountered; be that with patients, families and colleagues or within their own personal lives during vulnerable periods such as this.

NEED TO KNOW

- This stage is about **REGROUPING**—a time when you will settle into a deeper understanding of what nursing IS and who YOU ARE as a practitioner within the discipline.
- During the 8th to 12th month period of your initial year of transition, you will be primarily:
  1) **Exploring** where you are 'going' in your career and how the knowledge and skill base you have developed over the past 12 months has advanced your practice competence. You may also be delving deeper into any inconsistencies in the healthcare system and the nursing profession that you may have noticed previously. This exploration can lead to some disenchantment or disillusionment and should be carefully monitored by both you and your support network.
  2) **Separating** who YOU are as a professional from those practitioners you see around you. This is the time when the multitude of thoughts and actions that you have witnessed in others, perhaps over months, will be 'sorted' by you for their relevance and fit with your own evolving practice. The boundaries that frame your standards and ethics will be refined and decisions will be made about what you will or will not accept as ways of being, doing and knowing in nursing. At this point in your evolution, you may want to 'try on' more advanced practice experiences by requesting more complex clinical scenarios or contemplating a change in your practice setting. Just always keep in mind…it is the JOURNEY rather than the destination that makes the life

3) **Critiquing** your workplace for its resonance with your professional values, aspirations and expectations. This may include deconstructing some of the ways in which you witness your colleagues practicing, with the intent to further understand WHY they do things the way they do. While the motivation is not to find fault with anyone around you, the end result may be the exposure of practice improprieties of individuals, your unit, or your institution. Should you suspect a breach in practice standards or ethics, discuss your concerns or questions with the person/s in question FIRST, giving them an opportunity to explain, rationalize or justify their position. This is ALWAYS the best approach (it is process-oriented and respectful) to use in addressing issues of any kind. If you do not feel SAFE approaching an individual directly, consult a trusted peer with the intent of outlining next steps in your approach while maintaining confidentiality to the best of your ability. The intent in approaching someone outside of the individual/s directly involved in the breach should be to gain further **information and insight** while maintaining the highest level of integrity possible in accordance with the legal and ethical standards to which you are held. Ultimately, your responsibility is to REPORT any practice you have witnessed that puts either patients or practitioners at risk. There is no question that this can get uncomfortable, but it can also be done in such a way as to preserve the person's dignity AND prevent harm. Being a change agent in nursing is not easy; like many 'time honored' professions, we have traditions that are older than they are wise. There ARE ways to make change but they usually require grace, diplomacy, consultation and negotiation. Having said that, sometimes you have to take the Nike™ pledge and **JUST DO IT**!! You decide which approach works in your situation.
4) **Recovering** the energy, motivation and passion you once had for your life and your profession. Sometimes life gets the better of us and we feel like we have been 'left out in the rain without an umbrella'. The key is to get out of your wet clothes as quickly as possible, put on something warm (preferably flannel), grab a hot drink (in my case mulled wine would do) or if you prefer, a 'cool one', turn on the Golf Channel®, and let things settle. It's hard to talk, or even think straight when your teeth are chattering from the chill of an experience and we don't tend to make good decisions when our brains are numb. I suggest you remain in a stable place of work for the first year of your practice if possible—remember, this is a full, exciting, and energy-consuming 12 months that will challenge your mind, body and spirit. You WILL find your way to the place you want to be, but why rush? You have a lifetime of work ahead!
5) **Accepting** what you have gone through as a natural process of professional socialization and evolution. At the same time as you are accepting transition as a natural state, you must also accept that practice standards exist on a continuum. PERFECT PRACTICE does not exist, though there are situations and even

extended periods of time when we can say our practice is excellent. As a rule, you will have a few GREAT days, the rare REALLY BAD day and the rest of the time you will sit somewhere in the middle. If you practice competently and safely, learn something each day that enhances your practice, and TRY to give what you can to whomever you can for as long as you can, that is the most that anyone could ask.

NEED TO THINK ABOUT

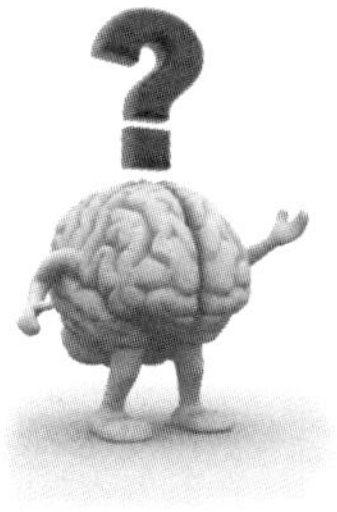

- Are you happy?
  a. What makes you happy personally? Professionally?
  b. When was the last time you laughed?
  c. When was the last time you 'played'?
  d. What or who brings joy into your life? Are you spending time in the company of that 'thing' or 'person'?
  e. Is there anything in your life that is preventing you from being happy or fulfilled? What? What can you do about it?
- What kind of a nurse do you want to be (attributes or professional characteristics)?
- What area of practice are you most interested in pursuing?
- What do you see yourself doing as a nurse in 5 years? 10 years?
- What do you need to do (ongoing education, skill acquisition, practice experience and knowledge) to get where you want to be? Who can help you get there?
- What does your career plan look like (what, how, when, who, where)?
- Are you being encouraged to take on leadership roles and responsibilities? How does this make you feel? Are you prepared to take on a charge nurse or preceptor role?
- What educational program will you be provided with to prepare for this advanced role? What rights do you have to negotiate these requests in your workplace?
- With whom can you have an honest and open critique of the professional nursing landscape?
- How might your experienced colleagues assist you to make sense of the questions you have about nursing?
- What does practice 'interdependence' mean to you? How can you achieve it?
- How have your needs changed over the past several months and what do you need now to learn and grow?
- What challenges or strains have surfaced for you at this time and how might you address them?
- How can you be supported to find your own unique way of nursing?
- What does a balanced life look like for you? How will you 'get there'?
- How do the nurses with whom you work balance their personal and professional lives?

NEED TO DO

1. Engage in **monthly dialogue** sessions with an experienced mentor who can assist you to work through the practice concerns or issues that may have surfaced for you.
2. Connect with someone (career counselor or interested manager/educator) who can help you create a **career trajectory/pathway** that will facilitate your growth and move you in your desired professional direction.
3. IF you feel that you are ready to begin preparation for an **advanced practice role**[4] (educator, preceptor, mentor or advanced clinical nurse), engage in **continuing educational opportunities** that expand your competency portfolio (i.e. taking *Advanced Cardiac Life Support* or acquiring your certification as a *Lactation Consultant*).
4. Find a way to **share your experience** as you are going through it (meet regularly with a good friend, a new grad colleague, a trusted mentor, write in a journal, take photographs, or tape your thoughts at the end of every shift).
5. **Take frequent outings** (stroll down a neighborhood walking path or go to an all-inclusive resort) AWAY from the workplace and **invite NEW people** (NON-nurses too!) into your life to give it flavor and perspective.
6. **IF you want to take on leadership roles (i.e. charge duty, preceptorship, or project development/management),** this would be a good time in your professional transition experience. Most institutions have programs that train you to take advanced practice roles so try not to get pulled into taking on a role because 'they need someone' and you happen to be available. As I said before, being in a formal leadership position is a professional career decision so make it carefully.
7. **Consider volunteering for work on a professional committee**, either in your place of work, your regional community, or in your state/province. Professional nursing and healthcare organizations are always seeking new insights and certainly have plenty of insights to offer YOU about nursing, healthcare and the political environment. Ask your manager or mentor how you might find a local or regional

---

[4]Like I have said a few times now, DON'T RUSH!! You have a lifetime of work ahead and plenty of time to pursue your dreams and aspirations. Advanced practice nursing is JUST THAT—it's advanced! In order to practice deeper and broader, we need a good strong base or it's like diagnosing and treating before we have adequately or comprehensively ASSESSED. Give yourself permission to COAST at this stage—making a decision to move forward can wait until your 2nd year at least. Why don't you close this book, head out to a movie with a good friend and have a glass of nice red wine for me (not that I am encouraging the use of alcohol as a coping mechanism)……

nursing or community organization and go to a meeting. You DO NOT have to make a commitment until you are ready, so 'shop around' for an organization with a mandate and vision that matches your values and professional aspirations.

8. **Pick up a hobby** that you always wanted to do, or return to one that you enjoyed!
9. Spend time with your **mentor** discussing the following:
    a. What made them choose their career path? How did it unfold?
    b. What do they think are your greatest strengths?
    c. Where do they feel your strengths would best be utilized?
    d. How do they deal with their frustrations and disappointments as a professional?
    e. Have they ever been burned out? What did it look like? Were there warning signs? How did they cope with it?

Appendices

- I. TRANSITION SHOCK Summary
- II. DOING Summary
- III. BEING Summary
- IV. KNOWING Summary
- V. Conceptual Model of Transition Support
  Framework for Transition Support Strategies
- VI. Senior Practicum/New Nurse Transition Schedule
  Transition Program Content
    - 1-4 Weeks
    - 5-8 Weeks
    - 9-12 Weeks
- VII. Finding the Right Job
- VIII. Working on a Team
- IX. Adjusting to Shift Work
- X. Taking Care of YOURSELF
- XI. Workload Distribution/Collaboration/Delegation
- XII. Managing Your Nursing Workload
    - Organizing
    - Prioritizing
    - Maintaining Professional Standards
    - Practice Ethics
    - Potentially Unsafe Situations for A New Nurse
- XIII. Thinking on Your Feet
- XIV. Conflict Management in the Workplace
- XV. Dealing with a Bully
- XVI. Communicating with Physicians
- XVII. CODES and Rapid Response Teams
- XVIII. Death of a Patient
- XIX. Nursing in Rural or Remote Areas
- XX. Working in High Acuity Areas
- XXI Generational Workplace Ethics/Behavior

Transition Shock Summary

RESPONSIBILITIES – Issues	RESPONSIBILITIES – Strategies
• **Connecting with other disciplines** collaboratively and autonomously for the first time; • **Integrating into an established healthcare culture** that has as its hierarchy with which you may be unfamiliar; • **Taking on additional responsibilities** such as delegation, collaborative care planning, leading and making decisions and clinical judgments; • **Managing ongoing personal responsibilities** to family, friends or partners	• ***Understanding that it takes time to establish yourself as a leader in patient care planning and directing***. While you have often been expected to plan, direct and evaluate significant patient care initiatives, you have likely NOT been fully responsible for the outcomes. But rather, you have been closely guided in the development, conduct and evaluation of those initiatives by experienced faculty or practicing nurse colleagues. Further to this, many new nurses are expected to work alone on relatively highly acute units with little or no consistent access to experienced preceptors or mentors. **WATCH and LISTEN** – spend time with an established nurse who has the kind of leadership attributes that YOU respect (i.e. organized, respectful, collaborative, etc.). Ask to SHADOW someone in charge and get a sense of HOW they enact their leadership characteristics. • ***Delegating to other practitioners.*** You may be expected to delegate roles and tasks to individuals who may be older in age and more experienced and this can be a significant stressor. This stress may cause you to take on tasks you would otherwise delegate to others, thinking that this will allow you to avoid having to deal with this uncomfortable responsibility. **Guidance and modeling** on how to approach staff to whom you must delegate, but to whom you must also look to for information about your patients or for experiential knowledge is available so ASK YOUR MANAGER OR EDUCATOR about

	this. **Understand that delegation and workload sharing are DIFFERENT**; delegating is about YOU being responsible for asking someone to do something 'on your behalf'(for which you remain partially responsible) versus workload sharing, which would be where 'licensed' caregivers (Registered Nurses, Registered/Licensed Practical Nurses, Enrolled Nurses, Physicians, Dieticians, Social Workers, Occupational and Physiotherapists, etc.) collaboratively decide who is the BEST individual/s to care for WHICH patients/communities/ situations and how best to work TOGETHER to accomplish what needs to be done. • ***<u>Making independent decisions and clinical judgments</u>***. You may be unprepared for, and experientially incapable of making complex patient care decisions in clinical/care situations with which you have little or no experience. Mentoring is a valuable tool for making this responsibility more manageable and learning occurs OVER TIME. Again, be aware of decisions being made by others (all team members) and 'go to school' on WHAT they decide, HOW they decide it, WHO they collaborate with and WHEN they reach out for assistance from others. It is always a good idea to ask questions and seek someone else's opinion on a decision you are making—over time, you will feel more confident making decisions on your own. Expertise TAKES TIME!! • ***<u>Balancing multiple responsibilities</u>***. There is ALOT going on for you during your transition to professional practice. Depending on the scope of responsibility, nurses carry varying roles and are afforded different levels of

decision-making and judgment responsibilities. Being introduced into your roles and responsibilities SLOWLY and sequentially is most effective, so try to negotiate this gradual integration with your manager and educator. If you can spend time 'buddying' with other healthcare professionals with whom you are to work (other nurses, support staff, other professional practitioners) you will have a sense of what THEY do relative to YOU; this allows you to take on only responsibilities that are YOURS to assume! There is enough work for everyone ☺

- ***Familiarizing yourself with practice contexts***. Being introduced into a professional practice role is often daunting when you feel completely responsible for the outcome of practice decisions you may never have made before. Access to a practitioner who has experienced the issues you are experiencing and worked through them over time can demonstrate for you how to balance all the roles and responsibilities. Even if you are in a rural or remote area or you are the ONLY nurse practicing in that center at any given time, make sure you have access to a senior practitioner by phone! As well, try to transition into professional practice in a familiar environment (i.e. take opportunities to do senior practicum rotations where you want to be employed) and try to remain in the area to which you initially transition for one year post graduation. It may be tempting to 'leave', particularly if you are struggling in your workplace, but remember—EXPECT to struggle—this is a MAJOR CHANGE in your life and there WILL be times of struggle. Changing your place of employment (unless you are being bullied and are unable to resolve the abusive situation)

	will only mean that you need to go through this AGAIN. The challenge with painstaking growth is that if we don't grow from it in one situation, 'life' will introduce it again….and again….until we learn whatever lesson it is trying to teach you. You have a LIFE TIME of work ahead—don't rush through your experiences!
ROLES – Issues • **Adjusting to additional roles** with primary responsibility for for patient treatment plans/multidisciplinary leadership roles/ collaboration on and implementation of appropriate physician requests (a.k.a. 'orders') • **Coping with role stress** particularly when roles are blurred, unclear or inappropriate for one's level of experience, knowledge or skill capacity • **Learning 'new' roles** related to specific workplace expectations, routines, and relationships that may be compounded by an overwhelming sense of responsibility for one's actions	ROLES – Strategies • ***Experiencing varying levels of stress***. Role stress is high, particularly during this first stage. The impact of this stress on your development depends on your perceived intensity of the stress, the supports and resources available to you as you navigate the environment (i.e. available colleagues and peers as well as prior and suggested coping mechanisms), your ability to experience success in your new role, consistency and predictability within the workplace and the time and opportunity you have to learn the roles, skills, routines, tasks and practices expected. • ***Progressively integrating into the role of a nurse***. Nurses function in varying but intense, dynamic and highly demanding contexts. New nurses, because of their limited experience in a variety of practice settings, should not be expected to make high-level clinical decisions or judgments unless provided with access to experienced collegial collaboration. Remember that much of your energy is being consumed by simply adjusting to a new reality that is both personal and professional. Expectations of performance without the provision of adequate support may result in unsafe practice situations that may go undetected by colleagues. The new professional's need to belong and feel

affirmed is highest during the initial months of their transition. As a new grad, you are developing a new professional identity during the first 12 months of practice, What you come to learn about yourself and others during the early stages of your transition will influence your experience for the remainder of your transition, possibly crystallizing your impressions of the profession as a whole. **Organize to be mentored** by an experienced practitioner who is as accepting and embracing as they are competent. That may mean you need to find someone who is an EXPERT practitioner to show you the skills you need to be proficient at, but a different individual to encourage you, listen to your concerns, challenges, and anxieties, support your ideas and strategize with you on how to accomplish the career path you have planned for yourself.

- ***Clarifying roles and responsibilities***. Role blurring and confusion (i.e. what does the social worker do and what do I do in this family crisis situation?) may be more prevalent if you have NOT been orientated (i.e. spent time shadowing colleagues in other disciplines as well as unit clerks, porters, nursing coworkers) to the roles and practices of your intra/professional colleagues. Spend time talking with and **shadowing** ALL colleagues with whom you will be working (including lab and pharmacy staff, your nursing partner [for LPN/RPN/Enrolled Nurses this would be an RN], nurse practitioners, physicians, receptionists, unit clerks, porters, allied health professionals and collaborating centers/organizations) so that you know WHAT they do, WHEN they do it and HOW to connect with them for support in your community or institution.

<table>
<tr><th>RELATIONSHIPS – Issues</th><th>RELATIONSHIPS – Strategies</th></tr>
<tr><td>

- **Establishing trust** and a sense of relatedness with new colleagues
- '***Trying out' or changing*** previously established roles and relationships

</td><td>

- ***<u>Learning to trust yourself and others.</u>*** If you were part of the 'culture' of your new workplace when you were a student, there will be some familiarity with power relationships and the established hierarchy of authority. Regardless of this however, you will likely experience a change in work relationships upon employment (i.e. the SAME people you worked with as a student may relate DIFFERENTLY to you once you are a fully responsible and accountable professional). Part of this stems from your own developmental adjustment to a new role and part of it arises out of altered expectations of colleagues who may feel you need to 'prove' yourself, or at least demonstrate to them that you can be trusted as a clinician. Establishing trusting relationships with new colleagues takes time. **Give yourself, AND YOUR COLLEAGUES time** to get comfortable with your new relationships. EVERYONE who comes into a new job feels the pressure of the expectations of others. The key is to focus on YOU—**learn something from everyone around you and be open to new ways** of approaching what you know, how you perform your roles and responsibilities, and how you engage with others in the workplace. Don't forget the **'Columbo' strategy**!!!! ☺ Ask LOTS of questions and know that things people say are RARELY about YOU and more about THEM…..dig for what is under the behavior to what might be motivating the behavior (yours and others).
- ***<u>Changing expectations</u>***. You know that you are expected to be directive and 'lead' the management of your assigned patient

</td></tr>
</table>

	load (after all you are a licensed professional!), but often new nurses do not have the clinical experience required to lead with confidence. This becomes more evident in clinical or relational situations that are unfamiliar, unpredictable or inconsistent. Moving from one unit to another in rapid succession (within 3 months) without adequate time to establish some familiarity, expertise or comfort with your professional colleagues, or to determine what support systems you have in your new area of work, may delay your progress through the stages of transition. In such situations, critical elements of success (i.e. consistency, familiarity, stability, and predictability) may be lacking. STAY PUT for 3 months, at the very least, so that you can get to know the people you are working with, the roles and responsibilities you are expected to assume, the kinds of patients you will be seeing and the work routines that are preferred! Working days AND nights can challenge your ability to cope with the transition experience so negotiate this with your manager. IF you have taken a 'float' position (moving between practice areas to relieve nurses who are sick or on leave), or if you have chosen to take two jobs, recognize that you will be adjusting and accommodating to many different sets of expectations, colleagues, routines and cultures. While moving between TWO jobs or placements isn't prohibitive, I strongly advise AGAINST rapid rotations between 3 or more areas of practice within your initial year. Spending time in a consistent area of practice/place of work for 3 month time frames allows you at least 'some' consistency, familiarity and predictability. • ***<u>Establishing respectful and collegial working relationships.</u>*** Delegation (transferring performance responsibility that is YOURS to unlicensed personnel or to a professional who

lacks expertise or training in the role, skill or responsibility you are delegating) is an advanced relational skill that requires both formal and behavioral mentoring. As a new nurse, you may be disoriented by your limited knowledge about various professional and ancillary roles and may hesitate to ask someone else to do something 'for' you. The tendency to 'do it myself' may be compounded by fears of appearing inadequate or incompetent, a lack of familiarity with the social and political underpinnings of the unit culture and a need to 'prove' to yourself and others (e.g. authority figures/seasoned colleagues) that you can 'handle' the role of a professional nurse. You may further assume that an enhanced level of function/task completion equals ***competence*** in the eyes of your colleagues and that expert ***performance*** will translate into respect and credibility by those individuals. As part of this, you may believe that getting your work done 'on time' (so that you do not stand out) is essential to being accepted. While it is always easier to be perceived as being 'a quick study', it is also **DANGEROUS to substitute SPEED for ACCURACY!** The key is to discuss with your educator or manager a **GRADUAL introduction/advancement of responsibilities** (it is better to have a reduced individual patient/case or community project load and PERFORM THE COMPLETE ROLE than do 'bits and pieces' of what you will be expected to do IN ITS ENTIRETY eventually). Once you are SUCCESSFUL at the modified load, add additional workload or complexity over time.

- ***Learning to work with others on a 'team'.*** As noted above, it is not uncommon for a new nurse to 'do it myself' rather than work through the uncomfortable process of asking for assistance or delegating a task to a colleague. This sometimes results in the unintentional crossing over of your roles and responsibilities into the work responsibilities and intellectual/practice territory of your colleagues (e.g. stepping on toes). Not meaning to, you may subsequently convey a lack of trust in your colleagues or you may appear arrogant, which can be responded to negatively. As well, not asking for assistance when it is appropriate can overwhelm you with work that is unnecessary or inappropriate. These are untoward outcomes of what may simply be socio-cultural naivety, but can serve to exhaust you physically and emotionally and add to your already taxed professional identity. Remember, **YOU ARE NOT ALONE** and it is always better to ask a colleague: '*Is this something that I should be doing myself*" OR '*Is there someone I should be working with on this*'? Again, spending time **shadowing all coworkers** with whom you are likely to engage in a working relationship can prevent these misunderstandings!

- ***'Getting' BACK a life!*** Your personal life may be undergoing significant change. You may be ending or deepening an intimate relationship or attempting to transfer your primary support network from family and school friends to your, as yet unfamiliar, colleagues. Understanding the impact of generational differences (Appendix XXI) on one's work ethic and values may influence the ease with which you integrate into your new work system. Remember that people of different ages come from different social, economic or political backgrounds and as a result, often have **different ideas about what constitutes 'work': HOW** to work (etiquette of taking breaks, working in isolation or collaboratively), **WHEN** to work (who works overtime and holidays, who

	has seniority, what the expectations are of shift work, and how work rotations are negotiated), **WHAT** work LOOKS LIKE (how to dress at work, distinction of 'personal' and 'professional' work, relationships with patients/clients/communities, professional values, physical labor vs intellectual capital) and **COMMITMENT** to the workplace (who works when, who does what kind of work—hierarchies of task performance). READ UP ON GENERATIONAL DIFFERENCES and be aware that we all have REASONS for seeing the world the way we do—each of us is as 'right' or as 'wrong' as the other!!! Being open to dialogue with your colleagues and supervisors will facilitate a complementary and collaborative working culture.
KNOWLEDGE – Issues • **Knowledge of the skills, tasks, routines, policies and procedures related to direct care provision** such as processing orders, communicating with multiple disciplines, distinguishing between LPN/RPN/Enrolled Nurse/RN/Reg Psychiatric Nurse roles • Learning about **professional and unit culture** requires significant time embedded within a workplace • **Knowledge of professional role transition** may be limited	KNOWLEDGE – Strategies • ***<u>Orientating to Skills and Roles</u>***. If you have not been previously exposed to the particular clinical workplace, patient/client community or population into which you are transitioning, you may not have specific knowledge or be versed in the roles, responsibilities, relationships or knowledge particulars required to function optimally in your new workplace (i.e. how orders are processed, how much autonomy you have in directing families during counseling sessions, how particular leaders in various communities have worked in tandem with their previous community nurse, how multiple disciplines in THIS institution navigate their boundaries of practice, or how nurses distinguish their roles and responsibilities on a team of caregivers). As a new nurse, you will BEGIN your transition focused on performing the tasks required of you—this is

natural as your 'competency' and acceptance by your peers is driven by their 'trust' in you. This is usually developed by what they can 'see' of what you are 'doing'. Hence, the focus you might have on your ability to 'perform' the skills and tasks of your practice area. Your progression to a focus on your larger role within the WHOLE of your workplace will advance more during the 2nd and 3rd stages of transition. Initially, it is what you SAY and DO that makes what you KNOW most evident.

- ***Preparing for role transition***. Many graduates are unprepared for the experience of professional role transition and are therefore unaware that their feelings and reactions to the changes they are experiencing are **NORMAL**. Educational institutions and health regions can provide this education in a way that both informs and allows new nurses like you to **role play** scenarios or transition situations. It is helpful to utilize experienced practicing nurses to assist you to construct responses to ethical or practice situations in which the 'ideal' doesn't quite match the 'reality'. This allows you to preserve the standard of practice you value while meeting the requirements of an intense, dynamic and fast-paced healthcare workplace. Encourage the educators in your nursing program to **TALK ABOUT TRANSITION!! Learn about the stages of transition and the phases of support** required to assist you to integrate into your new workplace in such a way that the needs of those you serve are met (patients/families/communities), YOU feel safe and supported and your colleagues know what they can EXPECT and how to facilitate your progression THROUGH the stages. This knowledge foundation can inform your managers and educators so that they can appropriately orientate, integrate and advance your knowledge, skill and practice capacity over time. Even just educating senior nursing students and new nurses about the stages of transition and providing formal and frequent feedback (i.e. sitting down with you away from the practice area to review your progress and give you constructive as well as affirming feedback) may be enough to open the door for you to share your feelings and move through the stages more easily.

- ***Acquiring cultural knowledge***. It is quite a different experience to be embedded in a professional practice culture as a working nurse than it is to see things through the lens of a student. Learning the nuances of nursing culture (i.e. how nurses relate to one another and to other members of the healthcare team) can be eye-opening and somewhat disconcerting. If you have not been in a previous professional role, you may lack the self-confidence required to advocate for yourself or your patients. This may make you vulnerable to misunderstandings as you socially 'engage' with your colleagues and may result in your behaving inappropriately, unintentionally offending others or crossing socio-political lines within the institution without knowing you have done so! **Having a mentor assigned to you who is a respected member of the community** to which you are transitioning will go a long way toward your own acceptance—kind of a 'you mess with my grad, you mess with ME' kind of thing. The 'bullies' on the unit are NOT the most respected individuals but they can be the most VISIBLE and VOCAL. Look around you for the 'quiet confident' type—they are often the informal leaders and will have so much to teach you about the ins and outs of workplace culture. The best way to take the temperature of a workplace culture is to spend time talking with the people you work with—just **ASK QUESTIONS** (personal ones!!!!!) like 'So how long have you worked here' OR 'What was your weekend like' OR 'I had a situation I was wondering if you could advise me on'. People ENJOY talking about themselves or feeling acknowledged for the level of knowledge they have. **NOTE TO SELF**: once a colleague shares something with you, FOLLOW UP with them: "*So how was your daughter's birthday party*"? As hard as it might be sometimes, **ATTEND ALL SOCIAL EVENTS**—the business deals that take place over a golf game are notorious and the same goes for social events and nurses. Bring food to work!!!! Go to a social event being planned on the unit or even S**IGN UP TO BE PART OF A COMMITTEE** on your unit!

- ***<u>Receiving frequent and consistent feedback</u>***. Getting feedback (and that sometimes means **ASKING FOR IT**) about expectations and role performance is critical. Because most students are accustomed to frequent and detailed feedback, NOT getting feedback during your initial transition experience can feel like you're swinging from a rope without a safety net! To ensure that you have both the insight and the growing confidence required to continue to progress and develop, you need to request feedback from your manager, practice educator, preceptor and nursing colleagues over the initial months. It is equally important to begin the process of self-evaluating, but this takes time and practice AFTER you have a sense of your level of performance as a practicing professional. While you might have had a good idea where you were when you graduated, it can feel like a NEW YARDSTICK is being used to measure your competency and it is NORMAL to want and need reassurance and constructive criticism. Listening closely to WHAT others say about your performance and requesting SPECIFIC feedback at SPECIFIC periods of time that gradually space out FURTHER and FURTHER from each other, offers you a framework to move your focus from what others think about your work to what YOU think about your work! Here is a **suggested schedule of feedback for the initial transition stage:**

1st and 2nd week of work 'on your own' (POST ORIENTATION) – **Feedback session after EACH WORKING DAY**

- ✓ What did you do well today?
- ✓ What did you miss or 'almost' miss today?
- ✓ Did you make any 'errors' – if so, what were they and what led up to the error?
- ✓ What did you NEED to prevent the error?
- ✓ What are the strengths you offered the workplace today?
- ✓ What might you work on tomorrow?

3rd and 4th week of work 'on your own' (POST ORIENTATION) – **Feedback session after EACH WEEK OF WORK/SET OF SHIFTS**

- ✓ What did you do well this week?
- ✓ What did you forget to do, or what mistake did you 'almost' make in your practice this week?
- ✓ Did you make any 'errors' – if so, what were they and what led up to the error?
- ✓ What did you NEED to prevent the error?
- ✓ What are the strengths you offered the workplace this week?

- ✓ What might you work on next week?

2nd to 4th MONTH of work 'on your own' (POST ORIENTATION)

– **Feedback session after EACH 2 WEEKS OF WORK**

- ✓ Do you have enough support at work?
- ✓ Who do you go to for consultation on work decisions and judgments?
- ✓ Describe a situation in which you felt GOOD about your practice. What felt good about it?
- ✓ Describe a situation that felt BAD in your nursing practice this week? Why did it make you feel bad?
- ✓ What is your greatest challenge at work right now?
- ✓ What support do you need to overcome that challenge?
- ✓ When do you want to meet next and what do you want to accomplish between now and then?

- ***Developing experiential knowledge***. As a new nurse, you are learning new patterns of practice and exploring new ways of 'being' as a professional by actually PRACTICING in clinical, relational, structural and organizational situations that add to, modify, verify or alter your pre-graduate knowledge and understanding of nursing and healthcare. It is through this 'hands on' practice that your tacit (from experience) knowledge is being acquired and developed. It is so essential that you 'practice, practice, practice', in an environment that provides you with feedback, support, reassurance and validation. If you are NOT having these needs met, speak with someone you trust in your life/workplace and seek out ways to GET these needs met!

New Graduate Stages of Transition
STAGE 1 - DOING

LEARNING

- At this stage you will be most comfortable in the learning role and least comfortable applying that knowledge—you will most likely feel insecure about what you know because the situations may '*look*' different than they did when you were a student.
- You will likely feel more comfortable with theory – you may find that you 'default' to theory when stressed because it is safe and familiar. Remember, it isn't as much WHAT you say or know as HOW you say or present that knowledge that people respond to. Consider using the following statements when responding to your colleagues:
  - o *That is such a great point. Can you show me what you mean?*
  - o *Thank-you so much for pointing that out to me—I do not have a lot of experience with this so could you tell me more about why you do it that way?*
  - o *I hope I didn't sound cocky/stuffy/presumptuous/like a 'know-it-all' with my answer just now—most of what I know and depend on right now in my practice is based on the theory I learned in school. I know that the theory is part of it, but I don't have the experience yet to ground that theory and make it 'real'. Can you help me understand how the situation in this case differs from what I know theoretically?*
- There is much to be learned in your new professional environment (who's who, what are the institutional policies and regulations, what are your professional responsibilities, etc…).
- Remember that you are likely a typical '*adult learner*' who does best when given a chance to apply what has been learned shortly after being introduced to the skill or theory – negotiate with the educator opportunities to move '*in and out*' of a classroom and clinical setting during your orientation so that you can immediately apply what you learn, returning then to the classroom to learn more. And remember that you are on a steep LEARNING CURVE in this stage of your transition—it will take LONGER to process what you are doing so give yourself that time. Try not to get caught up in the speed of what you are doing, but focus on doing it RIGHT.

Getting Support:

1. How can you get more comfortable with your new roles and responsibilities?
2. How can you 'learn' and 'perform' (i.e. get time to repeatedly practice and gain a familiarity with what is expected of you)?
3. Do those around you know about your stage of transition? Do they know it will take you longer to do most tasks?

4. What 5 skills do you need to be able to do WELL where you work (that are performed often)?
5. How can you practice them until you become competent in them?
6. How do you learn best (observing, reading about then doing, practicing first in simulation)?
7. How can you apply this to your learning during transition?
8. What can you learn about the colleagues you work frequently with (including allied health and support staff)?
9. How can you negotiate a gradual and progressive introduction into your roles and responsibilities?

PERFORMING

- At this stage you will likely be most concerned with your ability to '*perform*' the tasks and skills that are required of you.
- You may be aware that you are being '*watched*' and may feel you are being '*judged*' for how well you perform—acceptance of yourself is often dependent upon your colleagues' and mentor's acceptance of you.
- Your growing professional nursing self-concept depends on a healthy facilitation of your new roles and responsibilities. You will be expected to perform certain roles or skills as a professional nurse for which you may not have been prepared during your education, or for which you had not been given complete responsibility for when you were a student (it is virtually impossible to afford you opportunity to perform EVERY skill or give you EVERY responsibility of a professional nurse when you are a student).
- Graduates who are permitted and encouraged to '*practice*' their skills and thinking under the watchful eyes and ears of an experienced practitioner will do better overall.
- During this stage of your transition, it is very important to **ASK FOR FEEDBACK**: I recommend that you meet with your manager/educator and clinical support person at regular intervals. There are guidelines for the feedback process offered to you in the 'Transition Orientation Template' (see Appendix VI).

Getting Support:

1. What can your colleagues/mentors/preceptors do to facilitate your growing skill and confidence level?
2. How can you practice the skills you will need to do well in your workplace while you are still a student (i.e. can you perform the skills in a simulation setting before doing them in a clinical setting)?

3. How can you become competent at the 5 most frequently performed skills in the course of your work (i.e. if you are in acute-care could you organize to do ALL IV insertions on your unit for a 12 hour shift; if you are in the community, could you do NOTHING but immunizations for a month)?
4. How often can you turn a 'statement' ("*I have never seen anyone give an injection like that!*") into a QUESTION ("I *have not given injections that way but it looks like an interesting approach—could you tell me why you do it that way?*")?
5. Does your workplace facilitate feedback sessions? If not, how can you request this?

CONCEALING

- At this stage you will likely feel insecure about who you are as a nurse and what you know or are capable of doing.
- Depending on your age, your life experience and degree of self-confidence, you may be inclined to conceal feelings of inadequacy or concerns about your competence in different situations from the experienced people around you.
- Encouraging and understanding conversations will do much to '*bring out*' your feelings and concerns.
- Try to connect with nurses who welcome your questions and are genuinely interested in your growth and who understand what it is like to be 'new'. Talking with your colleagues and asking them a bit about themselves will likely reveal those who are interested in connecting with you and those who are not.

Getting Support:

1. What do you need to feel more comfortable around your senior colleagues/mentor?
2. How can your colleagues create a safe space where you can BE new but FEEL connected to the team?
3. What kind of support do you need to feel safe in your workplace? Who needs to know this?

ADJUSTING

- Remember that you are adjusting to many new roles, relationships and levels of responsibility.
- You may be adjusting equally to changes in your personal life as well as your professional life.
- Because there is a significant amount of energy being consumed by a variety of personal as well as professional adjustments in the initial 6 months of employment, you should really try NOT to accept overtime shifts, even though it is tempting to pay off all that debt!! Your 'down' time is critical during this rapid growth phase.

Getting Support:

1. What are the personal changes you anticipate making after you graduate (i.e. are you changing relationships, managing your finances for the first time – buying your first home)?
2. What plans do you have to make time for yourself? Where are you going to get YOUR support from?
3. If you are a parent, how are you going to re-engage in your family's life gradually? How can you negotiate a re-integration strategy that meets their needs but allows you the space to experience this professional role transition?
4. How might this transition affect your ability to focus, commit, and engage with friends, family or a significant other?
5. What discrepancies do you see between what nursing IS where you are working and what you thought it would be? How can you discuss these with a mentor, your educator or manager, or another new graduate?
6. What might assist you to bridge the differences between what nursing IS and what you thought it would be?
7. How have your colleagues adjusted to these differences?
8. What do you need from your friends, family, significant other and colleagues to help you adjust to your new life?
9. What do your family and friends need from YOU? How can you help them understand what you are going through?

ACCOMODATING

- New graduates at this stage often find themselves caught between a rock and a hard place. They have never experienced many of the things they are seeing and doing before. It is your developmental task at this stage to figure out what it is you need to 'accept' and what you can (and should) 'modify' according to your own way of doing things (perhaps a new theory that you were taught) or your own standard of practice.
- It is normal and healthy to seek counsel and modelling for how to 'be' in this new world. It is normal to need, and ask for, rationale for why things are the way they are so that you are better equipped to decide if that is something you should 'accommodate' in your thinking or if it is something that runs contrary to your thinking, ethics or standards of practice. These are tough decisions, particularly when you want to be accepted by those individuals with whose practice you might take issue. Figuring out 'who you are' at a time when you also need to 'belong' is one of the greatest professional adjustments you will make.

Getting Support:

1. Are you concerned about the level of practice where you work?
2. Who can you speak with about your concerns?
3. What can you change about the way nursing is practiced in your workplace?
4. What can you do to develop your own way of practicing as a nurse without alienating or discounting valuable input from others?

New Graduate Stages of Transition
STAGE 2 - BEING

SEARCHING

- Ever heard the phrase '*young enough to do it, but old enough to know better*'? Well, at this stage you have acquired some knowledge about nursing practice and you want to exercise it. You have 'been around' for a while now (albeit a short period of time in the grand scheme of things and when compared to your 'seasoned' colleagues) and you are getting to know what is expected of you. Slowly but surely you are making sense out of what a 'nurse' does and is—some of which you may find very satisfying, validating and rewarding. But NO JOB IS PERFECT and you may start to become irritated or frustrated with some aspects of your role as a nurse in the real world that may not be what you wanted or thought you would be expected to do.
- You may begin a search for meaning in what you are doing at this point. It is normal to want to UNDERSTAND why things are the way they are—not just that they ARE that way! You may experience a sense of dissatisfaction with just 'doing' what is asked of you without rationale, or just complying with sanctioned practices because 'that's the way we do things around here'. This is an important stage in your development and as you begin to look around, you will be searching for explanations that can answer the million dollar question - 'WHY'??? The search for reasoning behind accepted and common practices is a crucial step in the development of your own critical thinking. Just a caution—this 'curiosity' from a new graduate (NG), though rarely if EVER intended as a direct challenge or critique of the practice of their experienced colleagues, is occasionally misunderstood as such. As well, because it may require others to examine the reasoning behind their OWN practice, or require them to provide evidence for why they are making certain decisions or enacting existing policies and procedures, this period of critique can be variably received by more experienced nurses working alongside you. Be aware of how you approach others during this time and find ways to inspire THEIR curiosity as well!!!

Getting Support:

1. What can your colleagues do to facilitate your need to understand the rationale for what they are doing?
2. Who can you debrief with after every shift? When and where (i.e. maybe on the carpool ride home)?
3. How can you get to the 'so what' stage of your understanding of your workplace?

QUESTIONING

- Your thinking is rapidly advancing as you become comfortable with the routines, tasks and expectations of your workplace. You may begin to look around you and question why things are the way they are.
- Some of the questioning may be coming from a sense of frustration about why things ARE the way they are and your own lack of knowledge and understanding about the underlying rationale for existing ways of being.
- You may question the role of nurses in the healthcare system or the functioning of certain aspects of your workplace, institution/health center, or the healthcare system itself. **All of your questions are important**—this stage is about adjusting to and making sense of the environment in which you have chosen to commit your life's work. The fit between 'who you are' and 'where you work' is important to your evolving image of work and the profession of nursing. You may be struggling with aspects of yourself or the system that you see as the origins of a 'misfit' and need to be able to work through your thoughts and feelings about the incongruence. Questioning is a way to get the information you need to make sense of your world.

Getting Support:

1. How can your questions be verbalized so that you can engage in discussion about them?
2. What strategies can be used to encourage you to reflect on the incongruence between your own needs and professional values and those of your workplace so that you can make sense of both the origins of your struggles and the possible solutions?
3. Where do your experienced colleagues, your supervisor/manager and educator fit into this process? How can they be a part of this with you?

DOUBTING

You may doubt many things at this stage:

- You may wonder why you went into nursing at all (mostly because you may still not be sure what you offer to the profession);
- You may question whether or not you are capable of reaching the level of expertise you see in your more experienced colleagues or mentors;

- You may doubt that you will ever experience the professional respect as a nurse that you feel you should be afforded (this will be particularly evident in institutions or unit cultures that are hierarchical, where nurses of varying responsibility levels do not act in a collegial fashion, where nurses and physicians do not engage in a collaborative professional complement, or where nurses are not valued for their knowledge, skill, clinical judgement and decision making);
- You may doubt that your life will ever be balanced (you will likely be exceptionally tired at this stage and this exhaustion will feed your doubt) or that you will achieve the balance your experienced counterparts seem to have. These doubts are really about who you are—as a professional and as an evolving man/woman in a world that is 'new' to you. You may actually experience *grief* during this stage; while you are gaining so much as you grow, you are also letting go of ways of being and thinking that have framed your life until now.

Getting Support:

1. What can those who support you do to enhance your evolving professional self-esteem? What do you need to feel better about yourself as a professional?
2. Have you considered organizing a group of new grad peers to meet regularly for the purposes of discussing your transition journeys?
3. How can the nursing team you work with ensure that your doubts are acknowledged and that you have opportunities to reflect upon them with someone who has 'been through it'?
4. How can you be reassured that what you feel represents normal 'growing pains' and that time, experience and support will see you through?
5. What support do you need from your colleagues, family and friends right now?
6. Have you considered utilizing www.nursingthefuture.ca resources (e.g. blog/discussion board) as a source of support?

EXAMINING

- New nurses at this stage are even more aware that there are differences between what they are actually doing and what they were educated or prepared to do. Because you are not as stressed about 'doing' nursing as you were in the first stage, you can lift your gaze from the tasks and routines and begin to examine things for what they are.
- Your growing professional identity may well depend on your ability to engage in a critically reflective examination of your practice to date. What you need is to be guided by a mentor who understands that real practice is NEVER ideal, but that there are 'lines' that we all must decide NOT to cross when things get hairy. You need to understand where those lines are and how to negotiate the mine-field that

comprises the daily issues and clinical situations about which you are making judgements and decisions for those under your care.

Getting Support:

1. What support do you need to examine what you are doing and why you are doing it?
2. Who might be a good person to do that with and when can you plan to meet to discuss these issues?

REVEALING

- You have more time and energy now (the time and energy that was going into learning the routines, performing your roles competently, and understanding how to relate to others with whom you work has been greatly reduced as the familiarity with those aspects of your work has increased). This means you will likely 'see' more of the differences between what you expected from nursing or your work and what you are finding in the 'real' world.
- So much of what you didn't know (or couldn't be exposed to) as a student is being 'revealed' to you now. Sometimes the way we see things (and people!) is more glorified than perhaps it (or they) really are. This is what 'reality' is all about and there are elements of reality that simply need to be accepted once revealed. This is a critical time for you and it is a critical time in your relationships with colleagues and even yourself—you are looking for experts to whom you can go for guidance on how you balance 'reality' with your dreams and aspirations. Don't be afraid to ask the question: "*How do you maintain that very tenuous balance between striving for what CAN BE while working within what IS*"? There are MANY nurses around you who have done that successfully—LOOK around and you will SEE them. Connect with and LEARN from them.

Getting Support:

1. What can you do to get help in understanding what nursing is, why it is what it is, what it could be and how YOU can get it to where you want it to be?
2. With whom might you partner (educator, experienced colleague, another new grad) on your unit or in your institution to help you reach the goals you have for your career and profession?
3. Is there a colleague on your unit whose approach to practice you admire? If so, would you consider approaching them for further mentorship?

New Graduate Stages of Transition
STAGE 3 - KNOWING

EXPLORING

- As you recover your energy, you may begin to think about your future. Exploring one's nursing career trajectory or path is important, particularly for the newest generation of nurses who have grown up in a culture that is constantly '*moving*'. While we all live in, and have learned to adjust to, our contemporary society, the newest cohort grew up in a culture that values transportability, mobility and flexibility and considers knowledge or skill as the '*currency*' of success. Without always understanding why, graduates often feel the need to be '*on the move*'—this may be about advancing skills, knowledge or thinking, or it may be about moving your actions forward, changing roles, units, institutions or even geographical locations. Be sure to speak with your managers and educators about your ideas and aspirations—the place where you are currently working may want to be a part of your plans!
- This stage is likely a good time for your colleagues and mentors to assist you to think about your career path and plans.

Getting Support:

1. What kind of a nurse do you want to be (attributes or professional characteristics)?
2. What area of practice are you most interested in pursuing in the next 2 years?
3. What do you see yourself doing as a nurse in 5 years? In 10 years?
4. What do you need (ongoing education, skill acquisition, practice experience and knowledge) to get where you want to be? Who can help you get there?
5. What does your career map/plan look like (what, how, when, who, where)? Let's see some pictures or diagrams, people!!!!!

SEPARATING

- At this stage you likely **need some space**. The exhaustion of simply '*surviving*' the first stages of your professional role transition 'without killing anyone' ☺, accompanied by the intensity of emotions and energy that is consumed by adjusting to the differences in your life may cause you to feel like you need to withdraw a bit from your life and from your surroundings during the 3rd stage—you may need to separate simply to get some perspective.

- Because you are trying to distinguish and compare yourself as a professional with those around you at this stage of your development, you may need to '*try on*' a more advanced and independent level of practice. This means you may be looking for a different relationship with your mentor and the colleagues around you. You may want more give and take, negotiation and collaboration in your professional relationships and you may even put some distance between yourself and your senior colleagues. This is natural!! Letting your mentor know what you are doing and why will foster a healthier response from them and may dictate the future directions of the partnership. If you can, share with your colleagues how you are feeling and how your needs are changing—negotiate a different way of relating, informing them that as you become more independent they might need to let go of you a bit and be present but not 'sticking like glue' to you as they might have been before.
- This is also a good time to bring in other mentors or experienced colleagues, making room for different ways of practicing to influence you as you formulate your own professional identity.

Getting Support:

1. What does practice 'interdependence' mean to you? How can you achieve it?
2. How have your needs changed over the past several months and what do you now need to learn and grow?
3. What challenges or strains have surfaced for you at this time and how might you address them?
4. How can you be supported to find your own unique way of nursing?

CRITIQUING

- In order to explore, understand and reconstruct your vision of nursing, and then determine how that vision fits with who you are, you require a certain level of critique.
- Critique does not equate with '*criticism*'—just because you may be critiquing individuals with whom you interact or the situations in which you find yourself does not mean you are criticizing those people or those structures (units or institutions). But people may take your need to critique personally so you need to be careful about the way you approach it. Try to stick with 'I' as often as possible

or begin your conversation with "*This is not about YOU personally*" or "*I am not criticizing or even talking about what you personally have done, but....*" or "*Please know that I have absolutely no desire to offend you when I say this, but I am wondering about...*".

- What you are doing (and NEED to do) is deconstructing what exists in your world for the purpose of reconstructing it so that it is a better fit with your aspirations and expectations. You may need to help others understand why you are critiquing things and the ways they might assist you to move your concerns, questions, or the practice issues you are struggling with forward—they might have valuable experience or information on how best to make change in that unit or institution so be OPEN to the ideas of others!

Getting Support:

1. With whom can you have an honest and open dialogue about the professional nursing and healthcare landscape?
2. How can your experienced colleagues assist you to make sense of the questions you have about nursing and healthcare?

RECOVERING

- WHEW!!!!!!! What the heck happened there??????
- You might be wondering what on earth happened to you over the past 8 months and will need some time to recover from the draining experience of making your initial transition to professional practice.
- This process is related to '*separating*' in that the separation of your personal life from your professional work is important as you advance your identity AT and AWAY from work. You may want to spend more time with family and friends with whom you feel connected (in part because you may feel as though you have neglected them these past months as you have been absorbed in making the transition). You may well want to engage in personal activities (i.e. hobbies you want to reactivate) or just spend time away from the work environment. It is very important that you be encouraged to pursue activities OUTSIDE of nursing and NOT spending all your unscheduled hours working overtime! This distance will give you a more balanced sense of development, success and fulfillment.
- You may well be making decisions at this point about the meaning of your transition experience. Depending on the degree of adjustment you have experienced (this is VERY individual), your recovery will vary in intensity and duration.

Getting Support:

1. Are you happy? What is preventing you from feeling happy?
2. What does a balanced life look like for you? How will you 'get there'?
3. How do the nurses you work with balance their personal and professional lives?

ACCEPTING

- This process is about distinguishing, during the course of '*critiquing*', what you can accept and what you find to be unacceptable in both the practice and the professional relationships that surround you. This may mean that you have to reconfigure your expectations about something or someone (i.e. in order to accomplish your workload, you need to find a way to assess the patient and teach them at the same time) or it may mean that you need to initiate a change (i.e. approach the manager about staffing issues, request shift changes or targeted clinical experiences, or address a specific issue/conflict with someone in your work environment).
- Learning from a mentor about how THEY coped with their initial practice adjustments and integrated THEIR nursing standards into their nursing workload may assist you in generating your own strategies.
- It must be acknowledged that untenable conflicts may occur for you as you work your way through this process of accepting (or NOT accepting) what you find in practice. It is important to ensure that both you and your mentor steer away from perceiving all practice or work incompatibilities as a statement of failure on the part of you, your mentor, or even the institution where you are working. The responsibility of your support team is to recognize that IF an incompatibility exists, it is important to take steps to identify, understand and then, if possible, resolve it (i.e. meet with the manager or educator to strategize on resolution).
- *Resolution* may mean that the issue cannot be altered to your satisfaction and may require that you change your perception of the person or situation, or may mean that this is not the workplace for you. Again, just be OPEN to all possibilities!

Getting Support:

1. What issues about healthcare and nursing have surfaced for you?
2. What do you need from your mentor, manager, educator and colleagues during this final stage?
3. What are the triumphs of your transition?
4. What do you see for yourself in the future?

---

a) Conceptual Model of Transition Support
b) Framework of Transition Support Strategies

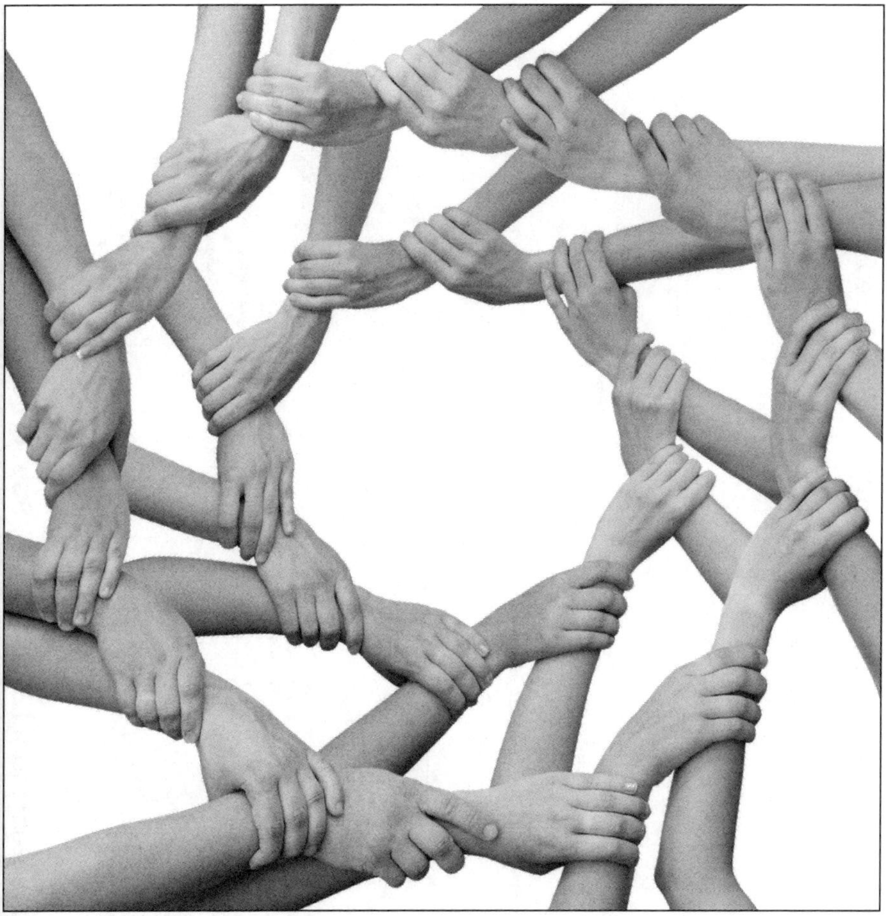

APPENDIX Va

New Graduate Entry To Practice Support Framework

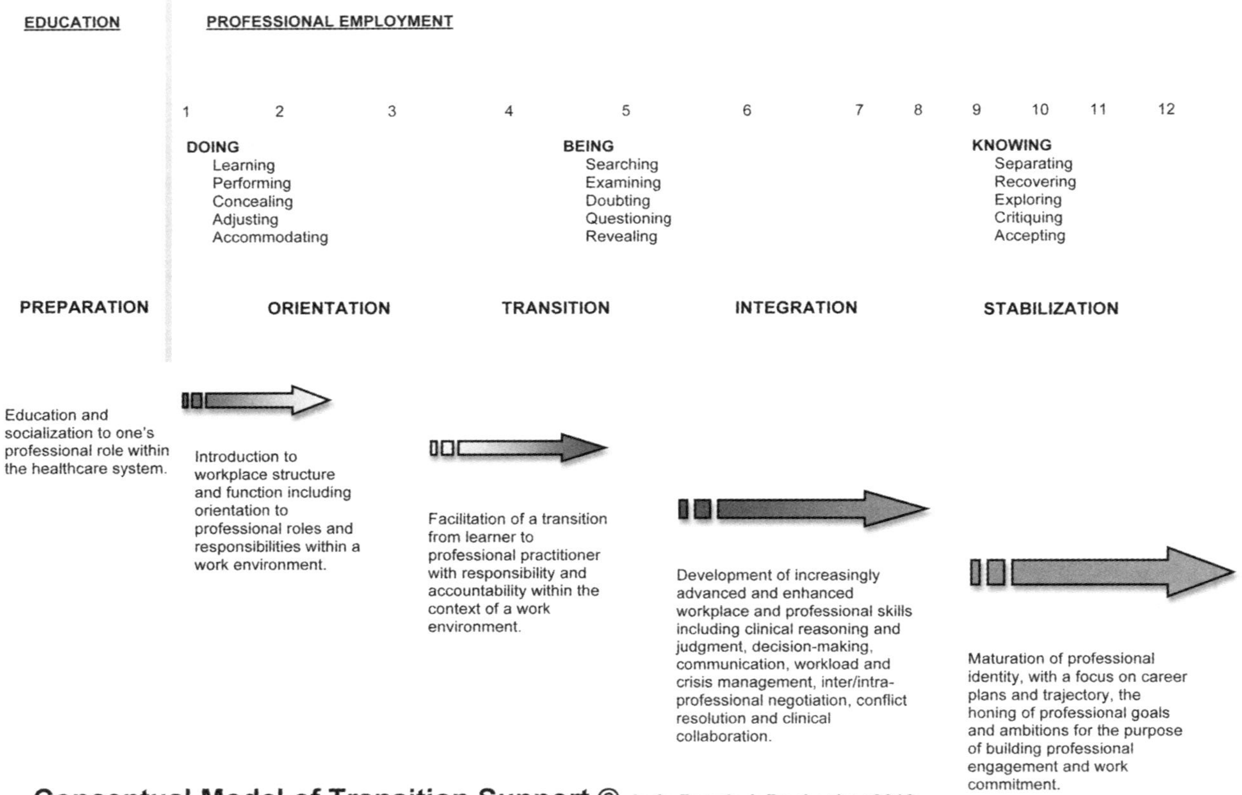

Conceptual Model of Transition Support © Judy Boychuk Duchscher 2012

New Graduate Entry To Practice Support Framework

EDUCATION | **PROFESSIONAL EMPLOYMENT**

1 2 3 4 5 6 7 8 9 10 11 12 →

DOING
Learning
Performing
Concealing
Adjusting
Accommodating

BEING
Searching
Examining
Doubting
Questioning
Revealing

KNOWING
Separating
Recovering
Exploring
Critiquing
Accepting

PREPARATION

- Professional socialization curricula
- Final practice in unit to which graduate will transition
- ***Mentor and Clinical Coach***: introduction and terms of relationship
- Professional role transition knowledge (stages/shock)
- Preparatory socialization exercises
- Healthcare/education transition facilitation partnerships
- Workplace engagement strategies
- Student work experiences
- Self-appraisal development

ORIENTATION

- ***Clinical Coach focus***: fundamental skill assessment, initial skill familiarity and performance confidence, and understanding work role expectations
- ***Mentor*** to facilitate personal connection q1-2weeks with a focus on encouragement, support and professional embrace
- Career intentions assessment
- Transition-framed orientation approaches
- Peer support programs
- Feedback/performance appraisal by manager/educator/clinical coach

TRANSITION

- ***Clinical Coach focus:*** progressive skill acquisition, time management, conflict resolution/coping skills training
- ***Mentor*** to facilitate discussion on professional culture, work relationships
- Clinical support team education on transition stages/transition shock
- Interdisciplinary knowledge sharing program initiation
- Supernumerary employment
- Creative scheduling options
- Feedback/performance appraisal move toward 'self'
- Optimize utilization of nursing

INTEGRATION

- ***Clinical Coach focus:*** development of advanced clinical judgment/reasoning/DM through experiential case study learning (debriefing)
- ***Mentor*** to facilitate discussion on coping strategies, self-care, 'big picture' thinking about healthcare system and relationship of micro-environment (workplace) to macro (healthcare system)
- Inter-institutional employment program initiation (option)
- Coasting and recovery strategies -- focus on personal balance
- Optimize utilization of nursing clinicians and charge nurses

STABILIZATION

- ***Clinical Coach focus***: 'guiding' decisions and experiences through 'clinical consultation' – graduate driven and directed – multiple coaches
- ***Mentor*** to facilitate professional development, practice introspection and professional perspective seeking
- Charge orientation >12 mos
- Advanced practice rotations (i.e. high-acuity rotations into ICU/ER)
- Career assessment update – professional trajectory planning
- Professional organization engagement – committee work
- Workplace committee work

NEW NURSE RESIDENCY/TRANSITION FACILITATION PROGRAM

Framework for Transition Support Strategies © Judy Boychuk Duchscher 2012

Senior Practicum/New Nurse Transition Schedule

The application of these senior practicum/new nurse transition suggestions will be most beneficial if you are a student intending to WORK on the unit where you are completing your final capstone course or final practicum/rotation OR if you are a new nurse approaching orientation. I am working on the assumption that this experience will last a MINIMUM of 12 weeks[1] and will consist of your being integrated into a full-time line[2] of varying 8/12 hour shifts beginning in the 5th week.

You will note that the *Senior Practicum/New Nurse Transition Calendar* at the end of this appendix infers a routine of Monday-Friday. I DO recommend that you STAY ON DAYS (this refers mostly to acute-care transitions or practica) until the end of your SUPERNUMERARY time. Supernumerary simply means that you are NOT included in the staffing quota for the clinical area.

Supernumerary status allows you to take on particular practice opportunities WHEN they arise. **For example**, as a new Outreach Nurse you could choose one day to spend time 'in the park' or 'on the street' talking with/seeking to understand the challenges of a homeless population; **OR** as a new (or wanting to find work in this role eventually) Cardiothoracic Rehabilitation Nurse, you might observe an open-heart surgery, follow the patient through to recovery and then visit with their family, gaining insight into the experience BEFORE this individual arrives to YOU as a nurse in cardiac rehab; **OR**, as a Med-Surg Direct-Care Nurse you might spend time with a dietician working with total bowel resection patients, or you might choose to observe the preparation of a Total Parenteral Nutrition bag by a pharmacist; **OR** you may ask to observe a radical head-neck resection in the operating room so that you can understand WHERE the drains are located when you are expected to change a dressing post-operatively. Supernumerary status allows you to take practice assignments like the ones described above because you are free to go to **where the EXPERIENCES are**.

The turnover required, particularly between day and night shifts, can be exhausting and will deplete energy that will be needed for your intellectual, emotional and physical transition adjustments. It will obviously be important for you to experience the differences in rhythm between shifts IF you will be required to work them as a professional. Having said that, the more important adjustments you will need to make during your initial transition will be easier

[1]Note that the suggestion of a 12 week transition program does not sanction nor recommend abbreviating existing or planned new nurse transition or residency programs of longer duration. Many established programs infuse similar components to what is suggested her, but over varying periods of time and in unique content combinations.
[2]A *line* is the staffing roster/schedule followed by your preceptor/mentor, who is assumed to be an experienced nurse working as staff in that clinical practice area.

if some stability, consistency and familiarity can be interjected into your 'routine'. Because the clear majority of students and new nurses are accustomed to a day-night circadian rhythm, disruption of these patterns AT THE SAME TIME as you are experiencing your transition can complicate things. While it is not recommended, if necessary, you can do several NON-day shifts during your supernumerary time as long as those shifts are done on the same line as YOUR PRIMARY PRECEPTOR/MENTOR (this is the individual with whom you are paired for the final 5 weeks of your transition program) (see schedule).

NOTE: Most centers refer to the initial introduction of new nurses into practice as a '*Transition*' or '*Integration*' *Program* but on occasion, it is referred to as '*Orientation*'. Please also note that the *Senior Practicum/New Nurse Transition Calendar* offered at the end of this appendix is modifiable—it is advisable to stay committed to the principles and the overall content, but the timelines and the order of the classroom content will need to be adjusted to meet the needs and requirements of the workplace. Take this information with you to your practicum, or use it as a basis to negotiate a transition program with your manager or educator.

Program Template (See Schedule Below)

1) **Shadow[3] your PRIMARY[4] preceptor/mentor for 2 days**—pay attention to *WHAT* the preceptor does, *HOW* this individual manages their workload, the *SKILLS* they do consistently and repeatedly and the *DECISIONS/JUDGMENTS* they make.
    a. **Identify a clinical situation** that you witnessed to use as the **debrief exemplar case**. Make extensive notes for yourself about it.
    b. **Consider at least ONE decision/judgment** the preceptor/mentor made that you would like more insight into—make note of the circumstances.
    c. Observe the process your preceptor/mentor uses in collaborating and delegating.
    d. **Make notes** that outline the routines you witness in the practice of your preceptor/mentor so that you can design a similar schedule for yourself—over time you will modify it to meet your own unique style but it is a place to start.
    e. **Note the primary 5 clinical presentations** (population health concerns) of clients/patients that are in that practice area (i.e. children with chronic lung disease/adult cardiothoracic surgery/older adults with chronic heart disease/young adults with fetal alcohol syndrome) and develop a ONE PAGE synopsis on each of them that

[3]To *shadow* your preceptor/mentor literally means SHADOW them. You do NOT do anything 'for' or 'with' them. Your role is to *watch INTENTLY* **what** they do, **when** they do it, **why** they do it (that can come during the debrief but make a note to ask) and **what result** they get from doing what they did. As long as you are DOING, you are not OBSERVING.

[4]You will likely require several preceptors/mentors (one of these individuals COULD be the educator in your practice setting) in order to accommodate the recommendation of supernumerary status and a strict day routine for the initial weeks. During your transition/practicum it is advised that you CHECK IN regularly with your PRIMARY preceptor/mentor for the purposes of consistency and follow-through.

includes pathophysiology, signs and symptoms, treatment, medications as well as health education and planning suggestions. Keep that information (along with other information you are gathering) in a small pocket binder, notebook, or mobile computing device such as a Blackberry®, iPhone®, iPad®, Android™ or some form of smartphone. Be sure you safeguard the confidentiality of any patient/client information stored on these devices!

f. **Debrief with your preceptor/mentor at the end of each of the 2 days**, and ask your preceptor/mentor the following questions:
   i. How did your day go?
   ii. Was this a busy day for you?
   iii. Was this a 'typical' day in this practice area?
      NOTE: this will give you insight into what a 'normal' or 'busy' day looks like for a nurse in your role in this practice area.
   iv. Tell me about this case (present the ***exemplar case***)? What went WELL in this situation and what DISAPPOINTED you about your care in this situation? What might you have changed and why?
      NOTE: You are trying to understand what 'well' means to this practitioner. You want to get a response from them around what they were disappointed in because EVERY situation can be made better and you need to understand the nuances of what COULD have been better in that situation. The more subtle the disappointment the better—there is more learning for you there as you could likely pick out the GLARING issues that needed resolution. As you discuss the case, note whether or not YOUR impressions of what went well are the same as your preceptor/mentor's. If they are NOT the same, explore this with them.

g. **Review your preceptor/mentor's exemplar decision/judgment**. What brought them to that decision/judgment? What was their thought process behind the decision/judgment? What other options did they consider? What ultimately made them lean in this direction?
   NOTE: You are trying to get a sense of the nuances of decision-making in particular clinical situations. Compare your OWN thought processes to your preceptor's to determine what is DIFFERENT in the way you are thinking. When you note discrepancies, ask your preceptor, "*Before we talked, I was thinking in this situation that I would have done _____. What would you think about that and would you choose your response over mine and if so, why?*"

2) **Shadow the Unit Clerk/Clinic Receptionist for a day** (review schedule). By lunch/dinner time, YOU should be admitting a patient, processing requests, answering phones or otherwise enacting the role of the UC/Receptionist.
   NOTE: If you haven't already figured this out, the POWER POSITION in any workplace is in the administrative/clerical role. These individuals are the gatekeepers of information and can make your life exceedingly difficult or a haven of joy. Spending

time with the clerical employees where you work demonstrates respect for their position and provides you with insight into what they DO and DO NOT DO. In order to anticipate the appropriate time and task to delegate to them, so that you do not need to DO something that is really someone else's responsibility, you need to KNOW what they do. This is going to save you a lot of time and energy.

DEBRIEF AT END OF DAY WITH PRECEPTOR/MENTOR

3) **Shadow the LPN/RPN/Enrolled Nurse/RN for a day** (depending on your role you would shadow your 'partner' role).

   NOTE: If your workplace utilizes a 'collaborative model' of practice, you will be working in partnership with someone from another practice scope within the nursing profession (an LPN/RPN/Enrolled Nurse will work with an RN). This will involve a significant amount of consultation and teamwork, which itself demands a comprehensive understanding of the 'other' role. Spending time with your partner in a shadowing capacity allows them to demonstrate to YOU what their role is. ASK QUESTIONS!!!! As well, there are often policies or job/role descriptions that outline the details of specific roles on the healthcare team. These would be available either from the manager or human resources upon request. READ THAT JOB/ROLE DESCRIPTION, and get access to any information from their professional regulatory body that speaks to their 'scope of practice' so that you understand what you CAN and CANNOT request or expect of your nursing partner. SHADOW this individual—watch how they engage and interact with the individual currently assuming YOUR role (remember, shadowing is about observation). Make notes for yourself about YOUR role and THEIRS.

DEBRIEF AT END OF DAY WITH PRECEPTOR/MENTOR

4) **Shadow the Care Aide/Certified Nursing Assistant/Nursing Aide for a day** (this is a NON-licensed, but perhaps '*certified*' individual working in a personal care role).

   NOTE: Many workplaces utilize non-licensed (but often *certified*) personnel to deliver personal care to clients/patients (particularly long-term care, rehabilitation and acute-care). The crucial point here is that these individuals have a job description as opposed to a '*scope of practice*'. Anything that is asked of them that lies outside of their job description is considered a '*delegated*' task, the responsibility for which lies with the DELEGATOR!!! BE AWARE of this so that you maintain safe practice standards in making requests of these caregivers.

DEBRIEF AT END OF DAY WITH PRECEPTOR/MENTOR

5) **Shadow the Hospital Porter for a day** to learn what it is THEY do so that you know how to collaborate with them, or when and what to delegate TO them.

NOTE: The role of the porter is usually limited to a hospital/acute care setting. Porters are valuable employees at hospitals around the world and work to assist doctors, nurses, and other hospital employees with any (or more) of the following tasks:

1. transporting patients/clients for diagnostics or ward/unit transfer (including morgue),
2. operating, cleaning or repairing equipment,
3. cleaning and sanitizing rooms,
4. assisting patients/clients with meals,
5. transferring laundry,
6. moving furniture and equipment,
7. elimination or biohazard waste cleanup,
8. delivery of mail, files, clinical samples,
9. picking up blood for transfusion.

DEBRIEF AT END OF DAY WITH PRECEPTOR/MENTOR

6) **Shadow the Clinical Nurse Specialist/Nurse Practitioner** for a day so that you begin to understand what their role is, how it is different from the direct-care nurses working in that practice area, and how this individual might assist you to optimize the care of your patient/client population.

DEBRIEF AT END OF DAY WITH PRECEPTOR/MENTOR

7) **Shadow the Intern/Resident/House Officer for a day** (attached at the hip if you will…), *while they make rounds* (if on an acute-care ward/unit), spend time seeing patients in their office, or as they move from one practice area to another (i.e. if they are a consultant in the clinic where you are working). This connection will help you understand why they might NOT respond to you when you call, or what they might need when they DO respond. As with the advanced practice nurses identified in #6, you will benefit from '*getting to know*' the practitioners with whom you are going to work on a regular basis. This can be an intimidating relationship for students and new nurses but spending an extended period of time with these individuals, during which *conversation* will naturally arise, is one way to connect on a less formal, but professional level. This familiarity will encourage both respect and consideration to develop on both sides of this relationship.

DEBRIEF AT END OF DAY WITH PRECEPTOR/MENTOR

8) In consultation with your preceptor/mentor, **determine the 5 skills you will be required to do VERY WELL and FREQUENTLY while on this unit**—spend the next week (1

day/skill[5] to ensure the repeated performance of ONE skill before moving on to another) doing NOTHING BUT THOSE SKILLS. You should be practicing these skills on any and every patient/client/population on your unit/ward/center regardless of where you and your preceptor are stationed (including neighboring units or centers if that can be negotiated by your educator and manager). Not only will you become quickly proficient such that you can move beyond the skills to the 'whole' of nursing practice[6] but you will develop relationships with your colleagues when you do some of their work!!! EVERYBODY WINS!!!

DEBRIEF AT END OF DAY WITH PRECEPTOR/MENTOR

9) Begin your **classroom[7]/clinical practice rotations that will TOTAL 8 WEEKS (see schedule)** and discuss with educator how to integrate 2 days theory/3 days practice X 4 weeks followed by 1 day theory/4 days practice X 4 weeks as identified in the schedule.

    NOTE: The objective behind the alternating theory/practice is to maximize learning while minimizing stress[8]/[9]. It is really in the 'classroom' that you feel safest because this is the environment that is most 'familiar' to your recent experience as a student. Along those lines, many students today learn effectively through simulation[10] and this

---

[5]It is recommended that ONE skill be performed at a time, repeatedly and consistently until proficient (including under duress or in a complicated scenario), but if necessary, overlap 2 skills to increase exposure to skill opportunity.

[6]The suggestion of repetitive skill performance at this early stage is NOT intended to reinforce the rather contentious claim that nursing is 'task-oriented'; quite the opposite in fact. My theory clearly identifies that in the early stages of transition, new nursing graduates are focused on what makes them VISIBLE to others. This arises from a strong socio-developmental need for acceptance and belonging within their professional group. As a result, graduates will perceive any skills, competencies, decisions, judgments or in a word PRACTICE, that is visible to others as of primary importance. In order to liberate their mind and activate their higher-level cognitive capacity, it is suggested that basic skill performance anxiety be eliminated. Any strategy that allows them to perform (to the point of ease), the skills that will be consistently and frequently required in their new practice environment is strongly recommended.

[7]Recommended classroom content is identified separately in this Appendix.

[8]Kolb, David A. (1984). *Experiential Learning: Experience as the Source of Learning and Development.* Prentice-Hall, Inc., Englewood Cliffs, N.J.

[9]Knowles, M. S. (1980). *The modern practice of adult education: From pedagogy to andragogy.* Englewood Cliffs: Prentice Hall/Cambridge.

[10]*Clinical Simulation Learning Centers* are advanced practice labs that host varying levels of constructed clinical case scenarios that SIMULATE 'reality' (actors or mannequins are used and scenarios are constructed that look, smell and behave like the 'real' situation). These are state-of-the-art, highly computerized (and expensive) environments that optimize experiential learning within a monitored and controlled context. This is an EXCEPTIONAL learning format, particularly if debriefing is comprehensive and consistent. It is recommended however, that students PRACTICE the skills they learn in a simulation setting IN A CLINICAL setting where the circumstances are NOT as controlled and the 'unexpected' 'human response' (something that no amount of simulation can offer) becomes integral to their experience.

approach may be very effective in systematically introducing you to new skills or advanced levels of performance expectation. Entering the clinical practice environment shortly after theoretical or simulated learning allows for the immediate APPLICATION of what has been learned. This level of synergy requires effort on the part of the manager and educator (i.e. a classroom day is spent learning how to admit and discharge patients/clients and upon re-entry into the clinical environment, you ADMIT AND DISCHARGE repeatedly), but it CAN happen!! A healthy transition to professional practice will require that we rethink the way we introduce new nurses into the practice context. While this approach may not be as easy as compartmentalizing 'theory' and 'practice', it is more congruent with both the cognitive and practical development of a new practitioner.

NOTE: **During your initial 3 weeks of practice**, you should be considered **SUPERNUMERARY.**

10) **Debrief at the end of every SUPERNUMERARY shift for those 3 weeks**, using the following questions as a guide:
    a) What happened today? What did you do? What are you thinking about what you did? How did you feel about what you did? What stood out for you? What questions do you have about what you experienced?
    b) What did you notice about the nursing practice you witnessed today? How is what you witnessed different than what you expected?
    c) What did you notice about your own nursing practice today? How is that different than you expected? What changes/growth have you noticed in yourself today?
    d) What most concerned you about what you experienced today? Why?
    e) What was the HIGH point of the day? The LOW point? What would you have done differently to influence the LOW point of your day?
    f) What do you want to focus on next?
11) **During the remaining 5 weeks of your transition program**, you should be taking your OWN assignment, **GRADUALLY** increasing your workload (see *Senior Practicum/New Nurse Transition Calendar*) for 3 weeks until you are taking a full load at 10 weeks. You should be doing EVERYTHING for your patients/clients/community that is required within your nursing practice role (be that acute-care, community, public health or clinic) —including processing orders if that is required within your scope of practice, teaching patients and families, developing programs for immunization, etc. You will collaborate with, or delegate to all individuals with whom you will be expected to work in your professional practice role. You should have a good sense of how your role 'works' from your initial shadowing experience—USE your notes!!
    a. Ensure that your preceptor/mentor knows that **their role is to 'debrief' with you** at the end of every shift or set of shifts, as well as during your practice day as needed. After you have taken full responsibility for your professional nursing

workload for 1 week without incident, encourage the preceptor/mentor to consume themselves with OTHER work, making themselves less available to you and only upon your request. Ask that they check in with you several times during your day (or as needed) to see how you are doing.

b. Request that the preceptor/mentor **use primarily a questioning (Socratic) approach when dialoguing with you**. Ask that they NOT do ANYTHING for you that you have not approved beforehand. You should BE the nurse responsible for this workload, sharing it as you normally would with your nursing partner (LPN/RPN/Enrolled or RN/Registered Psych Nurse).

c. Using the following questions as a guide, **follow the debriefing schedule** laid out in the schedule included in this Appendix:

   a) How did the shift go generally?
   b) What struggles did you have and why?
   c) What did your preceptor/mentor 'notice' about what you did really WELL and what suggestions do they have for improvements?
   d) What most concerned you about what you experienced today? Why?
   e) What changes are you noticing in your practice? What changes are you noticing in how you are thinking about/in your practice?
   f) What was the HIGH point of the day? The LOW point? What would you have done differently to influence the LOW point of your day?
   g) What ONE thing might you focus on improving?

12) **ALL practice decisions related to your workload should go through YOU**—request that your preceptor NOT do anything to 'assist' you that YOU do not approve—let your preceptor know what you need for assistance and check in a couple of times a day, even once you have assumed a full workload. Request that the preceptor watch you *from a distance* with specific direction to: 1) assess your workload management, 2) observe your level of organization and prioritization, 3) witness your decisions but DO NOT INTERRUPT you unless you are likely to make a significant ERROR[11] (remember that you WILL MAKE ERRORS as a new graduate AND as a practicing nurse. The KEY is to LEARN from your errors). Most errors in the practice of a nurse are NOT life threatening to the patient/client and are part of the growing process for any professional.

13) Over the course of the initial 12 weeks of clinical practice, you should **gradually increase YOUR workload** (see *Senior Practicum/New Nurse Transition Calendar*) while the preceptor/mentor decreases theirs (if you are SHARING a workload), until you are caring for ALL the patients you would normally care for as a practicing nurse in that role and practice area. **You should be caring for a full load 2 weeks before your practicum/12 week orientation period is complete.**

[11]You should be allowed to go to the VERY EDGE of the process of medication administration, being STOPPED just prior to the point at which you might make an error, with a statement by your preceptor such as: "*Let's review that order before we proceed*".

TRANSITION PROGRAM CONTENT

PRE-GRADUATE KNOWLEDGE

1. Transition as a Process
   - Duchscher's Stages of Transition
   - Duchscher's Transition Shock model
   - Kramer's Reality Shock/Anticipatory Socialization
   - Benner's Skill Acquisition Model
2. Bureaucratic organizational culture theory
3. Change theory and organizational dynamics
4. Conflict management
5. Debriefing in clinical practice
6. Role theory
   - Negotiation
   - Collaboration
   - Delegation
7. Workload management and organization
8. Stress and empowerment in the workplace
9. Social media etiquette
10. Multigenerational dynamics in the workplace

GENERAL EMPLOYEE KNOWLEDGE

1. Institutional/Workplace Culture
   - Organizational chart
   - Communication lines (i.e. nurse-physician communication OR nurse-charge-physician)
   - Use of social media in the workplace
   - Reporting structure
   - Mentorship/preceptorship structure

- Cohesion in the workplace (i.e. social events)
- Relationships in the workplace—who the most 'senior' nurses are and how they relate to new staff
- Formal and informal leaders in the workplace (access to clinical experts)
- Bullying/Respectful Workplace/Incivility/Harassment policy review
- Employee Assistance Programs
- Occupational health out-reach
- Payment structure and overtime/statutory work policies
- Parking, lockers, uniform/dress policy
- Work scheduling/Payroll/Benefits/Sick Leave
- Inter-institutional/regional transfer options
- Institution and practice area layout
- Organization of peer networks of support (storytelling and confidential sharing)

2. Workplace Expectations
    - Routines
    - Roles and role distinctions (Nursing, Administrative, Support and Allied Practitioners)
    - Practice area policies (salient ONLY)
    - Error reporting
    - Critical incident debriefing/near miss reporting
    - Communication and confidentiality (practice hand-off report methods/physician call roster & procedure)
    - Charting/documentation methods and standards
3. Skill Performance Requirements
    - 5 primary skills performed regularly
    - Use simulated learning and clinical practice
    - MOCK CODES and Rapid Response Protocol
    - Security/patient lockdown procedures

4. Competency Expectations
    - Required entry-to-practice competencies
    - Advanced practice options (i.e. ACLS/Charge)
    - Continuing education credit courses (CEUs)
    - Career planning/path counseling

NURSING PRACTICE SPECIFIC KNOWLEDGE

1. Practice-based case portfolio (5 most common conditions/presentations/situations that dictate nursing support or intervention)
2. Review of **basic**[1] practice scenarios (process-oriented approach to case situations)
3. Assessment, interventional, diagnostic and procedural routines (i.e. meds/vitals/police or social services reporting/assault protocol/restraint policies
4. Program development/facilitation expectations
5. Residential security protocols (homecare/home health)
6. Emergency response (codes, fire, aggression)
7. Review low-volume high-risk skills (i.e. chest tubes/blood administration)

INTERDISCIPLINARY EDUCATION

1. Classroom teaching should be facilitated by allied, clerical and support staff as appropriate for content whenever possible (i.e. housekeeping IN the practice area should report on cleaning routines and expectations)
2. New nurses should follow practice population beyond the direct care environment (community nurses should follow population into acute-care situations/acute-care nurses should follow population home)

[1]Knowledge should progress from basic to complex—increasing complexity should be presented in case reviews over 12 weeks

Senior Practicum/New Nurse Transition Schedule

WK	MON	TUES	WED	THURS	FRI
1	**Orientation to Healthcare Institution** *Focus* should be on NEED TO KNOW ONLY—revisit other information during classroom time (see ahead on schedule); computer system; documentation; pay sheets; illness requests; benefits; employee assistance programs; physical layout of ESSENTIAL locations (cafeteria, work center, parking, elevators, diagnostics) USE A GROUP SCAVENGER HUNT (3 per group of workplace-like employees)			Primary Preceptor/Mentor Shadowing Debrief	
2	**Orientation to Practice Area** *Scavenger hunt*—this is an excellent strategy for locating 'things' and should be constructed in consultation with educator and preceptor/mentor; spend time wandering through the practice area; open all shelves and drawers; read all PATIENT/CLIENT EDUCATION material; spend time talking to *clients/patients and staff (nurses, allied, support and clerical/admin)* about what it is like to work or spend time there. Find out what the employees, patients/clients/families LIKE and DON'T LIKE about being there and what they need (if you are in a community health center, spend time at community 'centers' where people gather). WATCH, LISTEN and LEARN.			Unit Clerk Receptionist Shadowing Debrief	Nurse Partner Shadow Debrief
3	Care Aide/CNA Nursing Aide Shadow Debrief	Porter Shadow Debrief	Nurse Practitioner CNS Shadow Debrief	Physician Shadow Debrief	EXTRA DAY Shadowing
4	Skill Performance				

1-4 WEEKS

Senior Practicum/New Nurse Transition Schedule

WK	MON	TUES	WED	THURS	FRI
5	CLASSROOM		SUPERNUMERARY		
6	CLASSROOM		SUPERNUMERARY		
7	CLASSROOM		SUPERNUMERARY		
8	CLASSROOM		SUPERNUMERARY		

5-8 WEEKS

Senior Practicum/New Nurse Transition Schedule

WK	MON	TUES	WED	THURS	FRI
9	CLASSROOM	PRACTICE ON LINE WITH PRECEPTOR/MENTOR			
10	CLASSROOM	PRACTICE ON LINE WITH PRECEPTOR/MENTOR			
11	CLASSROOM	PRACTICE ON LINE WITH PRECEPTOR/MENTOR			
12	CLASSROOM	PRACTICE ON LINE WITH PRECEPTOR/MENTOR			

9-12 WEEKS

Appendix VII

Finding the Right Job

Congratulations! You made it through your nursing education program!

Now it is time to find a job!

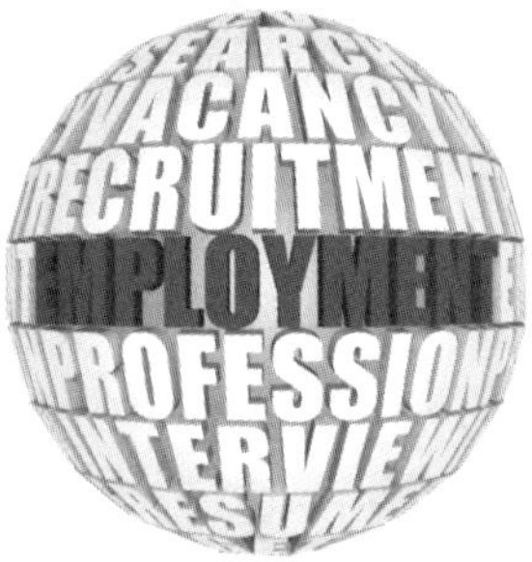

But how do you get a job?
Which job is right for you?
What are your employment options?

GETTING A JOB

The Job Market

- This is a challenging time to be looking for work in any profession, primarily because of recent changes to the stability of our economy.

> *"It seemed surreal that in a profession with an acknowledged shortage of human resources, that a 'hiring freeze' could occur. When I 'entered' nursing, the economy was sound, and we were told of the endless possibilities for career options. While I still believe there are endless possibilities, it hurt very much to graduate and only see doors being closed. I thought that I needed A JOB. That I ONLY needed A JOB. To the point where after I graduated I up and left to move thousands of miles away because, like many new grads I felt the pressure to begin paying off student debt. Even though I moved to a full-time position with a health authority that had a 'New Graduate Transition Program' in place, I lost familiarity, predictability, reliability and consistency in my physical environment, the culture of the community and province, immediacy of family and friends and regional nursing culture. It was SUCH a drastic change, which at the time I believed to be in the best interest of my identity and career in nursing. But in uprooting so much of what I identified with in the bigger context of my life, I experienced an EXTREME sense of disconnect and loss of self. In other words, when my nursing identity was rocked by transition shock, I didn't have any other part of my life (my prior 'self') to identify with. I literally did not know who I was or what I was doing....It was a hard process and difficult to dig my way out of, but with support from family, friends, Nursing The Future, time, and therapy I did make it through and came back to nursing 'on my own terms'. I have reconciled with nursing and made it to a place where I can continue my professional development. From this experience, I now share with new nurses and senior students that time with family & friends, and pursuing your interests outside of nursing are SO important. These activities build your identity beyond nursing, so that you can still recognize yourself when your nursing identity is challenged as you are moving through the stages of transition. If you do decide it is necessary for you to move for work, think VERY CAREFULLY about your pillars of support and*

acknowledge to yourself how that move will impact the REST of your life during your professional transition."

- I have personally lived through some LEAN professional years, but nursing employment is cyclical—the availability of work ALWAYS (and I mean ALWAYS) comes around... sometimes you just have to wait it out.
- If that frustrates you, LET IT OUT (punch a bag...not a person...) and then MOVE ON—ANGER EATS YOU UP!!! Sustaining a level of frustration about something you cannot control is just a waste of time, energy AND opportunity. It is quite possible that you won't see something DIRECTLY in front of you because your vision is either clouded by disappointment and anger, or you see ONLY what you are looking for and miss everything else.
- For the newly graduated nurse, this 'interesting' job market means several things:
  - ✓ The availability of work may depend on regional economics;
  - ✓ You may NOT get a placement in the practice area you desire immediately upon completing your program (for instance, community or public health) and you may have to take employment where the jobs are available (for instance acute-care or private home-care);
  - ✓ You may have to get CREATIVE;
  - ✓ You may have to work SEVERAL casual/relief positions or for a nursing agency;
  - ✓ It may be necessary to consider working (or volunteering) OUTSIDE of nursing TEMPORARILY. IF you do this, remember that REGARDLESS of what you do or where you do it, there are ways to develop your nursing capacity or capability through that experience:
    - o Work as a **waiter/waitress or in retail** (make contacts; practice speaking to strangers with the intent to get them to reveal something about themselves; practice your Socratic method...BUSTED...somebody needs to read Chapter 5 again!!!!);
    - o **Volunteer** at a shelter, hospital or clinic (or at public events like sports or entertainment—I volunteered for chili cook-offs (totally fun!), long distance running races, trade shows, exhibition/Shriner Circus (I made so many contacts, and even a few who wanted to '*introduce you to my son*' ☺);
  - ✓ Ask your previous instructors/faculty if they need anyone to assist them with teaching, act as a 'patient' during the students' practical examination time or offer to TUTOR struggling nursing students;
  - ✓ Consider enrolling in a continuing education course (Critical Care Nursing), completing an advanced certification program (ACLS/Ortho Technician/Wound Management Specialist), or starting a graduate degree (MN);
  - ✓ Work in a long-term care center as an aide, clerical assistant, or porter;
  - ✓ Attend job fairs and keep connected with the Human Resource Departments of your local healthcare institutions;

- ✓ Don't forget that healthcare organizations are not the ONLY workplaces that hire nurses!! Approach local industries such as power, electric or water companies, construction sites, schools, churches, or your own nursing professional organizations and unions—you never know who might be looking but just hasn't put their 'sign in the window' yet;
- ✓ Pharmaceutical and health supply companies are often looking for Clinical Specialists (nurses) and Sales Associates with healthcare background so get online and start 'trolling'!!
- ✓ If you know where you want to work, connect personally with someone who works there and make an appointment with the Nursing Manager or Administrator to ask for advice and MAKE CONTACT ('*dropping in*' to nursing practice areas is generally discouraged because Managers are often unavailable without an appointment and it is more respectful to provide them with some advanced notice—having said that I have 'dropped in' on managers and this approach has been effective…demonstrates initiative and interest);
- ✓ Consider being a *Research Assistant* (talk to your nursing program instructors/faculty) or contact a local researcher in ANY discipline and ask if they need any assistance with their work (they may be able to pay you but if they can't, VOLUNTEER a few hours a week! and you will have a GUARANTEED reference ☺);
- ✓ Reconnect with connections made during school (this is where the level of engagement you had with EVERY experience, interaction and placement you had is going to PAY OFF);
- ✓ Prepare a KICK-BUTT *Resume* (the web has all kinds of free sites that can assist you);
- ✓ NETWORK, NETWORK, NETWORK (get OUT THERE and meet people in the practice area that interests you);
    - o Think about leaving your state, province, territory or township for work in another region;
    - o Consider writing the National Qualifying Examination for a country outside of your residence or origin (just keeping your options open!);
- ✓ OR…..go plant some trees in the Rockies, spend the summer working at Starbucks™ or take a vacation and TRAVEL!! (remember what I said about debt being enduring….).

- Ensure that you have a professional portfolio (some schools now support their students to create e-portfolios that they can send to potential employers) which contains your resume and any other certificates/credentialing (i.e. Basic Life Support, Child Safe Environments, Manual Handling, etc.). When you initially enter the workforce, you can include particular projects or papers that demonstrate excellence in various ways but MORE is not always BETTER. Be selective (target what you send to the job you are applying for) or an employer might just find your presentation redundant and frustrating! Start a current, well developed but succinct portfolio during school and update it periodically throughout your work experience. It makes for an impressive document to take (or send prior) to interviews!

- While there has been 'some' flux in the availability of jobs, it appears that there has been a recent leveling out of employment opportunities. While the current fiscal *recovery* mode has slowed the job market in some places, the exit of the early baby boomer generation (currently >60 years of age) will result in a steady need for human resources over the next 10 years.
- What may change more significantly than the 'net' job availability is WHERE the jobs are located (geography and practice setting). It may come down to making a decision that favors either LOCATION (some of you may have families or working partners and may not be in a position to move) OR making a decision that favors a ROLE/POSITION/ PRACTICE AREA or desired hours or work (a preference for full time work). In both instances, your current stage of life (school-age children or a working partner who is unable to relocate) may impact your decision.
- Many parts of Australia recruit their own students to *Transition to Professional Practice Programs* (TPPP), which are 12-month government assisted, hospital-based 'temporary' jobs that provide an established program of transition support. This occurs through a centralized e-recruitment process and successful applicants receive a 0.84 or 1.0 full-time equivalent position. At the end of the year, they are able to reapply for any available positions.

FINDING THE RIGHT JOB FOR YOU

Evaluating Your Potential Workplace

- Consider the overall environment in which you are considering working. You will want to choose a job that fits you–try to match the '*culture*' and '*pace*' of the unit with your interests, your energy level, your home life and your family responsibilities (i.e. community health, public health, or homecare may be a better choice if you did not enjoy hospital nursing while in school, or if you are unable to work flexible and varying shifts due to child-care issues or personal intolerance of night shifts).
- Try to check out potential workplaces by asking to go on a tour. Some institutions/regions offer regular information sessions about their employment opportunities, so keep your eyes and ears open during your final study term).
- If you are not familiar with the practice setting, ask for an opportunity to shadow your partner nursing role (LPN/RPN/RN/Enrolled Nurse/Registered Psychiatric Nurse), unit aide and unit clerk (see prior Appendix for details)—this will allow you to become familiar with their roles and to better appreciate the distinctions between the roles of various nursing scopes of practice relative to other caregivers. This knowledge will be valuable to you when it comes to initially understanding, and then ultimately delegating responsibilities to, members of your practice team.
- When you are IN a potential workplace, observe the nurses in action. Spend time in the coffee room and chat informally with the nurses while they are working or on break, or

book a meeting with the clinical educator/manager/or supervisor to get a feel for how the unit is run. **Don't ever be afraid to ask questions**.

- Some considerations when looking for the right workplace 'fit' are:
  - ✓ **Staffing levels** (nurse to patient/client ratios and work organization in the practice setting) are often structured in accordance with client/patient acuity levels or nursing workload measurement, staff experience and staff mix. It would be fair to say that the nurse to patient care ratios vary between states, provinces and territories, but WITHIN those regions remain relatively consistent (so, 'theoretically', if you had experience in San Diego, California, USA, you could predict that the staffing ratios would be relatively similar in San Francisco, California but you could NOT transfer that assumption to Calgary, Alberta, Canada).
  - ✓ **Staffing schedules/lines** may be organized in advance by the manager, based on a set rotation (each nurse 'rotates' through a set schedule that consists of a 4-8-12 week schedule that keeps repeating itself), or flex-scheduling that is done by the staff themselves. Flex scheduling provides more room to modify and adjust your schedule on a rotational basis, but there are rules and regulations with this process–HAVE YOUR PRECEPTOR/MENTOR REVIEW THE FLEX-SCHEDULING PROCESS WITH YOU.
  - ✓ If you are taking a position in **community or public health**, the hours are generally prescribed; 8 hour day shifts are the norm with start times varying according to the particular clinic/center you are working in and the role you are assuming (i.e. a needle exchange out-reach clinic will have different hours than a well-baby clinic, a geriatric rehab program or an interval home for offenders transitioning into the community).
  - ✓ **Homecare positions** can be day or evening rotations and will depend on the caseload you assume. Generally, homecare nurses are required to provide their own transportation but are given a stipend for 'wear' on their car and reimbursement for fuel used. HOW this is provided will depend on the employer (flat compensation, gas receipts or mileage).
  - ✓ **Long term care and acute-care** are generally scheduled (that might mean flex scheduling) positions. If you are unable to get a full-time position (Full-Time Equivalent [FTE]), you can always consider part-time, casual, per diem, relief (these positions are dependent on geographical/country location) or agency positions where you have varying benefits but you get experience and perhaps even exposure to a particular practice area that you might consider down the road.
- How you are 'received' (embraced or welcomed) into your new workplace will depend on a HOST of issues, but the most important in my experience AND in my research is the

relationship between the Manager and the staff.

- Ask the nurses what kind of a relationship they have with the Manager, how 'visible' or 'responsive' that Manager is and how often they meet with him/her for 'performance reviews'.
- Be attentive to the visibility of the Nursing Manager, Clinical Coordinator or Clinical Educator—'*seeing is believing*' and if you don't SEE leadership, maybe it's not there. In my experience, the individual responsible for the daily practice of nurses in a particular setting is CRUCIAL to the culture of that workplace. Spend time talking with the Manager and with the nurses (if you are unable to do so, you might want to consider WHY—if you are unable to rationalize the lack of accessibility, rethink this workplace). Trust your instincts!
- Look for a work atmosphere where colleagues are helpful, seem to enjoy their jobs and can laugh. When you are 'trolling' the potential place of employment (walking around and generally taking the PULSE of the workplace), look in the break room and bathrooms. Do they have *humor boards*, locations where they post *social events*, or even areas where they post pictures of family and friends, sharing their 'lives' with each other? Maybe an 'Honor Roll' where individual staff have been recognized for their outstanding contributions to mentorship or nursing practice? Just remember that you have an equal part in this too. Nursing can be a stressful job so it is important to build one another up and help each other out to make those stressful times just a little bit easier.
- Just by spending time on the unit, you will get a sense of how the nurses relate to one other and to other disciplines, patients/clients, and physicians–pay attention to how varying levels of staff work together (LPN/RPN/Enrolled Nurses, RNs, Nursing Aides or Assistants), keeping in mind that NO UNIT IS PERFECT—there are always issues when people are working closely together under stressful conditions.
- You may want to discuss with the staff and manager how they organize meal and coffee breaks and, if this is a workplace that has varying shifts schedules, how staffing on nights accommodates for breaks. You will likely need to accept the process that has been adopted by this practice area for the time being (at least until you have the credibility and seniority to suggest changes and be HEARD), so you need to know up front what you are in for.
- Inquire as to whether or not there is access to experienced nurse consultation, or a *Rapid Response Team* for difficult clinical situations.
- In an acute-care setting, how flexible is the staffing for changes in patient acuity? Is there clerical and housekeeping support on ALL shifts? If you are swamped with admissions, how able is the system (and how willing is the Manager….) to respond to these changing needs by stepping IN, or calling in additional support (and ask the NURSES about this—they will usually be transparent about the degree to which their needs are met)?
- During your observation time with the nurses, don't be afraid to ask questions:
    - ✓ What is it like to work here?
    - ✓ What do they enjoy most about working here?
    - ✓ What frustrates you the most about working here?
    - ✓ How many, and what type of patients are you responsible for?

- ✓ What is the model of care and what are the roles of team members?
- ✓ Tell me what a typical day is like for you—walk me through from start to finish.

Finding the Perfect Job

- For those fortunate enough to have more than one offer to consider, how do you pick the best one? For those of you with limited job choices, how do you know if you are making the right move?
- We all want that 'perfect job' that can offer intellectual satisfaction, an environment that's conducive to our career development and one that provides a sense of fulfillment and joy while allowing time and energy for our family and social responsibilities. Here are some things to consider as you search for that perfect job:

  - ✓ THERE IS NO SUCH THING AS THE PERFECT JOB!!!
  - ✓ All jobs have their challenges. There will be good days and bad days—moments you will treasure and always remember….and times you wish you could just forget.
  - ✓ Stress exists in every job. As nurses, we deal daily with challenges in people's lives that threaten them at worst, and that compromise the quality of their health and well being at best. We accept the overwhelming responsibility that goes with the profession. But it is not difficult to lose track of the boundaries that keep us from becoming enmeshed in the tragedy and trauma that we are intimately connected to in our work.
  - ✓ BURNOUT is a term used to describe a point at which the coping skills of the nurse are inadequate to manage the level or degree of stress inherent in the work environment. The individual is incapable of separating work from home and the devastation of what is seen on a daily basis at work overwhelms the personal life experience of the nurse. Inappropriate coping mechanisms are often seen in this situation (i.e. withdrawal from patients, families, or colleagues, leaving you feeling '*cold and emotionally distant*', difficulty handling or appropriately expressing emotion, dysfunctional eating or sleeping patterns, dependence on drugs or alcohol). If you experience any of these symptoms, you should consult your physician or general nurse practitioner immediately. DON'T LEAVE YOUR FEELINGS BOTTLED UP INSIDE! Contact other new graduates and TALK TO SOMEBODY! Most workplaces offer FREE confidential counseling and psychological support for staff and their immediate families so check out your benefits! And remember that you can always contact *Nursing The Future* at newgraduates@nursingthefuture.ca). You might FEEL alone but you are never REALLY alone, so reach out!!
  - ✓ New graduates struggle initially with the differences between what they were taught nursing was going to be and what it is—sometimes what they see and what they come to know as their professional role is discouraging and disillusioning—if left unresolved, the resultant feelings of conflict between the 'ideal' and the 'real' can result in moral residue and ultimately in burnout. The new graduate, frustrated and

disenfranchised, leaves the job in search of another venue that better meets their professional motivations and aspirations, or leaves the profession altogether. The adjustment from the ideal to the real doesn't mean that you must leave your standards or high expectations behind and leaving one workplace for another may not change the underlying problem. You may need to adjust your expectations and the work environment may need to meet you half way. Talk with a mentor, your manager or your educator and construct a program of assistance that works for you.

✓ Job satisfaction and the quality of the workplace go together—you will need to give as well as get. Make the effort to get to know your co-workers (yes, go to that Christmas Party even though you are not a social person). Once you get to know them and they get to know you, there will be a significant difference in how you feel about work and you might be surprised at how much fun you have!!! Your co-workers will evolve into your new support system.

✓ Make conversation with your co-workers. Perfect the art of 'small-talk'—ask about their families and about what they did over the weekend.

✓ BEWARE OF NEWGRADUATE-ITIS!! This is a term sometimes used by experienced nurses when a new nurse with 3 months of experience gives the impression that they know more than a nurse with 30 years of nursing experience—REALITY CHECK!! WE DON'T! Be respectful of the senior nurses on your unit as they are a great source of nursing knowledge. Also be aware that some nurses are sensitive to how diploma/college, or hospital-trained nurses are received relative to associate or degree (university educated) nurses, or how LPN/RPN/Enrolled Nurses are received relative to Registered Nurses or Registered Psychiatric Nurses. Let's all try to remember that in a *practice* profession like nursing, theory and experience WORK TOGETHER and in the end we need to '*get our hands dirty*' to practice in the REAL work of nursing. We are all nurses and we need to stand together to move nursing forward.

✓ Some ways to get to know the nurses you work with, and for THEM to get to know and accept YOU, are:
    - Spend time eating lunch in the staffroom chatting with co-workers;
    - Attend social functions outside of work as they arise;
    - Take part in meetings and conferences. Try to strategically place yourself beside someone new each time;
    - If it is possible, arrange to car pool with a colleague;
    - On occasion arrive early to work to chat with the previous staff prior to shift change;
    - Join ward specific committees (i.e. social committee, Christmas decoration committee) or hospital-wide committees (i.e. interdisciplinary work collaboration projects) as your interest and time allows;
    - Bring an item of food along with the recipe to work one day (you may be surprised at how well received your cooking/baking is).

✓ Be proud of all that you know and have to offer—sometimes people are not as receptive to the '*new kid on the block*' because they believe that you have to '*earn*' respect over time. Continue to model excellent nursing practice and look to your experienced colleagues for what they have to offer your evolving knowledge (EVERYONE has something to teach EVERYONE!). This will contribute to building other nurses' trust in your skills, commitment, competence and communication ability.

✓ REMEMBER—you are a professional nurse who has much to offer your new workplace! YOU CAN DO THIS!!!!

EMPLOYMENT OPTIONS

To begin, you may want to ask your potential employer if they offer:

1) A Graduate Nurse Program;
2) A Transition Facilitation Program;
3) A Transition to Professional Practice Program;
4) A New Graduate Residency Program; OR
5) New Graduate Employment Incentives.

These programs (known by MANY names) are geared to the gradual introduction of, or support for, new nurses transitioning into the work environment. These initiatives generally include one, several, or all of the following:

- **Supernumerary** grad status (we reviewed this in the previous Appendix) where you are NOT included in the staffing quota but work alongside experienced nurses rather than by yourself;
- **Comprehensive educational programs** that use case scenarios based on actual complex clinical situations and include content related to professional role transition and nursing practice development;
- **Graduated practice integration programs** in various clinical specialties;
- **Access to a graduate nurse support person** or clinical consultant on call;
- **Gradual entry to practice** with educational support programs tailored to the new nurse transition stages;
- **Opportunities to 'rotate'** through several clinical areas (usually 4-6 months rotations) so that you can experience several different clinical populations and get a sense of what attracts you;
- **Preceptor or mentor support** for variable periods of time;
- **Employment options** upon completion of a 12 month graduate nurse program;
- **Extended orientation programs** up to 12 weeks with supervised clinical 'buddy' shifts.

Mentors and Preceptors

- Find out if the organization has a mentor or preceptor program where an experienced nurse (LPN/RPN/Psych Nurse/Enrolled Nurse/RN) can assist you in your new role as a professional nurse.
- ***Mentorship*** is truly a *relationship* between a novice and experienced practitioner and is intended to provide encouragement as well as support to the mentee, while simutaneously offering enhanced job satisfaction and fulfillment to the mentor. These relationships often last long after the novice outgrows the need for a formal relationship. Mentors are there to guide a new grad beyond the initial stage of graduation and there is often a bond that forms between mentor and mentee through sharing the experience of moving into professional practice for the first time.
- ***Preceptorship*** is more of a practical/clinical support person who can orientate you to the routines, responsibilities, skills and procedures related to your work area. A preceptor (often called a 'buddy') is usually an experienced nurse currently working in the practice area to which you are transitioning. This individual shows you the ropes of your job and will be scheduled to share a workload with you during your transition period. The ideal situation is if you and your preceptor work TOGETHER in completing your assigned nursing practice. '*Buddying*' does not mean "*you take half of the work and I'll take the other half*", though if your preceptor has not received prior training in this role or feels uncomfortable 'teaching', this may be an easier approach for them.
- It is very important that you and your preceptor/mentor work TOGETHER, so you have a chance to see the decision-making and clinical judgment process of this experienced nurse. If you want to go off and do something on your own as time progresses, ensure that you get together frequently during the day to discuss events that have taken place, how you dealt with them and how you might improve upon your practice.
- It is possible that the mentor and preceptor may be the same person—but they don't have to be.
- When meeting with the Nursing Unit Manager prior to employment, request shifts where you and your preceptor/mentor can work side by side (or at least the same shifts) for the 1st 6 months at least.
- Your preceptor/mentor can help you navigate the political environment that exists in any institution or professional unit, can inform you about those things you only find out about '*on the job*', and can be there for support and career development advice down the road.
- During your employment interview, ask what you can expect for preceptored/ mentored shifts–you should reasonably expect to have an orientation to the organization/institution that lasts 3-5 days, followed by an integration/transition program to your practice area that lasts a MINIMUM of 7 days to 3 weeks. As you know, from the previous Appendix, I recommend a much more extensive transition

program, so negotiate this with your manager! If you ENTER the meeting about your employment conditions with some sense of what is reasonable and what you would like, you might get it (or something close anyway!!). Your initial introduction to the practice area should be followed by at least 8-12 buddy shifts (a minimum of 4 nights and 4 days if you are working shift work or 2 weeks of 8-hour days if you are in a clinic, community or public health workplace). During this time your preceptor/mentor and you should be SHARING a normal workload for that position. YOUR workload responsibility should gradually increase, while YOUR PRECEPTOR/MENTOR'S gradually decreases.

- It is very important to have an experienced nurse to discuss your professional turmoil with and to receive advice from. Look for someone with whom you can create a personal bond and build a relationship based on mutual respect and collegiality.

Benefit Programs

- Benefit packages can vary from organization to organization if you are not part of a union that negotiates these packages on your behalf. **GET SPECIFICS** about those benefit packages and 'shop around' for which institution/company offers what—talk with the Human Resources Department.
- Most organizations that hire nurses into full-time equivalent (FTE) positions offer Health, Life and Disability Insurance plus a Pension Plan, but the level of coverage varies from country to country and region to region.
- Nurses are often automatically covered for Professional Indemnity Insurance and the employer usually protects against workplace injury.
- For those working in non-unionized contexts, salary packaging plans offer options such as reduced income tax, contributions to superannuation and medical health coverage.
- Contact the Human Resource (Benefits) Department of your workplace or read your union contract. Remember that the coverage you have as a part-time, temporary or casual employee may differ from that of the full-time permanent staff.
- Some institutions offer reimbursement for education debts you have incurred, but that is often a temporary 'incentive' bonus and rides the waves of staffing shortages. IF they are offering it, it could come in the form of a sign-on bonus or a contract that agrees to pay your loans in return for a specified period of work.
- Other 'perks' offered include paid continuing education (which may include time off) related to your field of work.
- Educating yourself on your options will help you and your family decide on the right fit for your individual situation.
- Salaries may vary if you are not hired under a union contract. The union or Human Resource Officer within your employment institution will spend time with you

during your orientation, so ask about how you will be paid and the salary grid you will be starting on.

- If the position for which you are applying is not supported by a union contract (more prevalent in the US), you should get your starting salary and bonus package committed to in writing along with a clear indication of how, when and between whom your incremental salary advancements will be negotiated.
- You should request information regarding sign-on bonuses, travel or isolation pay and any moving allowances when you negotiate your base salary and contract.
- It is possible to get sick as a nurse—even though you may feel as if you have developed immunity to every pathogen known to man through the course of your nursing education. Rest assured, your immune system will get stronger and stronger until it starts attacking squirrels in the park. BUT…..if you DO get sick, DO NOT GO TO WORK!! You will only make your co-workers and the patients ill. Ask your manager who to contact if you are ill and how many sick days you have allotted to you. There is also information on sick time and leaves in your union contract or, for non-union employees, in your employment contract.
- KNOW YOUR UNION/EMPLOYMENT CONTRACT—all workplaces will have a resource manual that outlines what you are entitled to as a contract or unionized employee but it is YOUR responsibility to access that information—ASK your Manager or a coworker! **YOUR UNION CONTRACT WILL SPECIFY THE CONDITIONS UNDER WHICH YOU WORK**[1] so if you are in a unionized practice environment, be sure to contact your local union representative (ask your Manager) to ensure you are working within the contract.

Employment Status

- Depending on the position you were hired into, you could be full-time or part-time. The other types of employment are permanent, temporary, and casual. There are benefits to all types of employment depending on your life circumstances.
    - ✓ **Full-time Permanent**—These positions are usually the most sought after upon graduating from a nursing program as your debts are often higher and, quite simply, you need the cash! Full-time status means that you are guaranteed full-time hours, benefits and some assurance of permanence. Countries have different representations of full-time equivalent rotations and hours, so check with your employment agency to determine what that means for you!

[1] If you work in a unionized environment, know your rights—if you don't know what that means, contact the union representative in your workplace (ask your manager or any of your colleagues who that is) OR connect with your manager in a non-unionized or 'employment contract' driven workplace. For nurses working in Canada, see: Canadian Federation of Nurses Unions (www.cfnu.ca), and for Australia, see: Australian Nursing and Midwifery Federation office in your state (http://www.anf.org.au/)

- ✓ **Full-time Temporary**—These positions are also good when there is not an option for permanence, as most are long-term appointments (many for a year). The unfortunate part of temporary positions is that you will not receive benefits (pension, health and dental) as quickly as you would if you were permanent.
- ✓ **Part-time**—In the posting for the position, it will tell you how many shifts per rotation are being offered this position. Always ask the Manager of the unit if there is an opportunity to have shifts added by scheduling extra shifts or by picking up casual work.
- ✓ **Casual/Relief/Agency**—If the area in which you want to work has no positions available and you want to 'get your foot in the door', an option is to work casual/relief or to apply to work with an external nursing agency that provides staff for that institution. This may work very well for you if you are a flexible, easy-going person who doesn't mind an unpredictable work schedule. A word of warning to the 'planners' out there—it is VERY DIFFICULT to plan your life if you work casual and want to work a lot. On the other hand, YOU are in control of what shifts you accept and what shifts you turn down. **SOME TIPS FOR CASUAL/RELIEF WORK**:
    - o Have a cellular phone with you so you are able to leave the house without missing 'the call';
    - o Plan time out to relax and re-energize;
    - o Have sacred family/loved ones time that cannot be interrupted with a call or calls for 'overtime';
    - o Decide on your boundaries and stick to them—if you made social plans that are important, try to honor them. That may mean saying 'no' to a shift—don't worry, there will always be another shift around the bend!

Vacation and Holidays

- Can you believe it? They will actually PAY you to care for patients/clients AND give you vacation time!!
- Yes, it is true that after approximately one year of employment you are entitled to somewhere in the range of 2-6 weeks vacation. Those lucky Auzzie's receive 6 weeks paid annual leave if they work a 7 day roster, and 4 weeks if they work a 5 day (Monday-Friday) roster. WOW, all that time to do as you please!
- Ask your manager when you are able to take vacation and how much can be taken at once. Usually summer vacation time is booked well in advance, so be warned—if you graduate in April-May, be ready to work through the summer or have your holidays agreed to before you start employment.

Working on a Team

- As nurses working in health care settings, we are only one part of a large team of health care professionals working together to care for every aspect of our clients' lives. Understanding the roles and responsibilities of each member of the team facilitates a collaborative approach to resource utilization and ensures that the expertise of all team members is available for the patients/clients/communities we serve.
- Knowing which member of YOUR team is the most appropriate person to deliver a particular aspect of care can help you to better understand your OWN role and can help you to draw upon the rest of your team members to optimize the care of the patient/client and their family or community.
- Below are job descriptions and responsibilities of many of the professionals you will encounter in your practice. It is difficult to include ALL varying job descriptions and diverse titling that come with allied and support healthcare providers (this book is targeted at new nurses from Canada, the United States, Australia and the United Kingdom). Consider this when you arrive in your workplace; clarify, validate and verify the particularities of roles and responsibilities as they apply to YOUR practice context.
- While the positions identified below were generated primarily from the framework of an acute-care setting (the majority of new graduates begin their practice in acute-care), similar positions with varying titles will exist in rural, public and community healthcare centers. Further to this, it is important to note that not all areas will have each of these professionals and the duties of each position may be divided differently based on the needs of the country, region, institution or healthcare facility, and client population you are serving.

Nurse Manager/Head Nurse

- ✓ Follows, promotes and upholds the unit/hospital's mission statement and the practice setting's standards and policies;
- ✓ Prepares, monitors, controls and evaluates the annual operating budget;
- ✓ Selects, hires, develops and evaluates all employees working within the practice setting for which they are responsible;
- ✓ Monitors staff attendance/absenteeism/sick time;
- ✓ Initiates employee disciplinary action and terminates if necessary;
- ✓ Participates in nursing, medical, administrative and allied healthcare committees to facilitate the operation of the nursing department; and
- ✓ Monitors the quality of nursing care clients receive, through audits and other means.

Nurse Practitioner/Nurse Clinician/Clinical Nurse Specialist

- ✓ Has advanced clinical preparation, most commonly at a Master's or advanced clinical practice level;
- ✓ Takes primary responsibility for the coordination of healthcare interventions and nursing care;
- ✓ Depending on the practice setting may write orders (nurse practitioner);
- ✓ May perform advanced interventional procedures (i.e. chest tube insertions, central line insertions);
- ✓ Coordinates clinical care follow-up during hospitalization or upon discharge if working within the community or in general practice;
- ✓ Writes discharge recommendations;
- ✓ Is usually practice based—functioning within a clinical specialty; and
- ✓ Generally spends significant time within the clinical practice setting and is quite accessible—often leads the '*Rapid Response Teams*'[1] within acute care settings

Clinical Coordinator

- ✓ Takes responsibility for the clinical aspects of the nursing unit operation - this is frequently an advanced practice nurse (Master of Nursing preparation) or a practitioner with extensive experience in that nursing practice setting or in that nursing specialty;
- ✓ Assesses staffing levels based on patient needs, ensuring staff are assigned and/or adjusted according to practice setting workload;
- ✓ Assesses and acts on clinical needs of clients;
- ✓ Monitors and ensures the quality, coordination and continuity of nursing care;
- ✓ Serves as a clinical resource person (particularly to new nurses) and/or supervises clinical care on the unit;
- ✓ Provides input into nursing staff performance evaluations;
- ✓ Advises nursing office of adjustments required in staffing – may actually find staff if required; and
- ✓ In the absence of the clinical coordinator, a charge nurse may be assigned to take temporary responsibility for the coordination of patient care.

[1]A *Rapid Response Team* (RRT), sometimes called a *Medical Emergency Team,* is a multidisciplinary team organized and coordinated to respond to ANY situation where clinical instability is noted. RRTs are usually activated by nursing staff but can be called upon by ANY member of the hospital staff.

Charge Nurse/Assistant Head Nurse

- ✓ Not all nursing units have initiated the role of clinical coordinator—they may, instead, designate one or several individuals as charge or assistant head nurses;
- ✓ Collaborates with, and offers assistance to, staff as needed;
- ✓ Recommends modification to nursing care when the patient/client's condition or treatment dictates;
- ✓ Takes client workload responsibilities as needed;
- ✓ May serve as primary liaison between direct-care/bedside nurse and physician/ medical staff;
- ✓ Coordinates staff workload commitments and care of clients during an emergency;
- ✓ Ensures proper staffing mix for each shift and replaces if there is an illness; and
- ✓ MAY assist with diagnostic, lab and consultative service requests, particularly on shifts when there is NOT a unit clerk or clerical support staff available.

Clinical Nurse Educator/Professional Development Nurse/Nurse Education Facilitator

- ✓ Takes responsibility for nursing orientation and continuing education in the practice area;
- ✓ Serves as an educational and clinical resource person for nursing staff;
- ✓ Assesses learning needs of nursing staff;
- ✓ Plans, implements and evaluates staff orientation/transition facilitation;
- ✓ Plans, implements and evaluates ongoing nursing education programs;
- ✓ Identifies and evaluates individual staff capabilities and readiness for practice; and
- ✓ Instructs staff on new nursing policies, procedures, equipment and practice.

Practical or Enrolled Nurse (LPN/RPN)

- ✓ A Licensed/Registered or Enrolled Nurse has a provincial/state/territory issued license to practice;
- ✓ Serves in a complementary role to Registered Nurses and other health discipline;s
- ✓ Shares responsibilities and functions with RNs, but is individually responsible for own nursing practice (i.e. if giving medications, Practical (LPN/RPN) or Enrolled Nurse is responsible to ensure appropriateness of medication delivery 'rights' and will be held accountable for the assessment, implementation, outcome and evaluation of medications given);
- ✓ Basic educational programs are designed to meet an established set of competencies for practice primarily in acute-care and long-term care facilities;
- ✓ Scope of practice can be expanded by acquiring additionally approved competencies or certifications (institution and practice area specific) through a post-basic education program;

- ✓ Held to legal and professional consequences commensurate with scope of practice; and
- ✓ Are required to provide annual proof of continuing education and acquisition of competencies in order to maintain their license to practice.

Registered/Graduate Nurse (RN/GN)

- ✓ A Registered Nurse is a practicing nurse with licensure from a province/state/territory—a Graduate Nurse is a recent graduate who has not yet become licensed and practices under a 'restricted' license (FIND OUT WHAT LIMITATIONS there are to your practice PRIOR to licensure);
- ✓ Serves in a complementary role to LPN/RPN/Enrolled Nurses and other health disciplines;
- ✓ Shares responsibilities and functions with their nurse partners, but is individually responsible for own nursing practice;
- ✓ Basic educational programs (Diploma, Associate Degree or Baccalaureate Degree) are designed to meet an established set of competencies for practice in a variety of settings, including, but not limited to, acute-care, specialty practice settings, community and public health, forensics and psychiatric mental health (particular to the Registered Psychiatric Nurse preparation);
- ✓ Scope of practice can be expanded by acquiring additionally approved competencies or certifications (institution and practice area specific) through a post-basic education program or post-secondary advanced degrees (Master/PhD);
- ✓ Held to legal and professional consequences commensurate with scope of practice;
- ✓ Are required (in some jurisdictions) to provide annual proof of continuing education and acquisition of competencies in order to maintain their license to practice; and
- ✓ Work collaboratively with LPN/RPN/Enrolled Nurses to determine what level of complexity is appropriate for the educational background, experience and permitted scope of practice.

Housekeeping or Cleaning Staff

- ✓ Answers telephones and refers calls and messages appropriately;
- ✓ These employees are VALUABLE extensions of the nurse's eyes and ears! Remember that the hospital is the temporary HOME to patients and their families;
- ✓ Duties involve regular cleaning of rooms and ward/units, changing of linen and the maintenance of hygiene within the clinical environment;
- ✓ Are frequently 'present' within the clinical environment and often 'chat' with patient/clients and their families. Because of their 'neutral' role in the practice setting, some patient/clients and their families disclose to these individuals information that they perhaps feel reticent to share with their primary healthcare providers;
- ✓ Called when discharges from acute-care are identified so that a cleaning of the room in preparation for the next admission can be completed expeditiously; and

✓ Will do isolation or biohazard cleanup in certain situations.

Ward/Unit Clerk or Clerical Administrator

✓ Answers telephones and refers calls and messages appropriately;
✓ Directs personnel and visitors to the appropriate practice areas;
✓ Maintains accurate and current patient/client charts;
✓ Files reports and memos;
✓ Contacts departments for patient/client admissions, equipment or general practice area required services;
✓ Orders supplies;
✓ MAY chart demographic and statistical data (practice area specific);
✓ Transcribes physician orders (practice area specific); and
✓ Prepares charts for client admissions and disassembles on client discharge.

Ward/Unit Aide/Certified Nursing Assistant/Nursing Aide

✓ Assists patient/clients with bathing and toileting;
✓ Changes and makes beds;
✓ Assists with lifting, turning and positioning patient/clients;
✓ Feeds patient/clients and/or assists with meals as needed;
✓ Assists with ambulating and transferring of patients/clients within the unit and/or to other institutional departments if porter is not available or not employed;
✓ Assists in care of a body after death;
✓ Sets up special rooms and carts (i.e. isolation carts);
✓ Cleans hospital equipment;
✓ Disposes of soiled linen and waste;
✓ Restocks supplies, including linen, in designated areas; and
✓ Runs errands, specimens, completes requisitions or transfers equipment to and from departments.

Hospital Porter/Patient Services Assistant

✓ Transports patients/clients for diagnostics;
✓ Transfers patients/clients between practice areas (including morgue);
✓ Operates, cleans and repairs equipment;
✓ Cleans and sanitizes rooms;
✓ Assists patients/clients with meals;
✓ Transfers laundry;
✓ Moves furniture and equipment;
✓ Cleans up elimination or biohazard waste;
✓ Delivers mail, files and clinical samples; and
✓ Picks up blood for transfusion.

NOTE: For the following allied health and interdisciplinary roles, nurse practitioner or physician orders for consultation MAY be necessary. Please check your workplace or institutional policies.

Social Worker

- ✓ Coordinates complex discharge planning;
- ✓ Counsels and supports client and family;
- ✓ Assists client and family to make adjustments in living context after illness and before discharge;
- ✓ Links client and family with community resources; and
- ✓ Assists client and family with transportation, accommodation or living needs at home.

Discharge Coordinator/Planner (this role will go by a variety of titles even within ONE city or country)

- ✓ Coordinates the implementation of home-based services for clients on discharge from their current acute-care setting. These services can include:
  - o Nursing care;
  - o Physiotherapy;
  - o Nutrition counseling;
  - o Home respite;
  - o Meal programs;
  - o Social work visits at home;
  - o Occupational therapy;
  - o Home intravenous and antibiotic program;
  - o Out of district/region patient/client transfers; and
  - o Eligibility assessments for long term care placement.

Dietician/Nutritionist

- ✓ Provides consultation, assessments and/or treatments for patients/clients who require:
  - o nutritional support such as enteral/parenteral feeding or oral supplements;
  - o diet instructions/counseling for diagnosed conditions (i.e. Coronary Artery Disease); and
  - o additional nutritional monitoring and guidance (i.e. malnourished or nutritionally deficient).

Spiritual Care Worker/Pastor

- ✓ Provides sacraments, religious rituals or celebrations;
- ✓ Informs client and family of spiritual reading and video resources;
- ✓ Links client and family with community spiritual resources; and
- ✓ Organizes follow-up visitation, counseling, and/or prayer.

Physical Therapy

- ✓ Provides consultation, assessment and/or treatment for patient/clients who:
    - o Require pre-operative education and post-operative preventative chest treatments (may need consultation to provide incentive spirometry);
    - o Have physical deficits that affect safe, independent mobility;
    - o Require education and/or treatment for breathing difficulties/clearing of respiratory secretions;
    - o Have or are at risk of developing musculoskeletal dysfunction; and
    - o Have mobility needs for discharge.

Occupational Therapy

- ✓ Provides consultation, assessment and/or treatment for patient/clients who require:
    - o Retraining for activities of daily living;
    - o Ordering of appropriate equipment (i.e. wheelchairs, cushions, splints); and
    - o Pre-discharge assessment of home access and mobility.

Respiratory Therapy

- ✓ Starts or changes treatment related to oxygen or ventilation;
- ✓ Performs diagnostic tests such as arterial blood gases and lung function tests;
- ✓ Supplies equipment for continuous monitoring of O_2 saturations or CO_2 levels, artificially ventilating, or instituting positive airway pressure intervention;
- ✓ Controls settings for, and monitors hourly functioning of, artificial ventilation; and
- ✓ Manages O_2 transport tanks in practice settings.

Speech Therapy/Language Pathology

- ✓ Provides consultation, assessment and/or treatment for patient/clients who have:
    - o Difficulty understanding and/or communicating in written or verbal language;
    - o Cognitive deficits which affect their ability to communicate;
    - o Slurred speech or difficulty with articulation of speech;
    - o Changes in voice pattern, cadence, pitch, tone or volume and
    - o Difficulty swallowing or at risk for aspiration.

Palliative Care

- ✓ Assesses, supports and educates patient/clients and families regarding a life threatening illness;
- ✓ Assists with symptom management including pain management (nurse practitioner/physician order may be required);
- ✓ Assesses and screens patients/clients for possible admission to the Palliative Care Unit (nurse practitioner/physician order required);
- ✓ Provides family counseling on 'do not resuscitate' orders;
- ✓ Organizes supplies and/or oxygen for home therapy (nurse practitioner/physician order required);
- ✓ Counsels patients/clients and family in dealing with death/dying and end of life issues; and
- ✓ Provides bereavement follow-up.

Adjusting To Shiftwork

This section will offer suggestions for minimizing the effects of shift work on your body AND your spirit and provides you with tips to effectively manage the inevitable disturbances that arise as a result of shift work.

- You may have never connected with the true meaning of '*working shift*' until your very first string of nights! Never fear—life will normalize somewhat after a few months of getting used to SHIFTING.
- We live in a society where shift work is not well accommodated. Our days turn into nights and our nights into days, while businesses and the '*social scene*' seem to roll along apparently oblivious to our scheduling chaos....go figure! You have chosen a profession where shift work is common, but remember that not all nurses work shift and you may decide that it is not for you (although I worked shift work for YEARS, and likely will again, it was never in line with my *'circadian rhythms'*). I remember one night shift I was particularly tired and before I got to work, I recalled that someone had once given me a bag of chocolate covered coffee beans (at this point I really didn't care how old they were...). What better time to try them! So I took one (ok, well maybe I took a couple.... they were chocolate after all ☺) and YEOWZA!!!! I definitely got through THAT night shift—in fact, I was awake for a WEEK!!!! Just sayin'.....

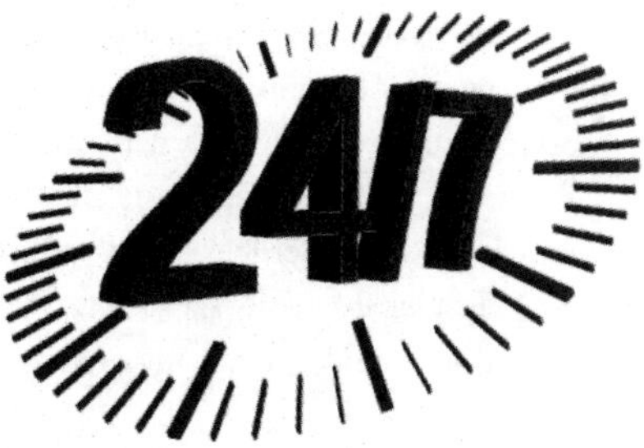

- There is little doubt that shift work will be a part of the first few years of your work (even if just part-time), so take it in stride.
- Shift work has been linked to a variety of health concerns. The most common health effects have to do with gastrointestinal and digestive disruptions, mood changes and sleep/rest pattern alterations.
- Other hazards of shift work include: stress; chronic fatigue; a general decrease in alertness and energy; disruption of family and social life; feelings of isolation; a greater risk of compromising safety on the job resulting in a potential increase in errors, miscalculations, reduced critical thinking and poor judgment; and a greater affinity for physical accidents while at work.
- Despite the rigors of working shift, the odd hours and lack of structure have distinct advantages!! You may find you are able to get more done on your days off because your friends, partners or family are working. As well, you will likely find shopping and errands easier because the commercial 'traffic' is less than during normal working hours and weekends.
- The most difficult time at work on the night shift is between 0300-0600. Try to have the more important/demanding tasks completed before this time and note

that you need to be more diligent and take more care when completing your responsibilities at this time—plan for this drowsy time and keep busy!

- Take your breaks so you can relax and get some rest. This translates into more efficient nursing. If the staffing allows, you might try to sleep on your breaks—these power naps WORK. While you may feel initially tired upon waking, you will find after about 30 minutes that you have increased energy and clarity of thought and this will enhance your effectiveness for the remainder of the shift.
- Some people find that exercising on their breaks is beneficial. It helps them relax on day shift, and alternately keeps them awake during nights. You can go to a gym if your workplace provides one, or just walk/run the halls. If you want, keep a resistance band or hand weights at work for strength training. Find a buddy and exercise together. It'll make exercising more fun and will also help keep you motivated.
- Adjust your workload to prevent boredom. If your nursing work is done, find something else that needs to be done. You could reorganize the lounge communication board, devise a strategy for communicating about practice issues amongst nursing staff, or draft a new policy or form for dealing with an issue related to practice in your work setting.
- Be careful when driving home after a 12-hour night shift as you are prone to fatigue—you may not even remember how you GOT home. Be sure to focus on the road!!!
  NOTE: I have actually slapped my OWN face to 'jolt' myself out of a night stupor—upon reflection, I could have approached a co-worker and given them this pleasure....

Managing Different Shifts

- Shift work is very hard on the body. It is often difficult to get adequate hours of sleep between shifts because of difficulty sleeping during daylight hours, managing life beyond work and the challenge of continually switching from days to nights. Your body often does not have enough time to establish a set routine. Let your friends and family know your work schedule. They will more than likely accommodate you for events and you won't have so many phone calls or people ringing your doorbell while you sleep. Here are some strategies that might help you to get your rest:

  Night Shift[1]

  ✓ Have a pre-shift nap 20-90 minutes before your shift. It can help you feel refreshed

[1]Evening shifts (3-11pm) are not generally a major issue from a sleep perspective but they can strain your social/personal life. It is possible to join events that continue to midnight, but otherwise you will have to forego social activities during working days. If you have children, you may not be at home when they arrive from school and you may not be available to feed them at dinner/supper, bathe or put them to sleep. If you are a single parent, this might be a challenge that you need to consider. If, however you have a partner who works primarily a day routine, this might work well once you coordinate who will care for them between the end of school and your partner's arrival home.

and more alert at work. Rouse yourself well before your shift starts, though, in case you feel groggy when you first wake up.

- ✓ Try to stay up late the night before your first shift starts. This way you are able to sleep in longer and hopefully get more sleep before you have to go to work. Afternoon naps are also beneficial before night shift.
- ✓ Talk with your Manager to see if it is possible to be scheduled in for a late 4-hour evening shift (7:30-11:30 pm or 1930-2330) the day before you begin nights—this will allow you to adjust yourself to the later hours. When you arrive home at midnight, watch a movie until 2-3 am and then go to bed.
- ✓ If possible, try to have your night shifts placed consecutively in your rotation so you do not have to keep adjusting between day and night shifts.
- ✓ Be aware that if you are sleeping during the day, you may wake up inadvertently because of hunger. Try to eat something (protein is best) before going to bed. The amount and type of food you eat will depend on your own body, but I suggest eating a small snack before going to bed such as a slice of toast and peanut butter, egg, salmon, tuna, or cheese as the protein may keep you from getting hungry while you sleep.
- ✓ If you are unable to sleep, don't continue to lie in bed and toss and turn. Get up, do a few things around the house, then try going back to sleep later on.
- ✓ Place dark curtains on your windows to help block out light (you may need to use the more 'cheesy' approach of putting tin foil on your window pane with the shiny side OUT)…hey, whatever works!!!
- ✓ Use ear plugs if necessary. Cover your alarm clock or watch, so you are not '*clock watching*'. Set the temperature to a comfortable level (cooler rather than warmer) and turn off the ringer on your phone (don't forget to turn off your cell phone!).
- ✓ If you have a basement, sleep there during the summer as basements are usually darker and cooler.
- ✓ Have a fan running in your room; the steady 'white' noise will drown out background sounds.
- ✓ You just spent a full day at work doing things that you don't want to dream about now (unfortunately this is the curse of being a new nurse…you WILL dream a lot about work initially)! It can help if you take some time to wind down when you arrive home in the morning. Use all the same tricks you would normally use to unwind and relax before bed like reading a book, watching TV, having a bath or soaking your tired feet. **WORD TO THE WISE**: Be careful about WHAT you read or watch prior to sleep—there is a tendency to replay what your mind has 'just' experienced (no horror movies!).
- ✓ Have a set routine, much like you do when going to bed at night. If there is something that might help to relax you, it will help you sleep better.
- ✓ Clear your mind of distractions. Pack your bag for work and have your clothes ready to go before you go to bed.

- ✓ If you are still unable to sleep—try a light workout routine at home. Invest in some yoga or Pilates tapes or do some light weight lifting. Stretching before and after you sleep is highly recommended as it loosens the tight spots and restores the body from the stresses and strains of work AND prepares it for another day on the job. The physical exercise may help take your mind off your thoughts and tire you out just enough to fall asleep.
- ✓ Speaking of exercise, I suggest that you consider exercising before work. Twenty minutes of aerobic activity, such as brisk walking, jogging or swimming, can help you stay alert on the job while keeping your heart in tip-top shape.
- ✓ On your first day OFF after working night shifts, plan to rest and recuperate. Try to keep that day clear of commitments so you can focus on yourself. You will need some '*turn around*' time. Generally I head to bed upon return from work, but I get up sometime around noon and then go back to bed around 10-11 pm. That routine has helped me transition back to a day routine more easily.
- ✓ Attempts to manage the exhausted sleeplessness associated with shift work may encourage you to turn to alcohol or drugs to cope. While there are times when medication may be necessary and therapeutic, you should discuss this approach with your nurse practitioner or physician first.

Day Shift

- ✓ Put your feet up at the end of the day and relax.
- ✓ Go to sleep early.
- ✓ Shower the night before your shift so you have more time in the morning to get ready for work.
- ✓ On days off package some left over meals and place them in the freezer to make quick grab and go meals.
- ✓ Try to follow as regular a schedule and routine as possible, on both work days and days off. For example, try to get up around the usual time you would get up for a day shift on your days off. This limits the amount of disturbance to your body's functions and routines.

Finding Balance

- In the upheaval of working long hours over consecutive days, it is easy to let other areas of your life get unbalanced. Always remember to take care of yourself first.
- The phone may ring every day looking for staffing, particularly if you work in acute-care or are working casual/relief, but remember, YOU CAN SAY NO! The workplace's primary interest is to manage ITS needs; YOU are the one who will feel burned out if you over-extend yourself. Set your own limits and your co-workers will respect that. Just a note about working casual or relief: there is a tendency to worry that if you don't take THIS shift (the one they are calling you about), there may

not be work tomorrow. While this is true, more often than not, I have seen grads working EXTENSIVE hours (and NOT getting paid overtime because they are casual/relief) in fear of not getting ANY hours. This can terminally exhaust you, so be careful.

- *Full time hours* (even less than full time) allow for PLENTY of practice experience when you are a new nurse. While it is tempting to take on overtime work to help pay off those school loans or get that car or that house you have wanted for so long, it will be hard for you to do this AND stay healthy during the first six months of your transition.
- Use nutrition to help you cope!!! It makes sense for shift workers to consume a lower fat, higher fibre diet that may help delay, avoid and/or treat some of the negative health effects of shift work. Keep the following points in mind when planning your meals:
  - ✓ Follow an established food guide for healthy eating and aim for the following number of servings per day from each of the four food groups:
    - o Grain products, 5-12 servings
    - o Vegetables & fruits, 5-10 servings
    - o Milk products, 2-4 servings (adults)
    - o Meat & alternatives, 2-3 servings
  - ✓ Decrease your fat intake by choosing leaner meats and lower fat-percentage dairy products. Choose lower fat snacks and eat out less often. Use small amounts of spreads, creamy sauces and salad dressings.
  - ✓ Increase your fibre intake by choosing whole grain breads and cereals, legumes, nuts, vegetables and fruits.
  - ✓ Choose high protein snacks like meat, eggs, nuts or cheese if you feel you are unable to stay awake.
  - ✓ Choose high carbohydrate foods like grain products or fruit to help you sleep. Bring raw veggies to munch on during the night and avoid high sugar content foods—they will prevent you from re-establishing a good sleep pattern when you get off the set of nights.
  - ✓ Limit your daily intake of caffeine to 4 cups of coffee. Avoid caffeine-containing drinks (pop) starting about 4 hours before the end of your shift.
  - ✓ Consume lots of water during your shift! However, cut back on your fluid intake as of 4 am (0400) to prevent unwanted trips to the bathroom while you are trying to sleep!
  - ✓ Plan ahead for lunches and snacks. Include lunch and snack items on your grocery list so you have them when you are packing for work.
  - ✓ Clean and cut raw vegetables and fruit, and wrap them in individual servings (or buy them that way!), so they are ready for your lunchbox.
  - ✓ Make extra food at lunch/supper for a few days before you begin your shifts. Leftovers are a quick and easy solution to the dilemma of what to take to work.
  - ✓ Pack your meals BEFORE you go to sleep—meal preparation provides your body and mind an opportunity to 'gear down' after a shift before you go off to sleep and

will ensure that you will have something to take back to work with you when you awake.

- The great thing about the profession of nursing is that its workplace diversity allows for movement. Shift work is only one option. You may want to consider talking with your manager to discuss a permanent shift schedule (days or nights), or you may have to contemplate a change in jobs if shift work is starting to affect your social and home life. If your health is changing or failing it may be time for a switch to something less stressful on your body or spirit. Please don't ever allow shift work to consume you. Try to listen to your body and learn to say no.
- Here are few tips from other grads who have '*been there, done that*':
  - ✓ Loneliness is common, because you may see other people participating in the 'normal' world. Make sure you schedule time with your family and friends.
  - ✓ There are changes in the way you socialize when you do shift work. Talk to your family and friends about your schedule so they know how to accommodate you and can keep you in the loop.
  - ✓ Get voice-mail installed on your phone! This allows you to know what is going on, without significant disruptions to your sleep-work patterns.
  - ✓ Use your family, friends and colleagues as support. You might find you are making new friends through co-workers that also work shift work and you may find new ways of socializing. If you and a friend are both trying to stay up late, go see a late-night movie together!
  - ✓ Be creative! Go out for BREAKFAST with friends instead of going out for supper/dinner.
  - ✓ Find an activity or hobby you enjoy or want to learn. This will help you feel less isolated when other people may be at work while you have time off and may help you to feel more fulfilled.
  - ✓ Regular exercise has been associated with better sleep and a more positive self-image. Integrate exercise into your normal routine. Walk or bike to work instead of driving. Climb the stairs instead of riding the elevator.
  - ✓ If you are struggling with the effects of shift work, seek help from your *Employee Assistance Program* or another professional support system. Do not sacrifice your health for your job.
  - ✓ If you are finding your rotation or schedule too demanding, talk to your Manager about making some adjustments or trade some shifts with your co-workers.
  - ✓ Make time for family and friends—socialize even when you don't feel like it.
  - ✓ Rest when you feel tired—sleep is good. The housecleaning can wait a day and you CAN ask for help from others you are living with. You may, however have to settle for a different standard of 'clean' while you are making this transition.
  - ✓ Over the next few months, things will come around and you will find yourself with more time and energy to return your life to a more comfortable state of balance.

- ✓ Talk with peers and friends from school about the changes you are going through. You will soon discover that you are not alone in your emotions.
- ✓ Find a new personal interest or hobby, or reacquaint yourself with what you enjoyed doing before being a student took over your life! You may find that you have 'free time' on your hands. Just a warning—you may question your drive, motivations, and purpose as you re-focus your time and energy. This is normal and natural. Things will sort themselves out—GIVE YOURSELF TIME!

Taking Care of YOURSELF

Nursing is an emotionally draining job at the best of times and if you do not allow yourself a recharging period you may suffer in the long run. YOUR EMOTIONAL HEALTH IS PARTICULARLY IMPORTANT AT THIS TIME.

Making Time for Family and Friends

- ✓ Provide family and friends with your schedule and let them know the best times to contact you. If you are working shift, they may be afraid to call you, thinking you might be working nights. You may assume they have forgotten about you, but more than likely they are just trying to be respectful of your schedule.
- ✓ Family and friends need time to adjust as well! They may have grown accustomed to having you around and perhaps you were more available for them when you were in school! EVERYONE WILL ADJUST WITH TIME!
- ✓ You may have established a student support group when you were in school. Now you may find you are working at different times and it may be hard to see each other. Schedule lunch dates, nursing review sessions, shopping trips or any excuse to continue those bonds. Your school friends are important to keep, as they can be a great support, especially in this transition year. It seems few 'outsiders' truly understand what this experience is like and those who have gone before you may have forgotten (or intentionally repressed their memory....or lost their memory....☺).
- ✓ Remember there are other services to access outside of friends and family. *Nursing The Future* is always available to 'chat' with you—it CAN get a bit lonely during transition, so REACH OUT!
- ✓ Schedule a regularly occurring date night with your partner, or quality time with your family or children. It is amazing how fast a week can pass by if you don't make special time for the ones you care about.

Taking Care of YOU

- ✓ BE CAUTIOUS ABOUT WORKING OVERTIME—a lot of energy is going into making this transition to your new life and you need to give yourself permission to take time off (we know bills are hounding you, but they likely always will!!)
- ✓ Some nurses find it helpful to plan a 'ME' day. Set aside a day where you give yourself permission to do whatever you would like to do. Go to a football game with a buddy or maybe even get a massage!
- ✓ A regular work schedule, or even just being in a consistent practice role is helpful when you are starting out—it allows you to plan other events in advance or change your schedule to get days off as needed.
- ✓ If you are working shifts, but able to self-schedule (also called *flex* scheduling), a WORD OF CAUTION... **learn how to do it first**. It may seem like a wonderful

opportunity to have as much time off as you would like, but it is a balancing act that takes practice and quite a bit of flexibility on your part. There are RULES to self-scheduling so be sure to connect with your mentor so you don't unintentionally break ALL of the rules the first time out of the gate!

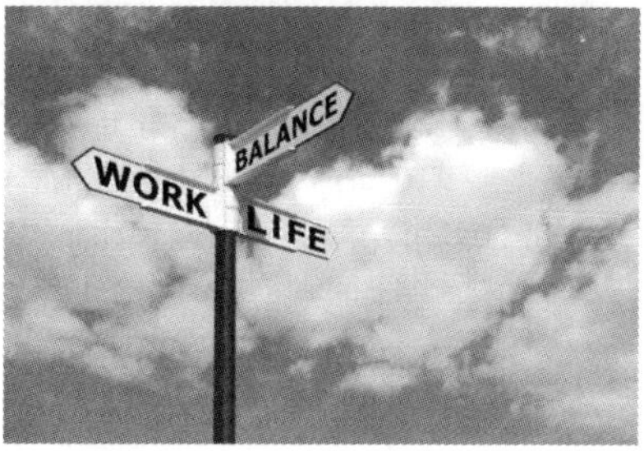

- ✓ Casual/relief or agency/temporary work may be necessary immediately following graduation. This may be a frustrating time for you as you wait for more permanent opportunities. This uncertainty can take over your life if you allow it to, so take note.
- ✓ DO NOT CANCEL IMPORTANT PLANS TO TAKE A SHIFT. Your personal life is equally important and making the transition can be difficult if you don't infuse time for yourself with friends and family. A cell phone can allow you to maintain a 'normal' life (without having to sit by the phone) while still making yourself accessible.
- ✓ You may need to be quite STERN (not rude….) with staffing clerks who call you daily for overtime work. It can be difficult, particularly if you work in a rural health center, because saying 'no' and then meeting up with someone in the local store can make for an uncomfortable dynamic. As well, there can be a sense of 'guilt' when you don't go in; knowing your colleagues are working 'short' is always difficult. But YOUR HEALTH is more important than anything else—nobody is going to look out for that except you. Be careful about taking on too much work!

Coping With Stress

Be patient with yourself! You ARE going to make mistakes because every nurse does—mistakes are part of life! '*This too shall pass*' OR '*Tomorrow is another day!*' are helpful phrases to remember right now! Being 'imperfect' is HUMAN—you can only do the best you can do with what you have to work with (both internally and externally). When you make a mistake, LEARN FROM IT and MOVE ON! Try to monitor the practice situations you are placed in and don't allow yourself to be put in situations that are beyond your experience, knowledge or comfort.

Stress IS a part of any new professional's life—you can't avoid it, but you CAN take some steps to deal with it:

1) Get Lots of Rest!

- ✓ Fatigue makes everything worse.
- ✓ Sleep will restore your sense of confidence and competence.
- ✓ Sufficient dream time will help your mind process and sort out problems.
- ✓ 7-8 hours of uninterrupted sleep is recommended for most people.

2) Be Good to Yourself!

- ✓ Laugh lots—it 'snaps' the grip of depression. Watch the comedy channel or treat yourself to a funny movie on your day off (I highly recommend '*Critical Condition*' with Richard Pryor!).
- ✓ Remember that negative emotions are linked to disease—think POSITIVELY!

3) Plan for Change!

- ✓ Nothing in life is permanent. It takes time to accept the dynamic state of nursing and healthcare today—change is the name of the game!!
- ✓ You can plan your day, but IT WILL CHANGE! That's OK and that's normal. Be fluid if you can—ROLL WITH IT! Everyone else is experiencing the same thing!
- ✓ Spend time journaling (or even blogging, but be careful about your level of disclosure) about your work—think about what has changed and why it has changed. This reflection will help you to see how much you have grown.

4) Resist Competition with Others!

- ✓ There are always going to be people who measure themselves against others—that can actually be healthy, in moderation.
- ✓ Better yet, we suggest you measure your progress by how much YOU have grown in the past week or month—go back to your journal and compare your entries.
- ✓ Speak with other new graduates—their perceptions may be a more accurate appraisal of what is 'normal' during this time of transition.
- ✓ Good work will be recognized for what it is—competing with others just causes tension.

5) Find Support!

- ✓ If support does not come looking for you—go looking for it!
- ✓ Good friends and family are VERY important to your survival, so make time to socialize—go out even if you don't always feel like it.
- ✓ Talk to people about your experience—seek out other new grads.

6) Work it Baby, Work it!

- ✓ Physical activity is critical to your mental health—go for a walk with a friend, exercise at the gym or take a yoga/meditation class. It will distract you and serve as an outlet for stress.

- ✓ You are NOT ALONE in your feelings! Try not to keep your feelings bottled up in those first few weeks—find someone you can confide in who understands this experience and who can listen without judging or trying to 'fix' your situation. Write about how you are feeling!!

7) Develop Yourself!

- ✓ Becoming the nurse you always wanted to be is a life long project! You are gaining critical experience every day and you need to be patient with your growth.
- ✓ Watch the experienced nurses around you and take '*the best*' from their practice and integrate it into your own. Remember that NO ONE IS PERFECT and even the most experienced nurses struggle with sustaining the practice they aspire to.
- ✓ DON'T GIVE UP ON YOURSELF—and don't think that you need to change the way YOU are in order to be accepted by your colleagues. Just be the BEST of who you are!
- ✓ Don't be afraid to bring your IDEALS and your IDEAS to the practice setting—start a new committee to help you make change in some area of practice that is lacking. Change happens when people commit themselves to making things better.
- ✓ Even though you are a new graduate, sometimes YOU are the model for others whose practice has become stale—YOU can show OTHERS the way by maintaining your standards and not accepting anything less.

8) Keep Learning!

- ✓ Attend conferences (like the NTF *Annual Nursing Graduate Conference*—see www.nursingthefuture.ca). Educational conferences are a great way to recharge your batteries and take a step back to reflect on your nursing path.
- ✓ Let your employer and co-workers know that you are keen to be put forward for new courses or certifications.
- ✓ Read articles—keep up to date on new nursing knowledge. If your workplace does not post articles for you to read, bring one to work and post it on the bulletin board yourself! Your colleagues will very much appreciate your efforts. In fact, why don't you start a reading club in your practice setting?
- ✓ Continue to write about your experience—I know that after all that journaling in school, you think you never want to see a journal again.... but it really is a great way to reflect on your progress as a new professional. And remember that recording your experience does not mean you have to write it; use your iPhone® and record your thoughts to listen to later!

- ✓ This is the age of information! There are lots of courses that you can take (and your practice area might even PAY FOR THEM!) that will keep you current in your skills and competitive in the job market.
- ✓ Advanced practice nursing courses are available at various colleges and universities though out the country—get online and start searching!
- ✓ If you are currently an Associate or Baccalaureate prepared nurse, advancing to the next level of your education might be the most appropriate step. If you are an LPN/RPN or Enrolled Nurse, taking an advanced certification program may interest you. There are COUNTLESS opportunities to advance your education and enhance the quality of care you offer!
- ✓ Once you feel you are ready to return to school, many programs can be done full time OR part time while you continue to work. Contact a mentor (or even one of your previous instructors/faculty) to discuss this possibility.

9) Ask for Help When You Need it!

- ✓ Your nursing education provided you with a broad overall knowledge of nursing, but cannot be expected to teach you all there is to know about nursing. There is a lot to learn in the 1st 12 months of nursing practice as well as throughout your career. Ask LOTS of questions!

10) Safety First!

- ✓ Patient/client safety is THE priority of a professional nurse. It is better to ask for information or clarification than put patients/clients at risk.
- ✓ THERE IS NO SUCH THING AS A STUPID QUESTION! END OF STORY (and I'm a nursing educator so I can say that!!!!). You will hear more experienced nurses commonly say, '*I worry about a new nurse who does not ask questions.*' We all know that nursing knowledge is so vast that no one person '*knows it all.*' That is why WE WORK AS A TEAM—TOGETHER, giving those under our care the benefit of ALL our expertise.
- ✓ ASK QUESTIONS!!!!! Learn from your peers, learn from your patients/clients, their families and the communities you work in.

11) Counter Peer Pressure!

- ✓ You may feel that others expect you to know it all. Unfortunately, some of the nurses you work with may not remember what it was like when they were 'new' and may not appreciate how important it is for you to ask questions. Sometimes you will ask the SAME question a couple of times—THAT'S OK!!
- ✓ On occasion, you may feel drawn into behaviors that are out of character for you, like engaging in workplace gossip or criticizing another team member. New

nurses can feel like in order to 'fit in' they need to comply with existing workplace culture. But there is NOTHING better than a cohesive, fun and embracing workplace (I mean SERIOUSLY—we spend a lot of time at work!!!).

✓ IF you see disrespectful or inappropriate behavior, DECIDE TO BE DIFFERENT! You can choose to say something or you can just WALK AWAY—that is a statement too! In the end, you WILL be respected for your unwillingness to contribute to a toxic workplace. There is NOTHING worth the price of your integrity.

Workload Distribution/Collaboration/Delegation

- Your workload as a new nurse (WHAT it is you are required to do and HOW you are going to manage it) will largely depend on: 1) your scope of practice (LPN/RPN/Enrolled Nurse/RN), 2) the setting in which you are practicing, and 3) the process of orientation, integration and transition into your work role and practice context.
- There are numerous documents available to you on 'collaborative' models of nursing practice and, while beyond the scope of this book, these are important for you to review IF these documents are applicable within your practice setting. Please consult with your Nursing Manager or Educator for more information on appropriate documents that you should review prior to engaging in your professional practice role.
- Nurses most often work in 'teams', interacting with *intradisciplinary* (within the realm of nursing as a discipline) and *interdisciplinary* (between nurses and 'other' practitioners who reside outside the realm of nursing, and in some cases outside of healthcare [i.e. law enforcement]). As a new nurse, you will be in a position to 'collaborate', 'share a workload' and/or 'delegate' or 'assign' care to other professionals. The following serve as general definitions:

Collaboration

- There are distinctions between a *Collaborative Practice Model*[1] and a *Collaborative Model of Nursing Practice*. A collaborative practice model is an overarching model of care that approaches the health of individuals, families and communities from a multidisciplinary, wholistic perspective. It is usually a community-based healthcare practice setting that utilizes a team of nurses, physicians, social workers, pharmacists, psychologists and other allied practitioners to manage the health of a population (usually geographic).
- A collaborative model of nursing practice[2]/[3] is defined through the principles that underlie it as an approach to care. Collaborative practice requires that patients/clients, employers, LPN/RPNs, Enrolled Nurses, Registered Psychiatric Nurses and RNs (or an appropriate collaborative team as determined per geographical location) determine together how to best meet the needs of individuals and families requiring nursing services. Not uncommonly there are state/provincial/territorial or national practice acts that determine scope of practice, collaborative and delegation responsibility. Scopes of practice will vary

---

[1]Casto, M. (1994). *Interprofessional care and collaborative practice.* Pacific Grove, CA: Brooks/Cole Publishing Company.
[2]Fowler, J., Hardy, J., Howrath, T. (2006). *Trialing collaborative models of care: The impact of change. Australian Journal of Advanced Nursing, 24(1)*, 24-28.
[3]Besner, J., Doran, D., McGillis Hall, L., Giovanetti, P, Girard, F, Hill, W., et al, (2005). *Nursing Scopes of Practice Study: A Systematic Approach to Maximizing Nursing Scopes of Practice.* Capital Health, Calgary Health Region, Saskatoon Health Region. Retrieved December 21, 2005 from http://www.cihr.gc.ca

from region to region, which is addressed by licensures (some reciprocity between states/ provinces/territories usually exists). The collaborative model of nursing practice approach is about optimizing the appropriate utilization of nursing practitioners. Collaborative models of nursing care are enacted within a framework that respects the following principles:

- ✓ care is practiced safely and effectively with the intent to maximize the health and well being of the patient/client/family/community/region;
- ✓ nursing practitioners act in a manner consistent with their scope of practice, ethical standards and legal guidelines as directed by their regulatory body; and
- ✓ decisions related to workload sharing and care distribution are grounded in a shared decision-making model that optimizes the skills, abilities and knowledge of all nurses.

- The process of nursing collaboration in YOUR practice setting will, in part, be up to YOU. Collaboration is fundamentally about transparency, mutuality, respect, negotiation and a willingness to put *care* at the center of the decision making process. Basic principles to be followed when collaborating on a shared workload are:
  - ✓ **WHO** is the most appropriate individual, taking into consideration the complexity of the workload and the knowledge/education/experience of the nurses, to take on **WHICH** of the practice roles and responsibilities?
  - ✓ **HOW** can you communicate consistently, frequently and accurately over the course of your day?
  - ✓ **WHAT** can each partner do to ensure a respectful, collaborative, effective and efficient utilization of the available nursing and support resources?

Workload Sharing/Distribution

- The outcome of a strong collaborative model of nursing practice is the appropriate sharing/distribution of the biophysical, cognitive, emotional, spiritual and psychosocial needs of patient/clients/communities/regions as these needs are 'translated' into the daily work requirements of a nursing team. Utilizing the knowledge, experience, skill capacity and competence of nurses from varying scopes of practice, collaborative decisions and judgments are made about how to OPTIMALLY 'share' and appropriately 'distribute' the work.
- This is NOT about a struggle for power between nursing credentials, but an authentic intent to provide the BEST nursing care.
- As a new nurse it is CRITICAL that you keep this intent uppermost in your mind as you integrate into a system that, like anything or anyone, can lose its way on occasion. I cannot tell you HOW the process of collaboration will work in your new practice setting but I can suggest that YOU be the one to begin the process.

Delegation

- It is important to understand the distinctions between '*assigning*' and '*delegating*'. **Assigning** care implies that you are collaborating with another healthcare professional who is licensed and works within a scope of practice for which they can be held accountable. IF you are 'assigning' care, it is assumed that you are transferring *responsibility* and *accountability* for care to the individual to whom you are assigning the task. Conversely, **delegation** encompasses requests for the performance of a task for which the individual to whom the skill or task is being delegated is NOT licensed and therefore is NOT able to be held ultimately responsible for the performance of that skill within their professional scope. In this case, YOU (the delegator) retain responsibility and accountability for the performance of that skill or task.
- As a new nurse, you may be working quite independently and autonomously, as is often the case in home healthcare, community or public health. In those practice settings, you are assigned a 'caseload' of clients for whom you take ongoing responsibility. In the broadest reference, you may be involved in program development, implementation and evaluation (community or public health) or responsible for a 'group' of individual clients and families (home healthcare) whom you visit daily, weekly or monthly. Your care responsibilities exist on a continuum, depending on the needs of the clients, your scope of practice and comfort level in your role (for instance you may be caring for a high-level quadriplegic, responsible to administer medication, perform wound care or intermittent catheterization; or you may be visiting new mothers to assess their situational coping skills and to do a basic assessment on their newborn).
- In some cases, you may be practicing in relative isolation, as in a rural or remote nursing context. In this case, your work with other practitioners may be by distance (telemedia/videoconferencing) or by monthly face-to-face interactions with another practitioner (i.e. a medical physician or nurse practitioner may fly in to your nursing station periodically). While the clear majority of new nurses transition within an acute-care practice setting, there is a wide variety of practice/workplace scenarios and contexts of practice that you might be transitioning into as a new nurse. This increases the likelihood that you will need to *delegate* or *assign* care early in your tenure.

What is delegation and how is it different from collaboration?

- While LPN/RPN/Enrolled Nurses and RNs are often required to *collaborate* with each other, the process of **delegating** involves a Licensed/Registered Professional requesting an unlicensed/non-registered care provider (such as a nursing aide, certified nursing assistant, porter, ward/unit clerk or other clerical staff) to perform a task or procedure NOT within that care provider's job description.
- The **delegator** retains RESPONSIBILITY for the care quality of the patients/clients AND accepts ACCOUNTABILITY for the delegated act.

Why is delegation important?

- Managing a patient/client workload within practice setting constraints is an increasing challenge for nurses in all settings.
- Delegation ensures that those for whom you are 'caring' receive the best possible attention, while also using nursing time, skills and education appropriately and efficiently.

How and when do I delegate?

- Delegating can be difficult for a new nursing graduate—you may not know the people to whom you are allowed to delegate and they may not be receptive to you because they don't know or trust you yet.
- There will be a tendency to '*do it yourself*', rather than ask someone else for assistance with your practice. That can be absolutely exhausting and others may conclude that you are not a '*team player*'.
- Sometimes it is difficult to delegate to someone who is older than you, who has been there longer than you, or with whom you sense a power struggle brewing. Rather than thinking of it as '*ordering someone else to do something*', think of it as facilitating a team approach—you are working together to get the job done.
- Remember, if you are delegating the right task to the right person, THEY are responsible for the quality of their practice. Having said that, YOU will be held accountable for the outcome of that task if the individual to whom you are delegating is NOT licensed, educated, trained or otherwise prepared to perform the task. Essentially you are being held accountable for your decision to delegate THAT task to THAT person.
- Being respectful when either delegating OR collaborating (remember that the difference between these is a matter of responsibility and scope of practice/licensure) is a sure way to succeed - use phrases such as:
  - ✓ "*I know that you are an established caregiver here, so please forgive me if I don't know exactly what you are responsible for. I am new, so I might ask you to do something you don't normally do, or I might forget to ask you to do something you normally do. If that happens, let me know*";
  - ✓ "*Jane, you've been around here longer than I have—who normally does vital signs on the post-operative patients?*" OR "*I understand you normally take vital signs on the clients. Would you mind taking Mr. Smith's vital signs for me?*";
  - ✓ "*I am unable to give Mr. Smith his pain meds. Could you do that for me?*";
  - ✓ "*When you do the assessment on Mr. Smith, could you please report any unusual findings to me right away?*"
- Be sure to sit down with your work partners immediately after report to sort out who is going to do what.
- When you are starting out as a new nurse and do not know the routines of the workplace, this organizational strategy can prevent slips and misses over the course of the day.

- Courtesy is always appreciated—offering a simple 'please' or 'thanks' or 'you did a great job with Mr. Smith today! I thought you were very efficient/caring/prompt' will go a long way toward establishing a solid working relationship with your co-workers.
- Leadership takes awhile to get used to—just try not to confuse good leadership with asserting power over others.

The 5 *Rights* of Delegation[4]/[5]/[6]/[7]

The Right Task

- ✓ Is one that occurs frequently
- ✓ Is usually technical in nature
- ✓ Has a predictable outcome
- ✓ Has a low potential for risk
- **Key Point**: Tasks that require sound nursing judgment or complex assessment, planning, or evaluation skills should not be delegated to unlicensed nursing staff.

The Right Circumstances

- ✓ The condition and needs of the client must be considered
- ✓ The appropriateness of the particular healthcare setting must be assessed relative to the task required
- ✓ Identify whether the proper time, resources, equipment and supervision are available for the safe and successful delegation of work
- **Key Point**: Safety of the patient/client is paramount. Delegation is undertaken ONLY when you believe that the safety of the patient/client would not be jeopardized if someone other than a Registered Nurse were to provide care in that particular circumstance.

---

[4]Document used to guide content: *Joint Statement on Delegation*. American Nurses Association (ANA) and the National Council of State Boards of Nursing (NCSBN). Retrieved January 6th, 2012 from https://www.ncsbn.org/Joint_statement.pdf

[5]Document used to guide content: Canadian Nurses Protective Society (2000). *Delegation to other healthcare providers*. INFO: A legal information sheet for nurses, 9(2). Retrieved January 6th, 2012 from http://www.cnps.ca/upload-files/pdf_english/delegation.pdf

[6]Australian Nursing and Midwifery Council (2003). *Guidelines on delegation and supervision for nurses*. Retrieved January 6th, 2012 from http://www.brisbanesouth.com.au/content/Document/Resources/Nursing%20in%20General%20Practice/ANMC%20guidelines%20on%20delegation%20and%20supervision%20of%20nurses.pdf

[7]Gillen, P., Graffin, S. (May 31, 2010) Nursing delegation in the United Kingdom. OJIN: *The Online Journal of Issues in Nursing 15*(2), Manuscript 6. Retrieved January 6th, 2012 from http://nursingworld.org/MainMenuCategories/ANAMarketplace/ANAPeriodicals/OJIN/TableofContents/Vol152010/No2May2010/Delegation-in-the-United-Kingdom.html

The Right Person

- ✓ 2nd RN?
- ✓ LPN?
- ✓ Ward Aide?
- ✓ Unit Clerk?
- ✓ Porter?
- ✓ Cleaning Staff?
- **Key Point**: You must assess the competence and appropriate skill set of the staff member to whom you are delegating. Does this person have the education, training, level of confidence and physical capability to perform this task? Is this particular task outside of the scope of that individual's job description? **KNOW YOUR TEAM MEMBERS**! You may want to take some time getting to know them in your work setting prior to delegating a lot of tasks to them—you should get a feel for their skill set, competence, and confidence after several weeks. Remember to consult with another RN if you have doubts.

The Right Communication

Appropriately and specifically communicate the:

- ✓ Methods and supplies to be used for the task(s)
- ✓ Any concurrently required observations/assessments/specimens
- ✓ Time limits or performance deadlines
- ✓ How and when the staff member should report back to you.
- **Key Point**: Most failures on the delegation process are due to inappropriate or inconsistent communication that is based upon inaccurate information—be sure you have the background information (role, boundaries, and individual competence) on the individual to whom you are delegating and communicate CLEARLY what, how, when, and why.

The Right Evaluation

- ✓ Was the appropriate task performed?
- ✓ Did it have the desired client outcome?
- ✓ You must give feedback to the delegated staff member on their performance and follow-up when expectations are not being met
- ✓ Remember to acknowledge and thank the staff member for completing a task and recognize them for a job well done
- **Key Point**: Both you and the individual to whom you delegated are responsible to reflect on what was done, how it was done, and whether or not the process could be improved upon. If any issues arise around delegation, discuss your concerns WITH THAT PERSON! If you are unable to resolve your concerns, approach your manager or educator for further advice on alternative approaches or strategies for conflict management in the workplace.

Managing Your Nursing Workload

The management of your nursing workload, as outlined here, will focus on new nurses working in an acute-care practice setting. Community or public health settings vary significantly in WHAT they do, HOW they do it and WHO DOES WHAT. If you are employed in one of these settings, you will receive an individual orientation to managing your workload from the preceptor/mentor in that setting.

Working in an Acute-Care Setting

When you first arrive to work, you may feel overwhelmed by all the work you have to do and everything you have to remember. You may not know where to start. When you are beginning your new nursing practice, it is difficult to know what issues are most important and what issues or tasks can wait until later. This section will assist you to navigate through your shift efficiently and effectively.

The **SBAR**[1] (**Situation-Background-Assessment-Recommendation**) technique is a way to organize and prioritize your practice, and acts as a framework for communication between members of the health care team. SBAR is easy-to-remember and useful for framing conversations, especially those requiring immediate attention and action. It allows for an easy and focused way to set expectations for what will be communicated, how and between whom.

Organization

How you go about organizing your work for the day will depend on the routine of the clinical setting in which you are working, but the following ideas can be applied to most acute-care ward/units:

1) Preparation

✓ Arrive early to work (about 45 minutes before your shift is to start), and review your assignment. Review the nursing ward/unit worksheet prior to receiving report on your patient/client assignment. This will give you extra time to familiarize yourself with what you might be expected to do that day, what clinical conditions you might need to know, patient/client mobility issues that could change your prioritization, and any special challenges such as pacemakers, legal blindness, feeding tubes etc.

[1]Michael Leonard, MD, Physician Leader for Patient Safety, along with colleagues Doug Bonacum and Suzanne Graham at Kaiser Permanente of Colorado (Evergreen, Colorado, USA) developed this technique. Information retrieved January 6th, 2012 from http://www.ihi.org/knowledge/Pages/Tools/SBARTechniqueforCommunicationASituationalBriefingModel.aspx

Adapted SBAR Tool[1]/[2]

S Describe **SITUATION**	My name is ____________ and I work ______________ (practice area) I need to talk to you about: ☐ an urgent safety issue regarding __________________ (name *of client)* ☐ a quality of care issue regarding __________________ (name *of client)* I need about ________________ (minutes) to talk to you If not now, when can we talk? I need you to know about: ☐changes to a patient status ☐changes to treatment plan, procedures or protocols ☐environmental/organizational issues related to patient care
B Provide **BACKGROUND**	Are you aware of ____ (specific *problem)* The patient is ____ (age) and has a diagnosis of ________ as well as ________ (including any relevant CHRONIC conditions) He/She was admitted on ______ (date) and is scheduled for discharge on ______ (date) His/Her treatment/intervention related to this issue was ______ ordered on______ (date) and the outcome was _______ He/She is being followed by _______________ (specialist) and has appointments for _______________________ (procedures) I am requesting that ____________ be ordered or that _____________ occur This patient/family/staff is requesting _________________________ (requests)
A Provide Client/Patient **ASSESSMENT**	I think the key underlying problem/concern is _________________ (describe) Key changes from last assessment regarding concern are: BELOW **Person Level Changes** ‰ Vital Signs/GI/ Changes ☐ Cardio-Respiratory ☐ Neurological ☐ Musculoskeletal/Skin ☐ Pain ☐ Medications ☐ Psychosocial/Spiritual ☐ Sleep ☐ Cognitive/Mental Status/Behav ☐ Nutrition/Hydration **Activity/Function** ☐ ADL ☐ Transfers ☐ Home/Community Safety **Environmental Changes** ☐ Org/Unit Processes ☐ Discharge Issues ☐ Social/Family Supports
R Make **RECOMMENDATION**	**Based on this assessment, I request that:** ☐ we discontinue/continue with______________________________________ ☐ we prepare for discharge OR extend discharge date ☐ you approve recomm changes to tx plan/goals including________________ ☐ you reassess the patient's_______________________________________ ☐ the following tests/assessments be completed by____________________ ☐ the patient be transferred to____________ /be moved to______________ ☐ you inform other team members/family/pt about change in plans ☐ I recomm we modify team protocols by doing_______________________ **TO BE CLEAR, WE HAVE AGREED TO______________ ARE YOU OK WITH THIS?** ☐ I would like to hear back from you by ___________________________ ☐ I will be in contact with you about this issue by ___________________

Modified with permission from the *Institute for Healthcare Improvement* January 9th, 2012 http://www.ihi.org/about/pages/contact.aspx

Trentham, B., Andreoli, A., Boaro, N., Velji, K. & Fancott, C. (2010). *SBAR: A shared structure for effective team communication. An implementation toolkit*. (2nd Edition). Toronto Rehabilitation Institute: Toronto.

- ✓ Using the practice area's clinical worksheet (or start another worksheet of your own), write down every task you anticipate having to do (i.e. like dressings, glucose monitoring and IV tubing changes) and each issue of concern you have in the care of your patients/clients. Cross these off as you accomplish or address them during the course of your day.
- ✓ Remember that many of the informal nursing worksheets used in practice ARE NOT LEGAL DOCUMENTS (you should ask about this), so use them like worksheets—they are intended to look 'messy'[2].
- ✓ During report, list every patient/client issue that needs to be addressed that day with a special designation (maybe you can use a highlighter): distinctly color code the issues that require consultation with varying professionals such as the physiotherapist, respiratory therapist, nurse practitioner, physician and remember to use SBAR to organize and prioritize your issues and information. This will help you get what you need from the appropriate practitioners.
- ✓ As you are getting report related to your workload, or even during your initial meeting with your work 'partner' (LPN/RPN/Enrolled Nurse/RN/CNA/NA), identify the priorities and required nursing care for each patient/client. This will also assist in collaborating and delegating as needed.

2) Implementation

- ✓ Take a moment to prioritize your tasks/responsibilities and number them in order of priority on your worksheet if it will assist you. Take into consideration when your breaks are scheduled so you can take them on time if at all possible (i.e. if you are on 1st break you may only have time to do morning vital signs and meds. You can do your baths and charting when you return from your break). When you take YOUR break often influences when others can take THEIRS.
- ✓ Evaluate who are your most unstable patients/clients and keep this in mind when going through your day. Usually the less stable the patients/clients are, the more time they will take out of your day. You should ALWAYS see these individuals FIRST!
- ✓ BEGIN YOUR DAY by laying your eyes on each patient/client (seeing the sickest individuals first)—this allows you to reconfigure your priorities if you need to.
- ✓ Multitasking is something experienced nurses do without even thinking about it. As you gain experience, you will find yourself more able to accomplish several 'tasks' at once (i.e. washing your patient/client's back AND listening to their lungs or assessing their skin).
- ✓ You can complete much of your assessment by asking questions like, '*are you having*

---

[2]While this work sheet may NOT be a legal document, it may contain CONFIDENTIAL information. Take care to ensure the identity and health information of your clients is safe. Dispose of this document appropriately at the end of your set of shifts (put in shredder)!

pain' OR '*are you expecting any visitors today*' OR '*are you passing flatus*' WHILE you are assessing things like surgical incisions.

- ✓ Try to reduce the number of trips in and out of the patient/client's room. This saves time and energy. Before you go into the patient/client's room to do a procedure or assessment, **stop and think** of all the things you might need, write them down, collect them and then take them with you into the room.
- ✓ Make sure you have frequently used supplies (tape, gauze, scissors, stethoscope and alcohol swabs) in your pockets so you don't have to run out of the room and get them when you need them.
- ✓ **ASK FOR HELP** from your nursing colleagues if you are feeling overwhelmed.
- ✓ Remember to delegate some of your tasks and responsibilities. When you are touching base/collaborating with your nursing partner (RN/Enrolled Nurse/LPN/RPN) at the beginning of the shift, discuss what it is you need from each other. Utilize your nursing aides/porter in your practice area (i.e. get them to help with baths, run for supplies, answer phones, etc).
- ✓ Be aware that sometimes you might not be able to complete all that is required of you in a day. Just make sure you have done all the ESSENTIAL care (i.e. assessments, dialoguing with your patient/client and their family, vital signs, medications and time-sensitive procedures).
- ✓ Let your oncoming colleagues know what you were UNABLE to accomplish so that they are not 'surprised' when they discover this later.
- ✓ **NOTE:** IF you get a list the next day of all the things you 'did not do', let them know that you are new and it is going to take you a few weeks to months to remember EVERYTHING. If they persist on criticizing you for your inability to complete your workload, you should discuss this with your preceptor/mentor or the Nursing Manager. It may be that you need to have your workload adjusted or it may mean that they need to better understand your challenges as a new nurse in transition.
- ✓ For the first while you may want to jot down a few points about each medication you are giving so that if questions arise from patient/clients or family members, you are prepared to answer them. After a while you may only need to write down notes on the unfamiliar or new medications you are giving.

3) Evaluation

- ✓ Over the course of your day (or more likely AT THE END OF YOUR DAY), reflect on your nursing practice—was it therapeutic, successful, lacking, did you have a good overall understanding of, and insight into, the patient/client's condition, challenges and clinical issues. Is there something you should have done that you did not do or did not have time for? This is where delegation comes in handy! **Remember to debrief with your preceptor/mentor about all of these things so that you can figure out how to balance expectations with your transition stress.**

- ✓ Don't forget to think about what you did WELL—things can get a bit unbalanced if all we do is remind ourselves of what we did NOT do well.
- ✓ Being organized means knowing your patients/clients, knowing what you have to do for them, and knowing what remains to be done for them at the end of your shift (so you can report this to your colleagues).
- ✓ As you become more comfortable with your own organizational patterns you will soon be able to integrate what happened BEFORE with what you want to do NOW, and you will be able to PROJECT further into the future of your patient/client's condition. For example, if you are working a few days in a row, let the patient/client know that their hair wash can be done the 2nd day (try to limit what you do the 1st day because that is usually the day when you are least organized). Honesty is always your best policy—patients/clients and their families are more likely to understand your busy schedule if you keep them updated and informed as your day unfolds.
- ✓ Organization takes time and practice and with a little of both, you will soon be an effective and efficient nurse. Be proud of what you have done each day. We never give ourselves enough credit!

Prioritization

During your shift, you will need to be constantly reorganizing and reevaluating your practice and collaborating with your nursing partners. The plan you start with will likely change because '*stuff happens*' that will force you to modify your priorities and your actions—it is NORMAL to feel a little scattered as you adjust to the highly dynamic context of nursing practice.

The following issues MUST take priority when they arise—STOP WHATEVER YOU ARE DOING and address them:

1) Airway and Breathing

- Is your patient/client in respiratory distress?
- Are they breathing abnormally fast or slow?
- Do they have an unusual pattern of breathing (i.e. irregular)?
- Is their color blue or gray?
- Is their oxygen saturation low (below 90%)?

2) Circulation

- Is the patient's heart rate or blood pressure too high or too low (relative to their normal)?
- Are they symptomatic with these readings (are they dizzy, having palpitations, chest pain, shortness of breath, is their color poor, or is their urine output low)?

3) Level of Consciousness

- Is your patient/client unresponsive or difficult to rouse?
- Has there been a major change in the patient's level of consciousness since you last saw them or are they presenting differently than you were led to expect in report?
- Are they able to converse or is their conversation illogical/inappropriate or their speech abnormal?
- Do they appear unusually sleepy?

4) Bleeding

- Is there a wound from which they are bleeding?
- Is the blood fresh?
- Are they on anticoagulants?

5) Pain

- Where is their pain?
- How does it feel (sharp, dull, squeezing, crushing)?
- When did it start and what were they doing at the time?
- On a scale of 0-10, at what level would they rate their pain?
- Is the pain worse now than it was 5 minutes ago?
- Have they ever had this pain before? When? What caused it?
- What relieves this pain?
- Do they have any other symptoms (nausea, sweating, shortness of breath)?
- Get a client's pain under control as soon as possible—it will only get worse!

The following issues are NOT LIFE THREATENING but require PROMPT ATTENTION:

- **Lab value changes** most commonly include CBC, electrolytes, coagulation studies and blood glucose (including chemstrips). Be sure that you respond by calling the nurse practitioner/physician as needed. Sometimes there are standing orders to deal with lab values (i.e. heparin and insulin nomograms). Remember to think ahead to what might be the cause of the change relative to the patient's condition (i.e. patient/client is receiving 40mg Lasix IV BID, their potassium level is 2.8 mmol, and they do not currently have a K+ supplement ordered).
- **Nausea and vomiting** may indicate a deeper problem and are very uncomfortable at best. The patient/client should be cleaned up and antiemetics given ASAP when appropriate.

NOTE: **Assessment of volume status in the elderly[3] is ESSENTIAL, but often forgotten!** Assess all of your elderly patients for diuresis, diarrhea or vomiting and TREAT THEM FOR DEHYDRATION if you are AT ALL suspicious. Symptoms of volume depletion in the elderly are often not as accurate but be on the watch for lassitude, fatigue, muscle cramps and dizziness. The most significant sign of volume depletion in the elderly is acute weight loss, muscle weakness and sunkenness of the eyes. Skin turgor, though a traditional method of assessing hydration, **lacks precision particularly in the elderly**—if you use this approach, test the inner aspect of the thigh or the sternum. Finally, vital signs can be a key assessment in their volume status so assess for postural hypotension and tachycardia.

- **Incontinence** can contaminate wounds, cause significant skin breakdown, be embarrassing to the patient/client or unnecessarily upset family members.
- **Patients going for surgery** or other procedures need to be prepped and ready to go on time. Vital signs, operating room checklists and pre-operative teaching need to be completed and bowel prep or contrast medium need to be administered so other department schedules can be respected.
- **Patients returning from surgery** and invasive procedures need to be assessed and their vitals taken as soon as they are received back. Frequent vital signs following interventions or diagnostic tests need to be completed to maintain protocol and quality care. There will be a protocol in your practice setting, but if you are unsure, take the V/S every 30 minutes if the patient is stable until you find out what the protocol requires.
- **Medications**, especially antibiotics, need to be given on time (you generally have a 30 minute window either way—early or late).
- **Discharges** need to be completed in good time so that the bed can be cleaned and you can accept a new patient/client when needed.

The remainder of your nursing practice can be completed in between these events.

It is important to constantly be thinking about your nursing priorities as you complete your work. You need to be flexible and you will need to readjust your plan several times throughout the shift. Prioritizing based on client conditions will contribute greatly to the delivery of safe, quality nursing care. It is an essential skill for any nurse.

Maintaining Professional Standards

When you begin your work, there will be times when you just want to get through your shift '*without killing anyone.*' While this is a reasonable objective ☺, in time you will be able to lift your gaze from what you are doing at any moment to see what is happening around you—we call it the BIGGER PICTURE.

[3]Larson, K. (2003). Fluid balance in the elderly: Assessment and intervention - important role in community health and home care nursing. *Geriatric Nursing, 24*(5). Retrieved January 11, 2012 from http://www.medscape.com/viewarticle/463744_print

- ✓ Know what the expected standards are in your practice setting and review your entry-to-practice competencies. If you feel the standards practiced there are not adequate, practice to the highest level possible and identify your concerns to the Manager.
- ✓ REMEMBER—UNSAFE PRACTICE ENVIRONMENTS VIOLATE YOUR CODE OF ETHICS AND ARE THEREFORE UNACCEPTABLE. You are OBLIGATED to complete a work situation report form (what this is called differs between geographical locations) and these should be readily available in your practice area.
- ✓ NEAR MISSES, or adverse events where '*nothing bad happened*' after all was said and done (but the risk was THERE), are equally dangerous to patient/client safety. If something 'nearly' happens due to an unsafe practice environment, TAKE THE TIME TO REPORT THIS. You cannot be penalized, harassed or disciplined for submitting a work situation report (well, I suppose you CAN be but you SHOULDN'T be as this your legal and ethical responsibility)!
- ✓ Further to this, you are obligated to report wrongdoing (practice performance or ethical conduct) of colleagues in the same fashion—this includes nursing, support staff and physician colleagues. This is what professional self-regulation means.
- ✓ Excellence and quality care exist on a continuum—there will be times when, despite your BEST EFFORTS, you will be unable to provide optimum care to your patients. THIS IS ACCEPTABLE ON A TEMPORARY BASIS ONLY and care must ALWAYS be SAFE!
- ✓ Being unsure is different from being unsafe—you may be put in situations where you have not performed a particular skill in awhile and you need additional time to perform it—THAT IS OK!!! You might need some encouragement from a senior staff member and that is also OK! We are all in that position at various points in our careers but there may be times when you are given an assignment that is beyond your education, experience or comfort level—while everyone is NERVOUS when taking care of patients they have not had before, or caring for individuals whose diagnoses/clinical situations we have not seen before, YOU WILL KNOW (deep in your gut) WHEN THE SITUATION IS UNSAFE.
- ✓ A NOTE about professional appearance....remember that the practice environment is not about YOU—it is about the individuals you are caring for. While YOU may feel that the way you are presenting yourself is appropriate, you need to '*check that out*'. You can start by looking around you—how are the more experienced nurses or 'leaders' (the most respected individuals) in your workplace presenting themselves. Taking generational variations into consideration and appreciating that people have preferences according to their personality, there IS a way to dress professionally in a clinical practice area. Dress according to the demographic you are caring for—that may be different if you are practicing in a forensics unit, a youth safe-house, a large urban med/surg unit, a client's home, an out-reach needle exchange van, or a geriatric rehabilitation unit.

- ✓ THINK about the care population and how YOU would want a nurse to present themselves if YOU were receiving care. And remember that you can always look to your preceptor/mentor for guidance.

Practice Ethics

- **Remember that you are responsible for the following ethical practice standards:**
  - ✓ Safe, Competent and Ethical Care
  - ✓ Health and Well-being
  - ✓ Choice
  - ✓ Dignity
  - ✓ Confidentiality
  - ✓ Justice
  - ✓ Accountability
  - ✓ Quality practice environments
- If there is an action or inaction that you believe **violates your code of ethics or scope of practice**, STOP… and explore things further. For further information on what YOUR scope of practice is, call or check the website of your local regulatory body or professional organization, or contact them directly. Remember, unethical practice (which includes an unsafe practice environment) threatens patient/client safety.
- If you witness or experience an unethical practice situation, you are obligated to speak to an experienced nurse or your nursing mentor—**if they seem unconcerned while you remain uncomfortable, this does not mean the situation is OK**. Use your critical thinking skills—approach another experienced nurse on the unit, activate the Rapid Response Team or page the Nursing Administrator on call.
- When you are able (likely AFTER things have settled), explore the situation more extensively with your Manager or mentor to discuss how they believe you should respond in the future. This advice also needs to be considered critically as you are responsible to the public through your professional association and union where applicable.
- If you are concerned about the standard of practice or with the state of professional relationships on your unit, and attempts to discuss the issues are not received in kind, contact your professional organization or your union.

Potentially Unsafe Situations for a New Nurse

- The following situations **MAY be considered unsafe** for a newly graduated nurse:
  - ✓ **Floating** to an observation/high dependency unit or critical care unit;
  - ✓ Working in an **observation/high dependency unit** or covering for breaks in these areas without experienced nursing access (**REMEMBER**: While there are FEWER patients to take care of in an observation unit, they are much sicker and require a high level of practice expertise);

- ✓ Caring for patients **beyond the scope of your practice** (i.e. being asked to remove a central line catheter on a general ward/unit) without prior certification;
- ✓ **Taking the lead** in a CODE, administering IV cardiac emergency drugs, or defibrillating (depending on the practice area, you may be certified in *Advanced or Intermediate Life Support* in which case you ARE permitted to defibrillate in appropriate circumstances);
- ✓ **Performing skills that require special certification** but for which you have NOT been certified—if you haven't done a procedure before, ASK a senior nurse if you are required to be certified to perform that procedure or look it up in the nursing care procedural care manual on your unit. If the procedure is not in there, or if it identifies itself as a 'special' procedure, you should be questioning it;
- ✓ It may be difficult for you to admit that you 'cannot handle' a situation—this is totally understandable and we have all experienced that. But **SAFETY of the patient, family and the staff on the unit is PARAMOUNT**. If you are EVER in an UNSAFE PRACTICE ENVIRONMENT or FEEL like you are in an unsafe practice situation, you must: 1) consult an experienced colleague, 2) ask for a change in your assignment, or 3) speak with your nursing unit manager, charge nurse, clinical coordinator or nursing educator;
- ✓ **If you are on nights and feel unsafe**, contact the patient/client care supervisor or nursing administrator on call (through switchboard) or, if this is a physical safety issue, **page security STAT through switchboard**;
- ✓ As a newly graduated nurse, **you should always have immediate access to experienced nursing staff for consultation**—if this support is unavailable, you must bring this to the attention of the nursing unit manager or patient/client care supervisor and an '*unsafe workplace form*' (may be termed variably depending on the institution) should be completed.

Thinking on Your Feet

- During the first few months as a new grad you will find yourself so busy in your new workplace that you will have little time to think about what you are doing and why. You will be satisfied with just surviving the shift and getting all the essential tasks completed. But critically thinking about your nursing actions is very important for quality care and patient/client safety. It is your responsibility to ensure that your practice is as optimal as it can be and to question any decision or action that you feel is inaccurate, insufficient, unethical, illegal or otherwise inappropriate. While at times physicians or experienced nurses may give you the impression that you '*should not have bothered them*', you are ALWAYS doing the right thing when you choose to address an issue you find concerning or confusing.
- To be able to think on your feet, try these tips:

  ✓ Several times throughout the day, find a quiet place, out of the hallway and away from the central work area to review your to-do lists, your worksheets, care plans, clinical or situational assessments.

  ✓ Think about each client's or community's overall status—does what you are seeing, thinking, hearing (or smelling☺) make sense? Is there anything you feel uncomfortable about or have a funny feeling about? If there is, DON'T IGNORE IT. Talk to a more experienced nurse or a physician about your concerns. Pursue the issue until you feel better about it, but above all TRUST YOUR INSTINCTS! They are rarely wrong!!!

  ✓ When you sit down to document your practice, try to go to a quiet corner or another room away from distractions. The time you take to document your assessments, interventions, evaluations and overall findings from your practice is a good time to think about what you have done that day and how effective it has been for the challenges faced by those under your care.

  ✓ Constantly reflect on your practice AS you are practicing—ask yourself repeatedly, '*is there anything I could be missing or may have overlooked?*' Once again, if you have any questions or concerns, tell someone. Everyone will be safer if you address an issue that, in the end, is nothing serious. But ignoring a problem that turns out to be something serious can put the situation, and those you are caring for, at risk. As you practice more, your judgment of what is significant will improve.

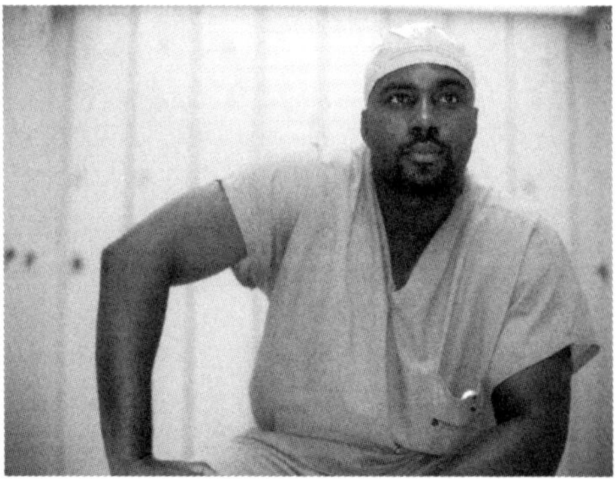

  ✓ If your day is crazy busy and you

find yourself overwhelmed—TAKE A TIME OUT. If necessary, forward your phone to another area, tell the nurse you are working with that you need a minute to gather your thoughts, or ask someone if they can cover your phone and, if in acute-care, your patient/client call bells for about 10 minutes. Go to a quiet place to collect your thoughts and calm yourself down. Unless it is an emergency, whatever is needed can wait the 10 minutes you need to collect your thoughts—you will refocus and be MUCH MORE EFFECTIVE.

✓ Remember that your years of school have prepared you to think critically—while this takes getting used to, your capacity for critical reflection WHILE you work will consistently improve if you 'exercise' that thinking. It is your capacity to think deeply and broadly about each nursing action, interaction and clinical patient/client situation, and to act on that thinking in a way that optimizes the care you give, that sets you apart from other disciplines and caregivers.

✓ Use the SBAR format (see Appendix XII) for identifying, describing and then addressing issues and challenges you have in the workplace—at the end of this Appendix, I have added a decision-making tool that I created for my students doing their senior nursing practicum. See if it helps YOU!

Reaching Out

- As a new grad, you need to be able to ask for help when you need it and admit when you are overwhelmed or over your head. It is not only a safety issue for your patients, it is a SANITY issue for YOU! There are several ways to reach out:

✓ Collaborate with your nursing partner (RN/LPN/RPN/Enrolled Nurse) immediately after your workday starts. Decide who should do what with whom and start working. Meet several times each working shift/day as a 'unit' or 'team' (if there are other allied healthcare practitioners working with you) to regroup; determine how each person's workload is evolving, what has changed and reconfigure the workload/roles/responsibilities as needed.

✓ Delegate tasks to other health care personnel (ward aides, nursing aides or assistants, clerical staff, housekeeping) and remember that we are ALL here to work TOGETHER—no nurse is an island.

✓ Inform your charge nurse or clinical coordinator that you are very busy and need extra help. If you need help IN A HURRY, yell, or pull the call bell cord out of the wall (most patient/client response systems are organized this way to prevent damage to the communications system if the cord is attached to the bed). Pulling the call bell cord out of the wall will set off an alarm and you WILL get help!

✓ Inform your Manager if your workload is overwhelming you and ask for assistance. But BE SPECIFIC ('*I need someone to demonstrate how to hold this child*' OR '*I need someone from the Head Office [of the industry plant where I am the occupational health nurse] to come to [city] and spend a week with me'* OR *'I need someone to discharge this patient' OR 'Can I have someone to do my 1000 vitals?'*). Remember that this is not a one-way street and someday you will be in the position to help your fellow colleagues who are also busy—what goes around comes around.

- ✓ Contact us at *Nursing The Future* (go online to www.nursingthefuture.ca) or write us at newgraduates@nursingthefuture.ca and we will organize to teleconference, speak with your colleagues and students, or give a presentation in your province/state/territory about professional role transition.
- ✓ If you have questions or need assistance with a clinical issue or procedure, speak to your preceptor/mentor, charge nurse, clinical nurse educator or another experienced staff member.
- ✓ BE PERSISTENT—sometimes you may feel as though your requests are not received as openly as you would like. This likely has more to do with the situation than it has to do with YOU.

CRITICALLY REFLECTIVE APPROACH TO PRACTICE

DATA

ASSESS — Has it changed? Is this normal for person/family/community? — ASSESS

LOOK AT/TOUCH/CONNECT WITH THE PATIENT/FAMILY/COMMUNITY BEFORE YOU DO ANYTHING ELSE

UNSTABLE | **STABLE**

TRUST YOUR JUDGEMENT !!
Don't do anything that doesn't feel right!
Pursue an ANSWER that satisfies you!

RED

- **Life threatening for patient/family**
- **Community is at IMMEDIATE RISK (i.e. fire, shooter)**
- **Alert** senior colleague – **CALL OUT**, pull call bell cord out of wall
- Press **CODE BUTTON, DIAL 911**
- **Page/Call** the NP/Physician/Administrator on Call

- Assess your patient/family/community
- Look at all prior documents – history and progress notes
- Look in the Medication Administration Record
- Read the care plan/community plans
- Access emergency plans
- Read your reference texts/doc/literature
- Ask a colleague their opinion
- Talk with the NP/MD/Nurse Leader/MD House Officer/ER Response Team

YELLOW

- **Concerned but situation stable**
- **Consider** *Critical/ER/Rapid Response Team*
- **Think—Connect—Collaborate—Act**
- **Connect with your nursing practice partner**

What is causing this?

- Is it part of a current situation/diagnosis?
  - Is this to be expected?
- Is it part of a past history/previous event?
  - Has this happened before? When? Why?
- Is it something we are doing/have done?
  - Medications? Intervention?
  - Treatments? A complication of?
  - Procedure?
- Is it something we are **NOT** doing?
  - Are we missing something?
  - Do we need a consultation?

ACT

Appendix XIV

Conflict Management in the Workplace

- Nurses work closely with many different types of people, so conflict is bound to occur. It is most often a result of the inability to express one's perspective or to FEEL that we are being heard; in other words, CONFLICT IS OFTEN ABOUT POOR COMMUNICATION.
- The challenges to communication may occur with your co-workers, patients, families or even the community leaders you deal with. It is important to recognize that conflict is NOT ALWAYS BAD! When dealt with effectively, conflict and the process of resolving it can result in an even greater understanding between people than existed before the conflict took place.
- Having said that, addressing and dealing with conflict quickly is critical—if ignored or handled ineffectively, conflict can damage interpersonal relationships, reduce workplace morale and productivity, and ultimately negatively impact on nursing practice and the quality of care.
- Remember, it isn't realistic to think that you will be 'liked' or that you will 'like' everyone you work with. Resolving conflict is not about maintaining friendships, but about finding ways of working together to deliver the best possible care you can.

How do I manage conflict in my workplace?

- There are numerous ways to manage conflict in the workplace: you can avoid it, accommodate it, compromise, or collaborate to resolve it. Whenever you are in conflict, there are always two perspectives—YOURS and THEIRS.
- Conflict resolution in any situation is about FINDING A THIRD PERSPECTIVE. You AND the other person(s) need to find MIDDLE GROUND where all perspectives are respected, honored and considered.

1) Avoiding

- Ignoring, withdrawing and/or suppressing thoughts and/or feelings
- Uses
  - ✓ In front of a patient/client and/or their family
  - ✓ If you lack time or an appropriate place to discuss the issue
  - ✓ As a 'cool-down' mechanism
  - ✓ When the consequences of confronting the issue outweigh the consequences of avoiding the issue
  - ✓ Issues of relative unimportance (but then again, unimportant to whom…)
- Advantages
  - ✓ As a short-term solution for complex issues
  - ✓ Provides time to think about the issue and devise a plan of action
  - ✓ Maintains the status quo

- Disadvantages
  - ✓ Issue does not get resolved
  - ✓ Stress and further conflict may ensue
  - ✓ Person who utilized avoidance may be taken advantage of

2) Accommodating

- One individual/group sacrifices their own needs and concerns to satisfy or appease another
- Uses
  - ✓ When the person accommodating admits they were wrong
  - ✓ When the issue is of more importance to one person than another
  - ✓ To achieve positive regard (i.e. to get 'in the good books' of someone)
  - ✓ To build status and credit for use at a later time
- Advantages
  - ✓ Resolves the conflict with little aggression and hostility
- Disadvantages
  - ✓ Self-sacrificing
  - ✓ Can build anger and resentment in accommodator

3) Compromising

- The ability to set aside difference, analyze both perspectives and derive a satisfactory solution. Sacrifice by one or both parties is usually involved
- Uses
  - ✓ Has the potential to solve almost any dispute, large or small
- Advantages
  - ✓ Issue resolution: attainment of closure on the issue
  - ✓ Shows cooperation and willingness to be a team player on your part
  - ✓ Demonstrates that you have concern for others' needs and feelings
- Disadvantages
  - ✓ Not useful unless both parties are willing to initiate and participate in the compromise
  - ✓ Each side sacrifices some of what they want

4) Collaborating

- All parties work together, merge insights and create a 'common' solution
- Uses
  - ✓ Dealing with unfamiliar circumstances
  - ✓ Political or high-profile decisions
  - ✓ Complex conflicts with multiple parties involved

- Advantages
  - ✓ Win-Win; no one has to sacrifice
  - ✓ Greater understanding between parties
  - ✓ Viewing multiple perspectives facilitates more informed decisions
  - ✓ Persons involved develop a commitment to change
  - ✓ Disperses responsibility and risk taking evenly
  - ✓ Provides long-term solutions

- Disadvantages
  - ✓ Time consuming
  - ✓ Complicated

Dealing With a Bully

- Workplace civility means being respectful, sensitive and considerate of other employees and colleagues[1].
- BULLYING is not only something that happens in the schoolyard—it CAN and DOES happen in the nursing work place (sad to say…).
- Nurses can be bullied by other nurses, nursing managers, physicians, families or patients.
- Most workplaces generally have a ZERO TOLERANCE FOR ABUSE and if they don't, THEY SHOULD.
- Harassment in your work environment is ***unacceptable,*** but intimidation of new nurses in the professional workplace continues to be TOO COMMON!! While we all know that the nursing workplace is intense, frequently changing and BUSY, this is ALL THE MORE REASON for us to work together collaboratively, respectfully and collegially—we need each other in the workplace.
- Some reasons why new nurses remain silent, or do not SPEAK OUT to STOP bullying behavior are listed here:

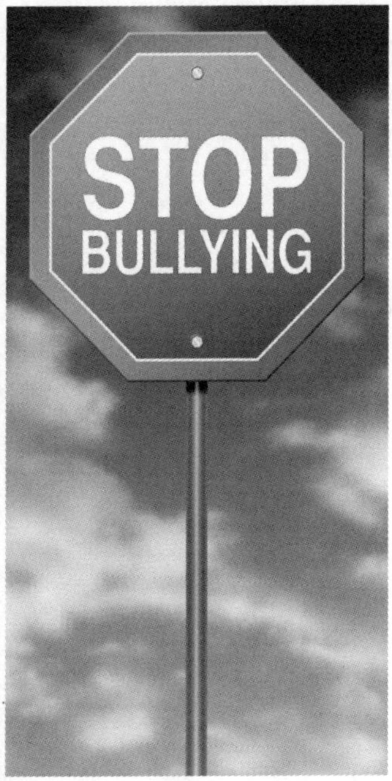

✓ I am already stressed enough—I can't deal with this;
✓ Maybe they just meant it as a joke—a little 'black' humor;
✓ I probably gave them good reason—I feel so inept right now;
✓ I can't really judge—I am sure they have their reasons for treating me this way;
✓ I'm not really sure what 'bullying' behavior is—what if they are just having a 'bad day'?;
✓ I think it's just a personality conflict between us;
✓ This is NOT my fight;
✓ He/She is normally such a nice person—I must have done something to anger them;
✓ If I say something, they'll know it was me and it will get worse;
✓ I'll never be accepted here if I make a big deal about this;
✓ I could lose my job if I speak out—what if the manager likes them?;
✓ Nothing ever happens when you say something anyway, so why bother?

---

[1]This document was created with the support of the *Nova Scotia Government Employees Union in Canada*. I am entirely grateful for their permission to use the '*Working Towards Bully-Free Workplaces*' participant workbook (2010) as I developed the tools and content of this Appendix. See www.nsgeu.ca/education for more information.

Literature on bullying in the workplace speaks about **MASTER SUPPRESSION TECHNIQUES** that bullies use to torment their victims:

1. Invisibility/Objectification

- ✓ To make you 'invisible' is to silence or otherwise *marginalize* you by ignoring or discounting what you say and do.
- ✓ To 'objectify' is to refer to you as a *concrete* or *separate object* for the purpose of scrutinizing you objectively and allows the bully to distance themselves from their oppressive behavior.
- ✓ **FOR EXAMPLE**:
  - i. The bully takes something you have said as if it was their own idea, or speaks OVER you (doesn't allow you to have a voice).
  - ii. When it is your turn to speak, people start to talk to each other, browse through their papers, essentially ignoring you.
  - iii. When you arrive at coffee, no one speaks to you or they choose not to 'include' you in 'their' conversation.
  - iv. "*These new grads are clueless aren't they*" (said within earshot of you).
  - v. "*Yeah, here comes our little 'baby nurse'*" OR "*Sorry (sarcasm), did you say something? (laughter)*" OR "*Whatever*" OR "*Go get me a real nurse.*"

2. Ridiculing

- ✓ In a manipulative way, the bully tries to portray you as 'foolish', 'stupid' or otherwise inadequate/incompetent.
- ✓ Spreading rumors about you (talking about you behind your back).
- ✓ **FOR EXAMPLE**:
  - i. When making an accusation of wrongdoing against someone, you are being told that you look cute when you're angry.
  - ii. The bully laughs at your accent or compares you to a character in a humorous TV show.
  - iii. "*You don't know that? What did they teach you in school anyway?*" OR "*They must have been pretty desperate when they hired YOU*" OR "*I need that NOW, not next week!*" OR "*Did you see Janet's (new grad) little nursing pin (laughter). She actually wears it—isn't that hilarious! Oh, to be so young and think 'Look at me, I'm going to change the world'…*"

3. Withholding Information

- ✓ Excluding you from the decision-making process around your client/patient/community, or knowingly not sharing information so as to make you less able to make a competent decision or judgment about your situation.

✓ **FOR EXAMPLE**:

i. Your colleagues have a meeting that concerns you or your patients/clients without inviting you.

ii. When expressing frustration about something the bully is doing or a behavior they are demonstrating, your colleague responds with the statement, "*So this aggression of yours, is that just a guy thing?*"

iii. Decisions that impact you are made, not in a collegial conference or gathering where everyone is present, but at a social event during the evening, and only some colleagues have been invited.

iv. While you are on a break, your patient/client requests something for pain but the nurse 'covering' for you <u>chooses</u> not to tell you. The patient/client feels frustrated at YOU because they believe you are neglecting them (this must always be distinguished from a colleague 'forgetting' to give you clinical information about your patient/client and can usually be discerned by the frequency of missing information and other behavior indicative of bullying).

4. Double Bind Situations

✓ Punishing or belittling your actions, regardless of WHAT you do.

✓ **FOR EXAMPLE**:

i. When you do your work effectively (focus on quality), you receive complaints for being too slow. When you do your work efficiently (focus on expediency), you are critiqued for not providing good care.

ii. "*You sure took a long time with that family. You know, this is the 'real world' and you don't have time to sit around 'bonding' with your patient/clients*" OR "*If you cry every time someone dies, you'll never make it here—you'll get used to it*" OR "*Wait until you've been here awhile—we'll work that compassion and enthusiasm right out of you.*"

5. Blaming and Shaming

✓ Embarrassing you, or insinuating that you are to blame for the situation (likely ANY and ALL situations), regardless of the bully's contribution to it.

✓ **FOR EXAMPLE**:

i. You inform your Manager that ____ is sexually harassing you, but are told it is your fault since you dress provocatively.

ii. "*If you knew what you were doing, I wouldn't have to correct you all the time*" OR "*I can't believe you did that! Were you even thinking?*"

6. Force or the Threat of Force

- ✓ Approaching you physically and entering personal space that makes you feel uncomfortable or 'threatened'.
- ✓ Raising a hand towards you in threat, throwing an object at you or grabbing your arm.
- ✓ Verbally threatening you or sending offensive/threatening emails/blogs/texts (ALWAYS keep a record of these for future reference).
- ✓ **FOR EXAMPLE**:
  i. "*If you weren't a woman, I'd....*" OR "*One more time and I swear....*"

- If YOU are a victim of bullying or you WITNESS a colleague being bullied, you should:

  - ✓ **DOCUMENT** your experience immediately:
    - o Date, time, location
    - o Who was involved
    - o What was the situation or event (remember to record words spoken, tone of voice, behaviors and gestures)
    - o Describe what happened (document the impact on doing your job or personal impact)
    - o What resolution are you seeking (what would restore dignity and respect to your work experience);
  - ✓ **Speak to friends or colleagues** to gain advice and support;
  - ✓ **Reach out** to a more experienced nurse in the workplace that you trust;
  - ✓ **Journal** (if this is a more 'public' blog, be careful NOT to disclose location, names or specific incidents publicly—you could be liable for character defamation);
  - ✓ **Reflect** on your Nursing Association Standards, Competencies and Code of Ethics as well as your Employee/Union Rights;
  - ✓ **Talk to the bully if you can**. Bullying, though ALWAYS unacceptable, may not be *deliberate*. If you can, talk to the person in question as they may not realize how their behavior has been affecting you. Work out what to say beforehand. Describe what has been happening and why you object to it. Stay calm and be respectful;
  - ✓ If you don't want to talk to them yourself, *ask someone the bully trusts to do so for you* or even have a colleague nearby/within earshot when you speak with this individual;
  - ✓ **Speak to someone** about how you might first deal with the problem *informally* (perhaps an employee or union representative, someone in the Human Resources Department, your Manager or Supervisor);
  - ✓ **Some employers have specially trained staff to help with bullying** and harassment problems. **CONTACT** your workplace *Employee Assistance Program* (they may have a *Harassment Adviser*), or visit the *Occupational Health Nurse*;
  - ✓ If the bullying is **affecting your health**, visit your doctor;
  - ✓ **Making a formal complaint** is the next step if you can't solve the problem informally. To do this you must follow your employer's/union grievance procedure;

- ✓ **IF the bully is your Manager** and the grievance procedure says that the Manager is the individual you should speak to about bullying, make the complaint in writing to that Manager and ask, within the complaint, to have your concerns further addressed by another Manager. If that doesn't happen, or isn't possible, send a COPY of the complaint to the individual TO WHOM your Manager reports, to the Human Resource Department department or to your Union Representative;
- ✓ **If you think that making a complaint will cause further bullying** or harassment, you don't need to follow normal grievance procedures. In cases like this, you can take legal action if you wish;
- ✓ If, after following normal procedures, **nothing is done to stop the bullying** behavior, you can think about legal action. Get professional advice before taking this step;
- ✓ **If you have left your job because of bullying**, you might be able to claim unfair 'constructive' dismissal. This can be difficult to prove, so it is important to get advice from a specialist lawyer or other professional.

Am I Being Bullied At Work?[2]

Is there someone I work with who repeatedly:	NEVER	RARELY	SOMETIMES	OFTEN
1. **Yells** at me, especially in front of others	1	2	3	4
2. **Ignores** me, either by not speaking to me in the workplace or not including me in workplace socializing; and/or not returning my phone calls or emails	1	2	3	4
3. **Dismisses** what I'm saying or puts me down either alone or in the presence of others	1	2	3	4
4. **Sabotages** me or makes me look foolish by withholding information and trying to make me look incompetent	1	2	3	4
5. **Gossips** or spreads rumors about me	1	2	3	4
6. Frequently **treats me like I'm incompetent**	1	2	3	4
7. **Blames** and criticizes me to embarrass or humiliate me	1	2	3	4
8. Tries to **intimidate** me by interrupting, contradicting, or undermining me or my work	1	2	3	4
9. Gives me the **silent treatment** but makes **rude gestures** (e.g. eye rolling, 'tsking', or communicating non-verbally to others)	1	2	3	4
10. **Teases**, ridicules, insults, or plays tricks on me to embarrass me in front of others	1	2	3	4
11. Always insists on getting their own way, never **considers my point of view** and never apologizes	1	2	3	4
12. **Takes credit or fails to give credit** for ideas or work	1	2	3	4

Add up the numbers for a possible total score of 48.

14 or below: you might want to consider how to address incidents of workplace incivility. If you are experiencing discomfort because of a work situation involving another person, conflict resolution or assertiveness training may help you.
15 to 26: there are indications of a repeated and persistent pattern of behavior. Talk to someone you trust to consider what action may be required.
26 or above: consider the health affects that you may be experiencing (physical, emotional, behavioral) from this bullying situation and talk to someone who can help you decide on appropriate action.

[2]Copyright permission received December, 2011 from the *Nova Scotia Government and General Employees Union.*

Health Effects of Bullying[3]

Check off those symptoms that you feel you may be experiencing as a result of a workplace bullying situation. If you find yourself checking off 'sometimes' to 'often', it is suggested that you discuss your findings with your family practitioner, *Employee Assistance Program*, or other trusted individual who can help you make some decisions about what you can do.

Psychological & Emotional impact		NEVER	RARELY	SOMETIMES	OFTEN
1.	Self-blame				
2.	Rumination, loss of sleep and nightmares				
3.	Loss of sense of humor				
4.	Loss of confidence and self-esteem				
5.	Severe anxiety				
6.	Fear				
7.	Panic attacks				
8.	Despair				
9.	Feelings of isolation				
10.	Becoming over-emotional, or easily losing control over my emotions				
11.	Feelings of powerlessness				
12.	Feelings of confusion				
13.	Forgetfulness				
14.	Hypersensitivity				
15.	Loss of concentration				
Behavioral changes/experience		**NEVER**	**RARELY**	**SOMETIMES**	**OFTEN**
1.	Crying				
2.	Irritability				
3.	Feeling vengeful				
4.	Nervousness				
5.	Shortened attention span				
6.	Ill health				
7.	Changes in sleeping, eating and work patterns				
8.	Loss of libido				
9.	Becoming obsessive				
10.	Memory lapses				
11.	Clumsiness				
12.	Withdrawal				
13.	Excessive focus on work or co-workers				
14.	Exhaustion				

[3]Copyright permission received December, 2011 from the *Nova Scotia Government and General Employees Union.*

15.	More prone to making mistakes, feeling less reliable at work				
16.	Drinking more alcohol/increasing medication use				
17.	Happier on days off but becoming edgy the night before going back to work				
Physical symptoms as a result of bullying		**NEVER**	**RARELY**	**SOMETIMES**	**OFTEN**
1.	Lowered resilience, taking longer to bounce back				
2.	Panic attacks on approaching the workplace or bully/s				
3.	Depression				
4.	Post Traumatic Stress Disorder (PTSD)				
5.	Betrayal Trauma Stress Disorder (BTSD)				
6.	Headaches and migraines				
7.	Sweating or shaking				
8.	Stomach and bowel problems				
9.	Raised blood pressure				
10.	Muscle spasm				
11.	Back pain and other chronic pain				
12.	Lack of energy				
13.	Loss of appetite				
14.	Nausea and vomiting				
15.	Skin rashes				
16.	Hyper-arousal				
17.	Hypersensitivity to external environments				
18.	Suicidal ideation				
19.	Suicide attempt				

Communicating With Physicians

- Let's clear the air—most physicians are great to work with. And you know what....THEY ARE HUMAN TOO!!!! They appreciate and value the role of the nurse and perceive the relationship between nurse and physician as highly complementary and collaborative.
- While you may not have had a lot of 'practice' speaking with physicians while you were a student, you do this all the time as a new graduate and IT WILL GET EASIER EACH TIME.
- A *Jursi, Intern* or even a *Resident* seems to be received somewhat differently than an *Attending Physician, House Officer, Staff Physician*, or even a *Fellow*[1]. Perhaps this is because the former are still considered 'students', and therefore on a more equal footing to the new nursing graduate with respect to their knowledge and experience in the 'real' world.
- You may be initially nervous at the thought of having to communicate with physicians—this is normal. But with the trend toward interdisciplinary education we hope to change that!
- Here are some strategies for you to consider when planning to communicate with your medical colleagues (AGAIN, use the SBAR Framework recommended in Appendix XII):

  ✓ Do you have all the information you need to present the issue over the phone?
  ✓ Have you consulted an experienced nurse to discuss the situation you are calling about? Particularly on nights, you will be extra nervous about contacting a physician, as you will likely wake this individual up! Be sure to connect with an experienced nurse before you call, just to help you prepare and boost your confidence.
  ✓ Do you know what it is you want from this physician? Do you have a sense of the orders you are expecting? This will save you a follow-up call—using the SBAR, write down what you want before you call!
  ✓ A change in the condition of your patient/client that threatens their health is an absolute indicator for physician communication—it is better to err on the side of caution!!!!

We do NOT Tolerate Disrespectful Behavior!

- On occasion, the new graduate will experience communication with a colleague (physician, nurse colleague, allied health practitioner or support staff) that is condescending, disrespectful or rude. In the rare situation (often a highly emotionally charged situation), one can understand a person being 'upset' or 'short'. But the use of profanity or professional slander is ABSOLUTELY UNACCEPTABLE!
- While we all have '*bad days*', it is expected that we will treat each other with professional respect and ethical consideration. Behavior of an inappropriate nature (i.e. throwing instruments in the Operating Room, or swearing at a nurse) must be reported to the

[1] *Fellows* are practicing physicians who have chosen to advance their level of specialty training. They are considered in the same realm, or at the same level as *Attending* or *Practicing Physicians*.

Manager, Clinical Educator and the professional association or union—all of the individuals representing these professional and regulatory organizations are available to you depending on the situation and your comfort level. Communications about relational ethics should be held in strict confidence.

Responding to Unprofessional Behavior

The following suggestions might help you as you consider your response to unprofessional behavior from a colleague:

- ✓ "*Your tone suggests that you are angry—is there something I have said to upset you?*"
- ✓ "*I have contacted you to report a clinical concern I have for your patient—I appreciate your professional consideration.*"
- ✓ "*I will make a note of your concerns for my Nursing Manager.*"
- ✓ "*Your* 'name the behaviour' *(i.e. swearing/yelling/sarcasm) is uncalled for and unprofessional—while I understand that you may be upset, I cannot accept that behaviour.*"
- ✓ If the situation is not urgent, you can say "*Please call me back when you have calmed down and wish to discuss this professionally.*" Contact the Nursing Manager, Charge Nurse, or Nursing Administrator-on-call to deal with the situation.

CODES and Rapid Response Teams

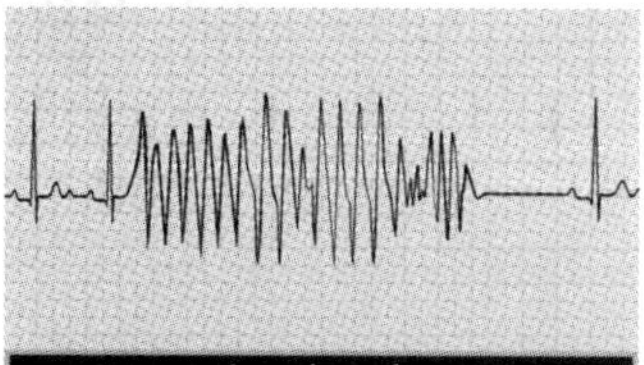

Ventricular tachycardia to sinus rhythm background

- Let's be honest—there is no such a thing as an EASY CODE. The problem with codes is that they are always different, always stressful and always unpredictable. Expect that you will be scared, shaky, unsure and that you will forget something or do something out of sequence—MOST NURSES FEEL THIS WAY unless they deal with codes on a day-to-day basis.
- **Advanced Cardiac Life Support (ACLS)** or **Intermediate Life Support** training will assist you to know what to do in the event of a code situation—they run you through '*megacodes*' that simulate the 'real life' situation. Ask your manager to support you to take either of these courses; they are likely offered through your institution or through the local community colleges.
- If you are unable to access these courses, ask that the clinical educator or manager organize a '*mock code*' for you, and for the other nurses on the ward—make sure that you get a chance to 'come upon' the situation and practice what you would do.

Approaching the Situation

✓ If you think something does not LOOK, SMELL, FEEL or SOUND right

GO DIRECTLY TO THE PATIENT

✓ **DO NOT PRESS THE CODE BUTTON YET**
✓ **ASSESS** the patient
✓ **Open their airway** by pulling their jaw forward and tipping their head back—are they breathing? Put your ear near their mouth and watch their chest.
- **Feel for their carotid pulse**—Do they have a pulse (FEEL FOR 5 SECONDS!!!!)

IF THE PATIENT

DOES NOT HAVE A PULSE

or

THEY ARE NOT BREATHING

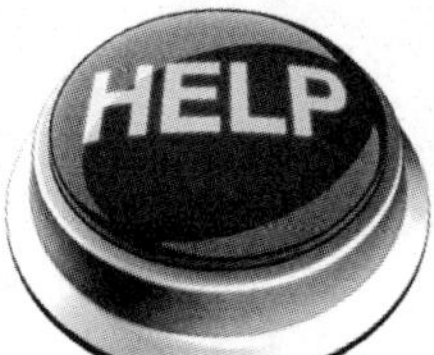

PUSH THE CODE BUTTON ON THE WALL

OR

PULL THE PATIENT CALL BUTTON/CORD OUT OF THE WALL

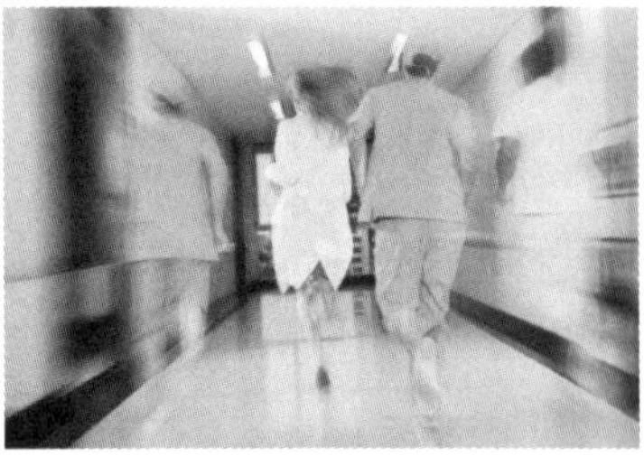

- ✓ **Holler out for help**—your colleagues will come running!
- ✓ When the code **cart arrives** OR if you have a crash cart ON YOUR UNIT

GRAB THE BOARD FROM BEHIND THE CRASH CART PLACE IT UNDER THE CHEST OF THE PATIENT

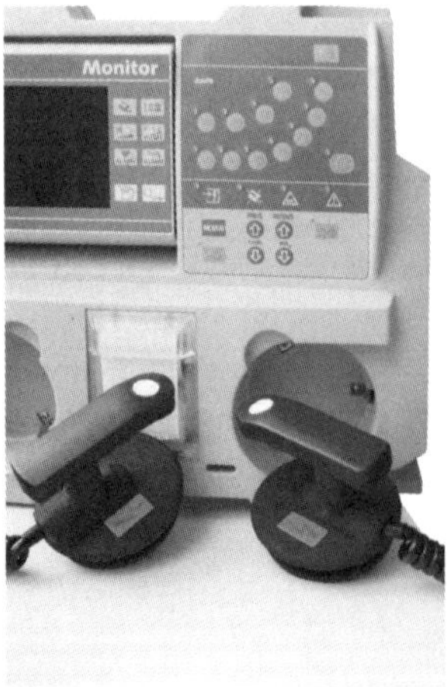

- ✓ If you are uncomfortable knowing what to do in a code, **BE THE RECORDING NURSE** or **DO CPR**.
- ✓ If you are taking on the role of recorder, remember to holler out a review of all that has been done every 5 minutes (i.e. meds given, tests and procedures done, etc.)

REMEMBER

- ✓ **ASSESS** THE PATIENT
- ✓ **ACTIVATE** CODE STATUS
- ✓ **START** CPR
- ✓ **CART ARRIVES**—PUT THE BOARD UNDER PATIENT
- ✓ **RECORD** AND REVIEW

Rapid Response Teams

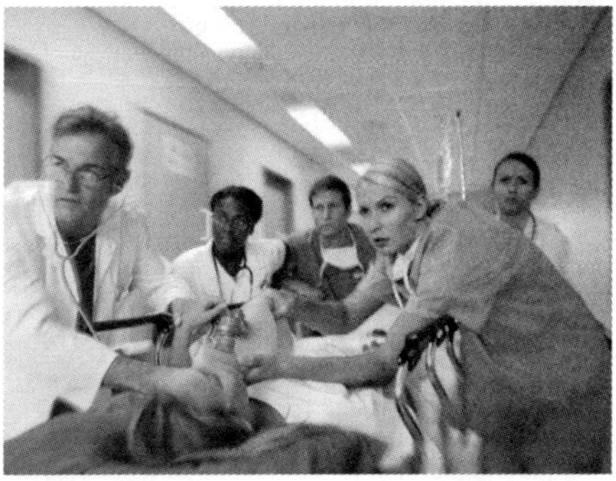

WHAT is a Rapid Response Team[1]?

A *Rapid Response Team* is an organized team of emergency healthcare professionals whose primary role is to respond to, assess and intervene in the urgent/emergent care of a patient.

WHAT Is the Role of the Rapid Response Team (RRT)[2]?

- Assess
- Stabilize
- Assist with communication
- Educate and support
- Assist with transfer, if necessary
- Follow-up of discharged patients

WHO Can Activate the RRT?

- Any staff member (nurse, physical therapist, respiratory therapist, physician) who is worried about the patient
- Family members (institution specific)

WHEN Do I Activate the RRT?

- Acute change in heart rate <40 or >130 bpm
- Acute change in systolic blood pressure <90 mmHg
- Acute change in respiratory rate <8 or >28 per min
- Acute change in saturation <90% despite O2

[1]Shapiro, S.E., Donaldson, N.E., & Scott, M.B. (2010). Rapid response teams: Seen through the eyes of the nurse. *American Journal of Nursing, 110*(6), Retrieved January 10, 2012 from http://www.nursingcenter.com/pdf.asp?AID=1018846

[2]McFarlan, S.J., & Hensley, S. (2007). Implications and outcomes of a rapid response team. *Journal of Nursing Care Quality, 22*(4), 307-313.

- Acute change in conscious state
- Acute change in urinary output to <50 ml in 4 hours

HOW do I Activate the RRT?

- Your institution will have an RRT Activation protocol
- Generally SOMEONE on the unit has a beeper and it is used to activate the RRT
- The activator dials in the patient's room number
- If not in a patient/client room you dial in YOUR EXTENSION—the RRT will call for a location
- Many hospitals are encouraging families to activate the RRT if desired

WHAT Does the RRT Team Do?

The most common actions are:

- Deliver supplemental oxygen
- Radiographic testing
- Administer fluid bolus
- Start intravenous
- Ventilate (possible intubation)
- Administer cardiac medication

Death of a Patient/Client

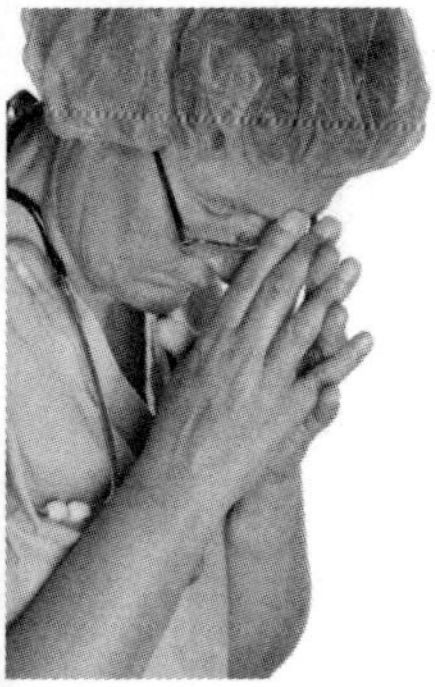

Upon the death of a patient, you may feel a range of emotions—you may feel ANGRY, DEPRESSED, or even DETACHED. All of these feelings are NORMAL grief responses and even nurses experienced in dealing with the dying patient/client feels them.

Find a colleague to speak with about your feelings and know that you might evolve through different stages of feelings as you process the death of your patient. Remember that the death of your patient/client is being experienced by you too!

Coping with Grief

The Nurse

- Because you may have tried to 'control' your feelings while you were IN the situation, you may find yourself overwhelmed by emotion once it is OVER.
- There is nothing inappropriate about sustaining a **CONTROLLED INVOLVEMENT** with a patient/client or family during an intense period of their life—in fact, this can be therapeutic both for you and for them. Remember that it is OK to share yourself with your patient, as long as your sharing has the patient/client and family in the *center*, and is **NOT ABOUT YOU**. If the emotions you are feeling ARE about you (the death of your patient/client reminds you of your own personal loss or the intensity and emotions brought about by the situation motivate overwhelming emotions for you), connect with a colleague, your Manager or Educator. In consultation with them, determine if you need to step away (temporarily) to soothe yourself and gain control over your emotions. If you are unable to do so (**grief is NOT a failure** on your part!), arrange with them to change your assignment. This is not uncommon and the majority of nurses will be overcome with emotion while caring for a patient/client/family or even community at some point in their career. You are a compassionate and caring human being, and your ability and willingness to respond with sadness and empathy to the suffering around you is part of what makes you a good nurse. It is the degree to which you respond, how you respond, the motivations for your response and how able you are to be therapeutic AS you respond that is important for you to determine.
- **Crying with a family** at the bedside of a patient/client is appropriate, as long as your tears fit the situation—sharing grief and sadness over the death of someone's loved one tells them that person mattered and that you are present with them in their experience. The important distinction in this situation is that the family is not there to console the care providers nor should they feel concern for any issues that this death has raised in YOUR life.

- **Reach out to your colleagues** to discuss the emotions that arise for you. Many workplaces have grief counselors or social workers who specialize in grief and who can be made available to assist practitioners significantly affected by the death of a patient/client. If there are extenuating circumstances around a death (i.e. severe trauma, death of infants and children, murders, death of a healthcare provider), trauma specialists (usually psychologists specializing in grief) may be brought in to assist healthcare personnel to deal with their feelings. This is strongly encouraged in workplaces that deal with death more frequently (i.e. palliative care, emergency, critical care, operating room).
- Occupational health nurses within your workplace or the *Employee Assistance Program* are other resources of support should you continue to feel the effects of this loss personally.
- A final comment about the coping of healthcare practitioners in the workplace. It is normal (and often healthy) to use **humor** when dealing with difficult situations—everyone approaches sadness and grief differently. While this may be an appropriate coping mechanism for you, it is important to be sensitive to how the use of humor might be interpreted or received by patients/clients and families—ADOPT THIS APPROACH BEHIND CLOSED DOORS.

The Family

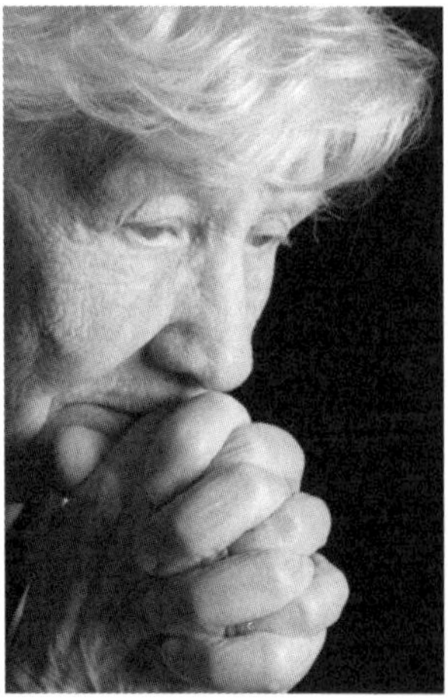

- Involve the family whenever possible—if you feel they can cope with it, encourage them to assist with the care of their loved one. Have them wash, or assist you to wash, feed or just sit with the patient/client.
- When I was a graduate of only 2 years I remember nursing the young victim of a motor vehicle trauma who was dying of multiple injuries. He was the husband of a nurse and together they had two young children. I sensed that she wanted to be close to him—connect with him, so I asked her to help me with his bath. As we worked, we talked....and I learned about *her* life, *their* dreams, and she shared her fears of not being able to go on without him. I left her alone for short periods of time because I knew she needed the space to say goodbye[1]. And while she navigated the miles that separated her past and future lives at warp speed, I monitored his status from the nursing station a few feet away. I am confident that what I did as a nurse in that one night helped this woman begin to process the rest of her life.
- BE FLEXIBLE WITH VISITING HOURS (of course I believe this generally)!
- Ask the family if they would like anyone from spiritual/pastoral care to provide support—

[1]I marvel sometimes at how my years as a nurse have fine tuned my senses (except apparently for the 'selective' hearing my husband tells me I have developed into a fine art), sharpened my instincts, and revealed to me the accuracy of my intuition when it comes to people and situations. Nursing has taught me to trust myself.

if they have a personal spiritual counselor (i.e. minister/pastor/priest), call THEM. It is interesting to reflect back on my own experience with this situation during the death of my father. At my mother's request, we called upon our Greek Orthodox Minister to come and deliver '*Last Rites*' (a tradition of my parents' religion). He arrived in relative pageantry, however solemn, with a tall black *kalimavkion*[2] and a long black outer *cassock*[3], chanting a prayer in Ukrainian (which, despite years of Ukrainian language schooling, I did not understand) over my father's bedside. I personally found this ceremony to be morbid, and it both disconnected me from, and aggravated, my sorrow. While my father was unable to share his perceptions of this experience with us, my mother expressed her gratitude to the minister for his presence and I believe it helped her in her grief. It was an example to me of the diversity in religious and spiritual needs and serves to remind me to stay connected to the patient/client and family's wishes with regard to religious or spiritual matters, regardless of how those beliefs make ME feel.

- Be careful about 'assuming' that families, or even dying patients/clients, WANT spiritual counsel—as my story above alludes to, there are few things as intimate and private as one's spiritual or religious beliefs. Tread carefully on this ground.
- If the family is struggling to cope with the death, you might call in a social worker (most healthcare institutions assign a social worker to a ward/unit or set of practice areas). Alternatively, ask the family as a group to meet with the primary physician or nurse practitioner so that issues of concern can be discussed and clinical expectations (i.e. imminent death) of the patient/client situation can be presented to, or discussed with, the family.
- Ask the family for their advice on certain issues (i.e. "*Is there anything you think 'patient/client name' would want at this point that we are not doing?*")
- Utilize your co-workers to counsel you on how to deal with death as a nurse, to advise you on clinical or family care issues, or to debrief with you as the situation unfolds—this reduces the stress of making decisions and judgments on your own. It would be highly unusual (unless you are alone in a practice area [remote nursing contexts]…which of course I hope you aren't as a new graduate!) for your colleagues not to know exactly what is going on for you in this situation. Nurses always seem to come together during periods of calamity and because you are a new graduate, you will likely have more support during a crisis (a 'formal' one that is) than at any other time in your practice. And so it should be….

[2] The *kalimavkion* is a stiff cylindrical head covering, similar to a stovepipe hat but without a brim. It is worn by monastics or awarded to clergy as a mark of honor. Retrieved January 10, 2012 from http://en.wikipedia.org/wiki/Clerical_clothing

[3] The *cassock*, an item of clerical clothing, is an ankle-length robe worn by clerics of the Eastern Orthodox Church. Retrieved January 10, 2012 from http://en.wikipedia.org/wiki/Cassock

Honoring the Body

- You will need to prepare the patient/client for viewing by the family. Sometimes family are required to come from long distances on short notice so you may be asked to keep the body on the ward/unit until they arrive.
- Viewing the body of a friend or family member in the morgue is usually a distasteful experience, so when you can, allow the family to complete their viewing in the practice area.
- **BEFORE THEY ENTER THE ROOM**, assess both the situation and each individual about to enter the room. Explain the following:
  - ✓ their loved one may feel cool to touch
  - ✓ there may be tubes present and why they cannot be removed
  - ✓ if there is blood, bandages, marks, bruises or wounds that you are unable to cover prepare them for this
  - ✓ Wash the patient's body carefully, removing all evidence of excretions on the bed linen.
  - ✓ Change the gown or cover the patient/client with another sheet if necessary. Comb their hair and close their eyes. If you need to, tape the eyes shut until the family arrives—this will allow the skin to adjust to being pulled over an edematous sclera so that the eyes do not '*half open*' when the tape is removed.
  - ✓ If they do not have too many marks on their arms, pull the arms out from under the sheets and pull the sheets up on to the patient's chest—this allows the family to touch them and hold their hand.
  - ✓ If there is not one already on, put a gown on the patient/client and do it up at the neck. Put a pillow under their head, dim the lights in the room (leave only one over-bed light on) and roll the head of the bed up about 25 degrees. This gives the body a more natural appearance. Lower the bed height to a normal level so that the family has easier access.
  - ✓ If the patient/client has tubes in place (IVs, NGs, catheters) you will need to know if the coroner has mandated a post-mortem PRIOR TO REMOVING THEM (**the coroner makes the decision on removal of any care devices in the case of a mandated post-mortem**).
  - ✓ Put chairs around the bed so that family can visit or pay their respects to the deceased person.
  - ✓ Ask the family about any cultural nuances of post-death care of the body and attend to those particulars BEFORE the viewing.

- Once you have spoken with the family/friends, **go in with them** and assess their response—you may have to hold on to a family member or bring them a chair if they are queasy or feeling faint. Be vigilant.
- It is also VERY IMPORTANT to let the family have time **alone** with the patient/client IF THEY WANT—**ASK THEM**! Remember that the policy and procedure manual will

have instructions on how to care for a deceased patient/client according to protocol if you are not sure how to proceed.

- Always use the deceased person's name when talking to the family. Try to avoid using the term 'body' in place of the patient's name when the family is present.
- A '*coroner's case*' is not the same as a request for a post-mortem examination. A coroner is usually consulted in situations of unexpected death, or any death that occurs within 24 hours of a hospital admission. ALL tubes, drains, and care devices MUST BE LEFT UNTOUCHED. Make sure you consult your policy and procedure manual to determine the institution's criteria for a *Coroner's Case.*
- In the case of a regular post-mortem request (a decision made by either the family or through a collaborative decision between the family and the health-care team), you are permitted to remove tubes, drains and care devices in accordance with your institutional policy.

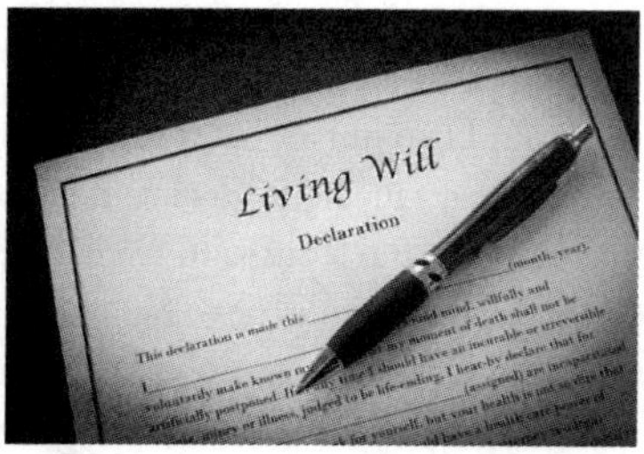

- If the patient/client has open cuts or wounds, you may want to place a dressing over them and ensure you are appropriately protected (i.e. head injuries or blood in the hair can be addressed by wrapping gauze around that part of the head).

Preparing the Body

- You will need to wrap the body and prepare it for delivery to the morgue. BE PREPARED!!!! When you move the body to place it on the plastic wrap sheet, there may be a release of air (sounds like the person is 'letting out a breath'). This is the process of air being expelled from the lungs by virtue of the pressure from the abdominal cavity pushing on the diaphragm during the turn. IT IS NORMAL!
- Each institution will have a standard 'wrap' package—this contains the documentation and the physical materials required to adequately prepare the body for post-mortem or for the funeral home.
- It is customary to roll the patient/client on one side like you were making an occupied bed—then you place half of the plastic sheet under the patient, roll them to the other side and fully extend the sheet under the patient.
- Wrap the remaining sheet around the patient, tying it around the neck and around the ankles—you will use the rope ties provided in the wrap package to secure the plastic sheet. While taping the sheet is not favored by the pathology staff, there are times when the body is too large to be accommodated easily by the wrap and tape assists to secure it in place.
- The morgue will have a special gurney that allows you to 'hide' the fact that you are carrying a body inside it (the body goes 'underneath' the gurney so the 'form' of the body is not visible).
- Once the family has viewed the body, take it to the morgue, sign in, and leave the body with an attendant or in the refrigerated section of the morgue as per the direction of

institutional policy. Deaths often occur at night when there is no attendant, so you will have a unit policy on how to deal with this situation—ask a senior nurse if you are unsure.

Debriefing After a Death or CODE

- Experiencing the rapid decompensation, cardiac arrest or death of a patient/client is never easy—no matter HOW LONG you have been nursing or HOW MANY DEATHS you have witnessed.
- Ask to leave the unit to regroup if you need to—go somewhere private where you can cry (i.e. chapel) or seek out a colleague to talk to about your feelings.
- If you feel traumatized by the death (difficulty refocusing or controlling your emotions), request relief to go home and don't be afraid to speak with your Manager about the situation. I remember having to do that after a young woman died in our critical care unit. I had nursed her for several days but she died of an overwhelming infection for which we were unable to determine a cause. She was 30 years of age and left behind 2 young children and a husband who was clearly struggling to comprehend what was happening. I recall him asking me to remove her wedding ring, which I did with some difficulty because she was so edematous (not uncommon in end-stage sepsis). As though it were a movie playing in slow motion through my mind, I see her husband walking toward me, looking as though he was 'afraid' to come too close. He gingerly held open his hand and I put a single gold wedding band in his palm. Like it was yesterday, I remember him looking at it with utter confusion and disbelief, then looking up at me, then looking back at the ring.... as though doing so might bring some insight into, or awaken him from, the nightmare that surrounded him. We never spoke. After a few moments he turned and walked away. I wept for a while in my now quiet corner of the unit. Then I went home early. Everyone understood because many of us have been there.
- It is important NOT to BLAME YOURSELF when a patient/client dies! Assuming that you have given all you can for as long as you can to whomever you care for, there are some things you simply can't stop, change or prevent.
- IF you feel there was something that could have been done and wasn't, that is a discussion you should have with your Manager, the Nurse Practitioner or the patient's Primary Care Physician.
- If you feel you are NOT COPING with a clinical event with which you were directly or indirectly involved, I encourage you to let your supervisor or educator know or CONTACT YOUR *Employee Assistance Program*—they are there to assist you at any time and will do so CONFIDENTIALLY if that is your preference.
- For many years I worked as a critical care nurse, coordinated several heart and lung transplant programs and was responsible for the clinical management of hundreds of multiple-organ donors at centres throughout Canada and the United States. Then, one day, my 'motor' just up and stopped!! I could NOT get it started again....YUP, I had burned out BIG TIME. In retrospect, it is clear to me that I simply could not see all that I had seen, and do all that I had done for all those years, without eventually experiencing

some 'push back'. As I reflected on what had preceded this 'set back', I realized that in all my years as a critical care trauma, cardiac and transplant nurse, I was NEVER debriefed about the horrific tragedies I witnessed. Nor did I seek counseling for what was clearly expressing itself as *Post-Traumatic Stress Disorder*[4] (PTSD) until I was well into my decline. As the saying goes, those were the 'old' days and I believe (and certainly HOPE) that it IS different now.

Dealing With Families in Crisis

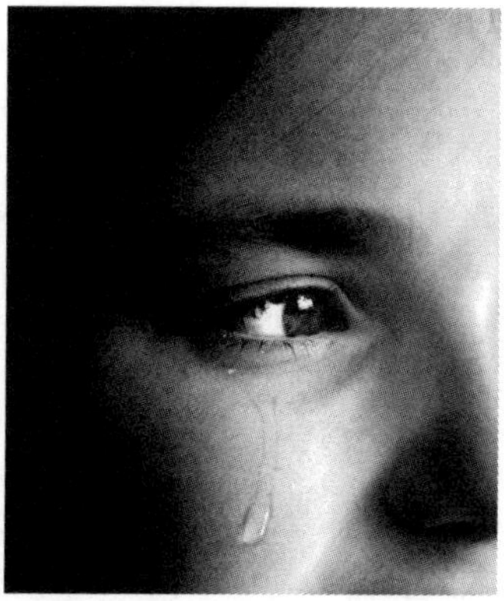

- Distraught families really want to be heard—SO LISTEN!!! You DON'T have to necessarily SOLVE their problem (unless of course you can), because often times you CAN'T. Let them talk and respond with, "*I appreciate/understand/can see that you are upset*" OR "*You have every right to feel the way you do.*"
- Take the distraught individual/group to a quiet, preferably isolated room (multi-purpose room, quiet room, report room, lounge) where you can sit down with them. Get THEM to talk while YOU listen.
- Ask them: 1) how they are feeling, 2) what it is that is most upsetting them, and 3) what you can do to help.

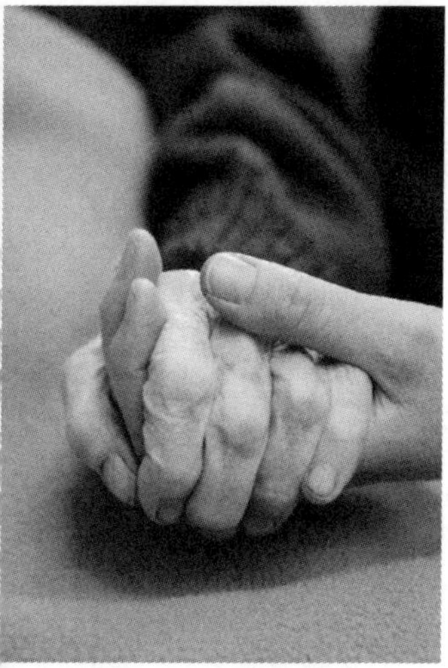

- When possible, ask them if there is another family member you might call to support them—if one is available, encourage them to accompany you into the room. Remember that they will usually trust their family or friends over you—know the situation and the players so you will know WHEN, HOW and through WHOM you will be able to diffuse the volatility that often comes with trauma, grief, stress and sleeplessness (all contextual elements of families in crisis).
- If at all possible, don't make 'promises' to family members. Using phrases such as "*I will see what I can do*" OR "*I am going to follow-up on that/find out and get back to you*" OR "*I will contact_____to find out what options we have*" are acceptable ways of offering hope and optimism without instilling false security.
- Remember that an experienced nurse, your Manager or Clinical Nurse Educator are good resources in situations you feel have gone beyond your experience or comfort level.

[4]See http://www.ncbi.nlm.nih.gov/pubmedhealth/PMH0001923/

Appendix XIX

Nursing In Rural and Remote Areas[1]

The decision to take a nursing post in a rural or remote (RR) practice area as a new graduate is as critical as it is complex. The primary reasons most nurses choose this practice setting are:

1) The nurse or their partner were born and/or raised there and want to return 'home' to provide care for their community.
2) The nurse completed a practicum in a RR community and the setting appears to be consistent with their personal characteristics, attributes and lifestyle preferences.

The most common reasons nurses STAY in a RR practice setting are: 1) the need for professional services in northern communities, 2) the career opportunities that exist for both the nurse and their partner, 3) the resonance of a rural lifestyle with their personal lifestyle preferences, and 3) the potential for clinical practice growth within a community-based and collaborative multidisciplinary approach to care.

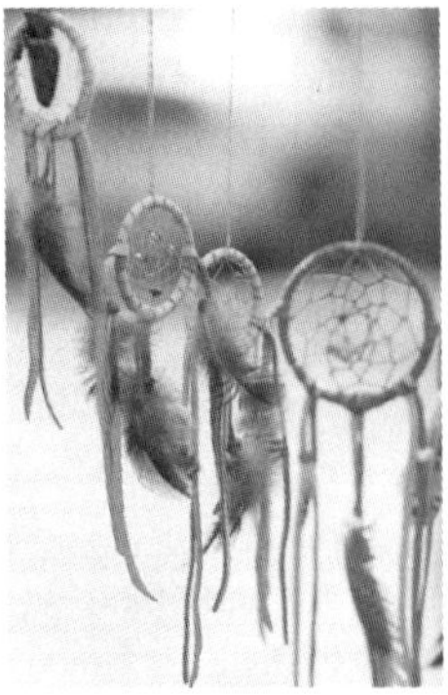

New graduates can be particularly challenged in RR practice settings due to their limited clinical experience (particularly as it applies to the broad range and scope of potential issues that can arise) as well as their limited independent decision-making and clinical judgment of complex individual, family and community situations. The unpredictable, inconsistent, or potentially unstable and highly complex scenarios that can present in these practice settings make this a demanding setting for a new nurse.

Some RR practice settings DO employ new graduates. If you choose this setting it will be CRITICAL for you to discuss the availability of an extended and comprehensive (mentored) transition program.

Consider the following points as you make your decision:

- There is a large scope of responsibility and, depending on the staff complement (availability of nursing, support and allied health practitioners), a new nurse may be required to take a Charge Nurse role immediately (this is particularly relevant to Associate Degree/ Registered/Registered Psychiatric Nurse graduates).
- Highly developed collaboration and delegation skills are critical because of the relative independence of the nursing role and the need to assume leadership responsibilities within a short period of time.

---

[1]Particular acknowledgement goes to *Anna-Marie Offiah, Kendra Ayers* and *Lorisa Earnshaw* from the All Nations' Healing Hospital inn Fort Qu'Appelle, Saskatchewan, Canada for their contribution to the insights revealed in this Appendix.

- RNs may be the only nurse in a rural facility during late evening and night shifts, while LPN/RPNs are most frequently paired with an RN during the day or evening.
- There are often minimal diagnostics, staff and equipment, requiring that the nurse have exceptional assessment, diagnostic, implementation and evaluation competencies.
- Responses to a diverse set of individual, family and community issues demand significant ingenuity and creative problem solving. There may not be access to advanced practitioners such as nurse practitioners or physicians (i.e. sometimes only by phone or videoconference, or during onsite visits weekly/monthly) and the availability of allied health professionals and emergency support (i.e. CODES) is often minimal.
- Because of the broad range of possible clinical situations that present in this setting, nurses need to know '*a bit about everything*' or, put another way, they need to '*be an expert at things they rarely do*'. The nurse may be expected to be proficient at a host of skills that may lie outside the immediate purview of a basic nursing education (i.e. phlebotomy, housekeeping, autoclaving, human resource planning and management, clerical duties, obstetrical emergencies/births).
- Relationships between nurses and RR communities are usually quite strong; it is not uncommon to be called at home for advice about personal issues that may or may not relate directly to 'health' (i.e. how to unplug a toilet, repair a leaking roof or assist in getting out of a snow drift).

If you HAVE chosen RR as a new nurse here are some TIPS FOR SUCCESS:

- **Choose a GOOD** mentor and do it QUICKLY—rely on them to ask questions, solve problems and debrief with you frequently. Model your practice after them.
- Negotiate with your Manager to **be certified in as many advanced practice skills as you can** (i.e. obstetrical emergencies, Advanced Cardiac Life Support, Advanced Trauma Life Support, Pediatric Advanced Life Support, intra-partum nursing, rural acute-care nursing certification, community and emergency mental health certification).
- Ensure you have **access to an experienced practitioner** at all times (hopefully your mentor!) that you can contact any time of the day or night when you are working alone in a leadership role (by phone if necessary). **Have their cell phone on YOUR speed dial** ☺
- **Plan ahead** as best as you can for what you will do IF someone calls in sick, is unable to GET to work (i.e. weather) or if you have an emergency (large and small scale). Know **WHO** you will contact, **HOW** to contact them and **WHAT** you will do when confronted with the most common situations. This is when having a '*what to do when________ happens*' manual that **you prepare yourself**, would be GREAT!
- **Build relationships** in the community and LEARN FROM all the professionals, support staff and administrative people you work with. They will be your support in times of need.
- **DEBRIEF** with your mentor or an experienced nurse FREQUENTLY (car pooling is particularly helpful, as the ride to and from work provides opportunity for in-depth and confidential discussion).

- The Managers or Charge Nurses in these RR locations are critical to your success: **STICK TO THEM LIKE GLUE** for the first year!!!
- Ensure that you spend time during your transition and integration program with **staff from ALL departments** (i.e. housekeeping, lab, x-ray)—you never know when you will need to DO THEIR JOB!
- If you are practicing in a rural setting **try to start by caring for the most stable, predictable and consistent patients on the *floor*.** GRADUALLY work your way into more urgent or emergent situations if possible, though in a small rural health center this is challenging to control. Many new nurses are simply put where they are needed.
- Most **remote practice settings DO NOT HAVE inpatient beds** and therefore the practice is largely community-based public health and emergency care—situations requiring admission are usually transferred to the closest tertiary health center.
- **Work hard at valuing and promoting the people you work with**—these are 'tight' communities and you often '*make it or they break you*'. Remember, this is THEIR community (the residents), so it is YOU that will need to do the adjusting and accommodating initially—over time you will establish your credibility and influence, allowing you to make the changes you believe are necessary to enhance the health of the population.
- Access as much **continuing education** as you possibly can—with online courses and remote resource knowledge access (handheld computers and mobile devices) so easily available, your only 'limitation' might be wireless access in the more remote centers. In RR nursing, you need information to be **ACCURATE** and **AVAILABLE**—and yesterday isn't soon enough!
- **Guard the safety of your practice**—it may be tempting for administrators or more experienced practitioners to launch you into roles you are not yet comfortable with or adequately prepared for.

Working in High Acuity

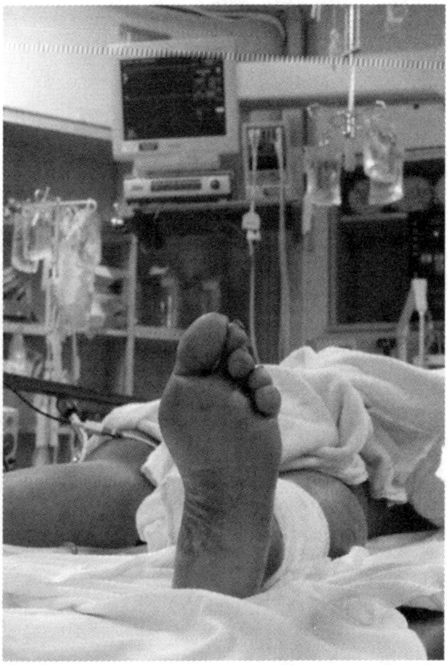

The recent downturn in our economy has been reflected in nursing staff shortages and reduced practice support resources EVERYWHERE. Some of the hardest hit are high-acuity practice areas that see the most unstable, least predictable and sickest on our health continuum; *emergency* departments and *critical care* units. Quite simply, it is difficult to recruit and retain nurses in these areas.

It is not surprising to me that the fast-paced, dynamic and largely independent practice context of these areas attracts the intellect, creativity and high energy of some of our new grads (hey.....that is what attracted ME to critical care!!!). But, as a rule, there is a lack of predictability, stability, consistency and familiarity in these patient/client populations that does not match with the knowledge, practice or development needs of a new nurse.

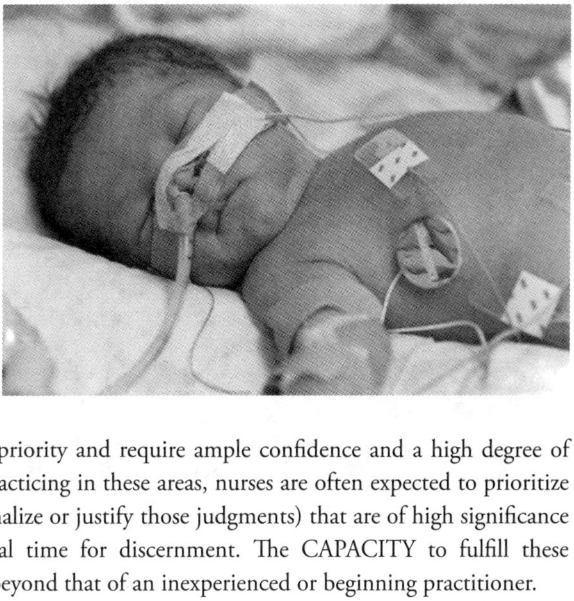

In fact, until a few years ago, nurses hired into these practice areas required a minimum of 2-5 years of experience, advanced skills in clinical assessment and experience with a variety of complex clinical situations. These protocols for hiring were based on the assumption (and I do not think this has changed) that practitioners in these areas manage multiple demands of often equally high priority and require ample confidence and a high degree of professional capability. When practicing in these areas, nurses are often expected to prioritize judgments (and be able to rationalize or justify those judgments) that are of high significance and for which there is minimal time for discernment. The CAPACITY to fulfill these expectations was thought to be beyond that of an inexperienced or beginning practitioner.

I believe it is important to clarify that this does not speak to the CAPACITY of new nurses; they have obviously completed a rigorous and qualified nursing program.

CAPACITY=POTENTIAL
CAPABILITY=ABILITY/SKILL

With advanced knowledge, the appropriate level and type of experience and sufficient professional support, most nurses can be developed into EXCEPTIONAL high acuity practitioners. The issue that appears most contentious (particularly in discussion with experienced practitioners IN these practice areas) is whether or not a newly graduated nurse is READY to meet the expectations required in these often volatile and high-risk practice areas. I believe it is more appropriate for new practitioners to be exposed to ranges of ABNORMAL within a relatively controlled environment prior to intentionally exposing them to the clinically UNSTABLE. The ability to witness the steady but slow(er) 'decompensation' of a patient/client situation and then participate in the assessment, recognition, notification, intervention and evaluation protocols that follow, allows for a 'logical' ordering of ABNORMAL>UNSTABLE within the evolving cognitive development of a new nurse's thinking.

This isn't personal…it is about standards of practice and patient/client safety.

This is not an issue that is unique to nursing. If you explore other professions (law, medicine, accounting, journalism, engineering, dentistry to name a broad few), you would be hard pressed to find the most junior of these professionals charged with carrying out the most contextually difficult and precarious assignments. And in many of those professions, life and death are not part of the equation as they are in this discussion.

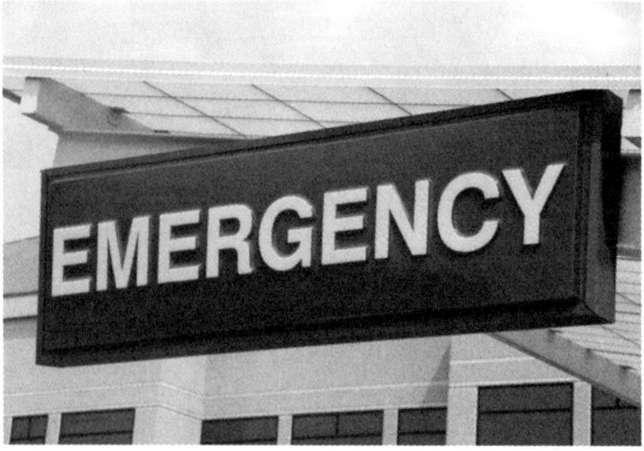

My extensive research into the experience of transition for new nurses (including my research of new nurses in emergency), combined with my own personal history of working as a 'relatively' new practitioner in critical care inspires in me a relative CAUTION when it comes to this issue. While I appreciate that I am not '*the sharpest knife in the drawer*', I am also not the dullest—and I KNOW I made some scary decisions as a critical care practitioner with only a year of nursing experience. Recognizing the potential for patient risk that my inexperience might bring to that role, I left (temporarily) to gain some experience and returned with more knowledge, confidence and insight into the nature of my responsibilities. As a result, I am hesitant to recommend or support (without significant conditions) the hiring of new graduates into emergency, adult or pediatric critical care (though I do not necessarily feel this way about *Neonatal Intensive Care Units* as they are MUCH MORE discriminating, judicious and graduated in their integration process and timelines) PRIOR TO the graduate having A MINIMUM of 1-YEAR experience. I think even that is being somewhat liberal….. but times are tough everywhere.

Here is what I would suggest if you are INTERESTED in **pursuing a high-acuity career** (thinking about a **CAREER PATH** or **CAREER TRAJECTORY** in Emergency or Critical Care):

- If you're looking to develop expertise in a **specialty** area (not necessarily high acuity) either now or down the road, research the hospital or community health center's reputation in your area. Be sure to ask about opportunities for transitioning you into the positions that interest you the most. Also, check into any options for *additional schooling or courses geared to that specialty* that you might be required to take. Many institutions are willing to pay part or all of your advanced education for some promise of return employment once completed.
- Asking to **spend some observational time** in a nursing area where you are interested in working is a great way to gather inspiration and find mentors that you can look up to. Further to this, working in a more general practice area (i.e. medicine, surgery, long-term care, geriatrics) assists you to know whether or not you want to continue a nursing specialty in this field (i.e. nurse specialist or nurse practitioner).
- **Meet with a Manager or Educator** from the area of practice where you would like to ultimately work. Collaborate with them to determine what skills and competencies you need to function competently in that high acuity setting (see *Skill/Competency Profile for High Acuity Nursing* below).
- Begin your nursing practice (initiate your professional role transition) in an **acute-care practice environment** (working in a larger rural setting would also be beneficial for gaining many of your basic skills and competencies but it would need to be highly supported/mentored to be an effective 'learning' experience).
- Once you have determined the skills and competencies required to function competently in the high-acuity environment where you want to practice, **TARGET those skills and competencies** by practicing them in an environment that maintains an 'active' census but is not as unpredictable, inconsistent or unstable as that seen in high acuity. Learning how to perform these skills and competencies in a SAFE context is paramount to your success and to the safety of patients/clients.
- Ideally, the **Managers and Educators** from the high acuity unit would **COLLABORATE WITH** experienced nurses/mentors and leaders from the practice areas where the skills and competencies you require are most common. This approach **BUILDS A WORKFORCE**, utilizing numerous clinical settings as 'incubators' of development and advanced practice workforce preparation and facilitates a more strategic approach to meeting the needs of ALL practice settings.

- If it is possible, while you are establishing your experience and 'settling' into your new role as a professional nurse, **discuss the possibility of 'rotating' into the high acuity specialty area you are interested in.** This should NOT occur until you are in the 3rd stage of transition as it may be too disruptive to the foundations you are developing if your transition experience is 'interrupted' prior to that time.
- If you are able, take one of the **high acuity specialty training courses** WHILE you are establishing your basic skill base—this will provide you with some of the theoretical constructs you will need WHILE you are strengthening your performance (i.e. Critical Care Registered Nurse [CCRN], Emergency Nurse Certification [ENC], Canadian Association of Critical Care Nurses [CACCN], Australian Credentialled Critical Care Nurse [ACCCN], Critical Care Nursing Certification [CCNC/UK]).

Skill/Competency Profile for High Acuity Nursing[1]

The following is a list of skills/competencies most commonly required of high acuity nurses. Refer to these when planning your path toward practicing in this setting:

1. **Professionalism**
    a. Presents an appropriate image of nursing
    b. Understands and respects confidentiality and privacy
    c. Demonstrates basic nursing competence
    d. Recognizes own limitations, requesting assistance appropriately
    e. Appreciates the importance of privacy in care
    f. Practices ethically and legally with employer, colleagues AND patients/clients
    g. Identifies and responds appropriately to stress
    h. Incorporates contemporary evidence into practice
    i. Understands the role of nursing relative to other professions
2. **Competence**
    a. Excels at and maintains currency in direct-care practice
    b. Takes steps to move from novice to expert practice competence
    c. Initiates and participates in ongoing performance appraisal
    d. Demonstrates interest in advancing high acuity nursing standards
3. **Safety and Risk Prevention**
    a. Practices according to current policies and procedures
    b. Attends to safety in interactions with colleagues, patients/clients
    c. Demonstrates commitment to continuing education

[1]Ontario Critical Care Steering Committee (2005). *Critical care nurse training standards task force report.* Toronto: Ministry of Ontario. Retrieved January 11th, 2012 from http://www.caccn.ca/en/files/mohltc_report_ccn_stds.pdf

4. **Therapeutic Relationships**
    a. Communicates respectfully, accurately and comprehensively with all members of the healthcare team
    b. Includes family and community when appropriate in the care of all patient/clients
    c. Plans holistically and inclusively
    d. Optimizes communication (verbal, non-verbal, age-appropriate, electronic, interprets patient/client messages appropriately)
    e. Optimizes family dynamics (demonstrates appropriate concern, boundaries, information sharing, language appropriate to level of comprehension, expressions of empathy, crisis intervention, consultation referral, facilitates family decision-making)
    f. Provides realistic hope
    g. Identifies differences between expectations and anticipated outcomes
    h. Advocates for family
    i. Establishes therapeutic relationships in limited time period
    j. Facilitates adaptive coping of family as situation changes
    k. Maximizes family decision making involvement
    l. Shares relevant data on health progress with patient/client/family
    m. Demonstrates capacity to teach and understands readiness to learn
    n. Facilitates optimal participation of patient/client in own care
5. **Knowledge and Critical Thinking**
    a. Demonstrates capacity to think critically
    b. Understands basic data and health information as it relates to the evolving clinical situation
    c. Able to appropriately gather and facilitate diagnostics
    d. Considers pathophysiological, psychosocial, cultural, developmental and spiritual data when planning care
    e. Obtains a comprehensive health history in the absence of patient/client's ability to communicate
    f. Gathers and responds to data concerning family coping during crisis
    g. Appropriately channels own responses to stress and grief
    h. Understands relative risks of infection and takes appropriate steps to minimize
    i. Interprets data accurately and rapidly under duress
    j. Demonstrates knowledge of biological, physical and behavioral sciences, and analyzes same to formulate nursing diagnoses
    k. Functions independently and interdependently as appropriate

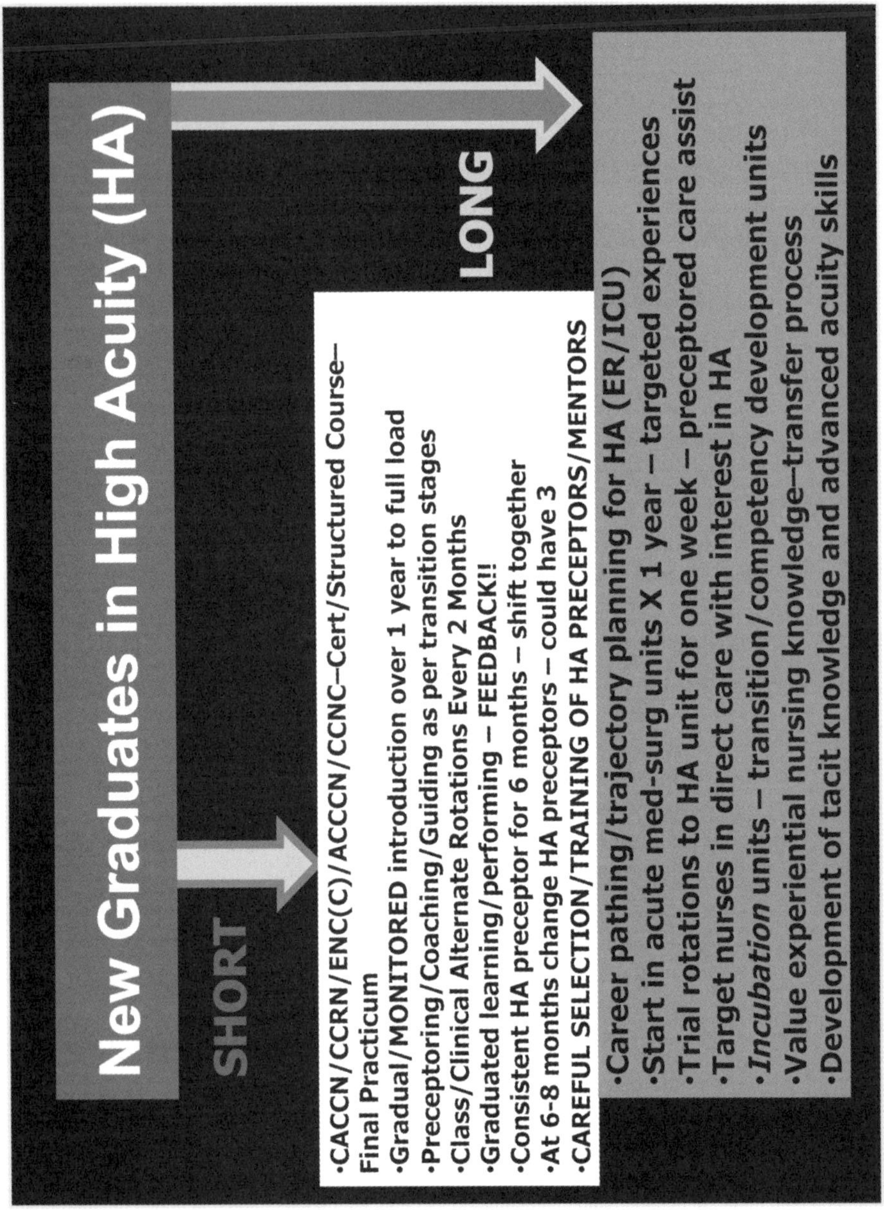
New Graduates in High Acuity (HA)
SHORT
LONG
•CACCN/CCRN/ENC(C)/ACCCN/CCNC–Cert/Structured Course–Final Practicum
•Gradual/MONITORED introduction over 1 year to full load
•Preceptoring/Coaching/Guiding as per transition stages
•Class/Clinical Alternate Rotations Every 2 Months
•Graduated learning/performing – FEEDBACK!!
•Consistent HA preceptor for 6 months – shift together
•At 6-8 months change HA preceptors – could have 3
•CAREFUL SELECTION/TRAINING OF HA PRECEPTORS/MENTORS
•Career pathing/trajectory planning for HA (ER/ICU)
•Start in acute med-surg units X 1 year – targeted experiences
•Trial rotations to HA unit for one week – preceptored care assist
•Target nurses in direct care with interest in HA
•*Incubation* units – transition/competency development units
•Value experiential nursing knowledge–transfer process
•Development of tacit knowledge and advanced acuity skills

Generational Workplace Ethics/Behavior

VETERANS (>65 YOA)	BOOMERS (45-65 YOA)
• Grew up in 'hard times' • Have 'old-fashioned family values' • Loyal and disciplined • Believe in teamwork and reward for hard work • Support seniority-driven entitlement – respect authority • More comfortable with rules and structure • Less familiar with diversity in the workplace • Expected a bright and predictable future • Frugal and rigid – loyalty is to the institution • Orientated to the 'collective' – utilitarian perspective • Consistent, uniform and compliant *WORK PRIORITIES*: hard working with moderate expectations for advancement, respect & trust authority, hierarchical, positive, loyal and disciplined, work for the greater good of the institution and work well on a team with directive leadership	• Currently dominate the workplace demographic • Raised in post-war affluence • Brought up to believe the world was safe • Inherited a sense of uniqueness and privilege • Idealistic, self-indulgent and socially righteous • Rebel against authority, question the status quo • Value integrity and immediacy – 'one strike and you're out' • Believe self above others • Support contributory-driven entitlement • Live to work • Highly competitive, strong-willed and self-sacrificing *WORK PRIORITIES*: driven and highly competitive, expect rewards based on work, little regard for or trust in authority, cautious and skeptical, loyal to self first, effort relative to outcome, idealistic, work well on a team but likely want to lead it and work best with leadership not direction
GENERATION X (28-45 YOA)	**MILLENNIALS (23-28) YOA)**
• Raised with an abundance of choice and minimal direction • Pragmatic and street smart – grew up under-protected and under-directed • Have learned to 'fend for themselves' – have a determined level of independence • Self-reliant but somewhat pessimistic about the future – world 'downsized' and 'corporatized' • Have few traditions, have lived with political uncertainty, and witnessed unprecedented social improprieties • Have lost faith in institution of 'work' and have little trust in 'reward for hard work' concept • Divided between work and life focus • Aware of their limited career mobility prospects • Teamwork driven – collaborative but interdependent • Demand balance between work and home *WORK PRIORITIES*: self-determining & highly adaptable, flexible & mobile, unwilling to sacrifice for the greater good, loyal to self, 'rights' oriented, distrusting of authority, like to work 'alone' or independently and come together later (interdependence with peers)	• Born into unprecedented prosperity • Raised in a culture of unparalleled social, political and economic change • Grew up with designer drugs and AIDS • Are intimate with the concept of 'uncivil war' – surrounded by conflict • Hyper-educated, ethnically diverse and technologically accomplished • Have inherited a deeply divided world • Grew up in eclectic social structures - highly pluralistic, inclusive, and integrated • Have a keen social conscience – 'repair mode' • Believe strongly in upholding individual rights • Embrace diversity in all life spheres • Technology is like 'breathing' • Know the world as 'virtual' – socially delayed • Expect balance between work and home – seamless relationship between environments • Loyal to principles, not institution • Work to live *WORK PRIORITIES*: feel comfortable in environments of change, conflict is normal (may not work to resolve it, but adjust to it), access to technology assumed (cognitive extension), seamlessness b/w work and home lives, socially conscious, inclusive, collaborative, multi-task well, accustomed to high speeds and highly informed but relationally naïve (social interdependence)

Used with permission from Duchscher, J.E.B., & Cowin, L. (2004). Multigenerational nurses in the workplace. *Journal of Nursing Administration, 34*(11), 493-501.

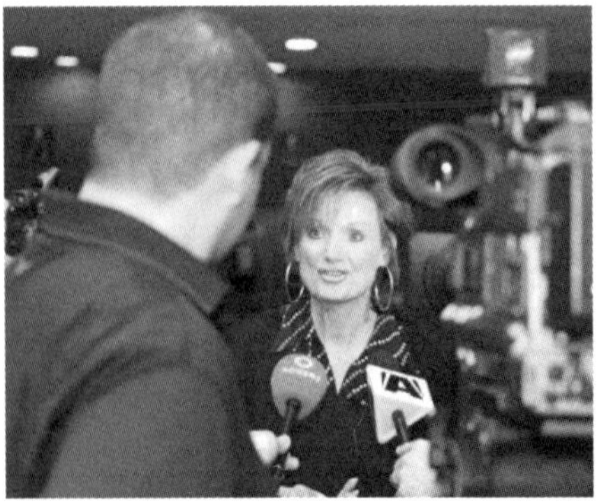

Judy E. Boychuk Duchscher began her nursing career in 1979 when she graduated with a Nursing Diploma. After practicing nursing in critical care for 2 years, Dr. Duchscher obtained a Post-Graduate Diploma in Intensive Care Nursing from the University of Manitoba, a diploma in Cardiovascular Nursing from Stanford University in California, and completed her Critical Care Registered Nurse examination (CCRN) through the American Association of Critical Care Nursing.

In 1983, her studies in heart and lung transplantation at Stanford University took her to the University of Alberta Hospital (Edmonton, Alberta) where she taught cardiovascular critical care nursing and coordinated the health-care team responsible for initiating the heart and heart-lung transplant program at the University of Alberta. In 1985, at the Toronto General Hospital (Toronto, Ontario), she developed a multi-organ donor referral and management program, and then continued on to Barnes Hospital (St. Louis, Missouri) where she initiated and coordinated a single and double lung transplant nursing program. Dr. Duchscher completed her American hiatus in 1989 by coordinating the United States clinical specialist operations for a coronary angioplasty company in Minneapolis, Minnesota, after which she returned home to Canada to complete her Bachelor of Science in Nursing Degree and return to staff nursing in Intensive Care.

Between 1990-1998, while completing both her undergraduate and graduate degrees at the University of Saskatchewan, Dr. Duchscher developed the Out-Of-Province section of the Saskatchewan Transplant Program in Saskatoon and taught with the University of Saskatchewan College of Nursing. In 2007, she worked with Dr. Netha Dyck and over 40 of her nursing faculty to develop the conceptual, philosophical and organizational framework for an Institute for Nursing Scholarship in the SIAST Nursing Division. In 2009, Dr. Duchscher joined the University of Calgary nursing faculty professoriate where she works today, concurrently holding professional Faculty Associate, Adjunct and Affiliate positions with the University of Saskatchewan, the University of Alberta and the University of Western Sydney in Australia.

In what she identifies as her most meaningful career achievement, on July 25th, 2004, Dr. Duchscher launched a new non-profit nursing organization entitled *Nursing The Future*. This initiative (www.nursingthefuture.ca), initially sponsored by Saskatchewan's Ministry of Health and supported by local industry and educational stakeholders in many Canadian healthcare communities, continues to serve as a bridge between the ideals taught in undergraduate nursing education and the realities of the 'real' world of professional practice. The over 3000 international members of this organization receive this book as part of their membership, along with onsite and online support that connects them with other senior students, new graduates and nursing and healthcare leaders in their communities.

Dr. Duchscher's long-standing devotion to this topic has been informed and inspired by literature that recounts the traumatic socialization to the role of professional health care practitioner that is experienced by the new nursing graduate. Her doctoral work built on her 1998 graduate (Master of Nursing) research on new graduate transition as well as a major qualitative study in 2001 that explored the experiences of new graduates integrating into a busy emergency/trauma unit. She continues an ongoing program of research in the area of professional role transition, with studies currently focusing on the professional role transition experiences of non-traditional (accelerated track or 2nd degree nursing graduates) and male graduates, with grants submitted to study the experience of transition for medical physicians newly licensed for independent practice.

The findings of her research have generated a theory of *Transition Shock* and a model of the *Stages of Transition* that underscore the essential nature of mentoring relationships between seasoned and novice nurses, identify the importance of feedback, balance and a gradual introduction to the workplace, while drawing attention to the multiple dimensions of the new graduate experience that include physical, intellectual, emotional, developmental and socio-cultural factors.

As a scholar, Duchscher has received numerous awards for her research, teaching and study of nursing over the course of her 32 year career. During her PhD program (2001-2007), she studied hospital nursing in Canada, focusing her efforts on furthering the understanding of the new nursing graduate transition experience as it influences, and is influenced, by post secondary educational preparation and programs of support within the healthcare industry. Duchscher has been recognized by the Saskatchewan Ministry of Health, the Saskatchewan Nurses Foundation, the Saskatchewan Registered Nurses Association, the Izaak Walton Killam Foundation, the University of Alberta Faculty of Nursing and the Faculty of Graduate Studies and Research, the Alberta Heritage Medical Research Foundation, the Social Sciences and Humanities Research Council of Canada (SSHRC) and the Canadian Nurses Foundation for her contributions to, and potential for excellence in, qualitative research and nursing scholarship. In 2008, Duchscher received the Sigma Theta Tau International (Mu Sigma) Award for Community Leadership, was inducted into both the Cambridge and Strathmore's Who's Who Directory, was recognized for her work with new graduates and the development of *Nursing The Future* by the Saskatchewan Ministry of Health with the 2009 Healthcare Excellence Award for Leadership and was most recently awarded the 2010 Outstanding New Investigator Award from the Canadian Association of Nursing Research.

Dr. Duchscher has established strong professional relationships with international scholars in the topic of new graduate transition. She has published numerous peer-reviewed articles and several book chapters on this subject, several of which have been collaborative efforts with nursing and educational leaders across North America and Australia. Currently, Duchscher speaks on issues related to the contemporary climate of acute-care nursing, new graduate transition to professional practice in hospitals, leadership succession in new nurses and understanding and working with multi-generational nurses in the workplace.

Dr. Duchscher resides in Calgary, Alberta, Canada with her husband, Eldon Duchscher.

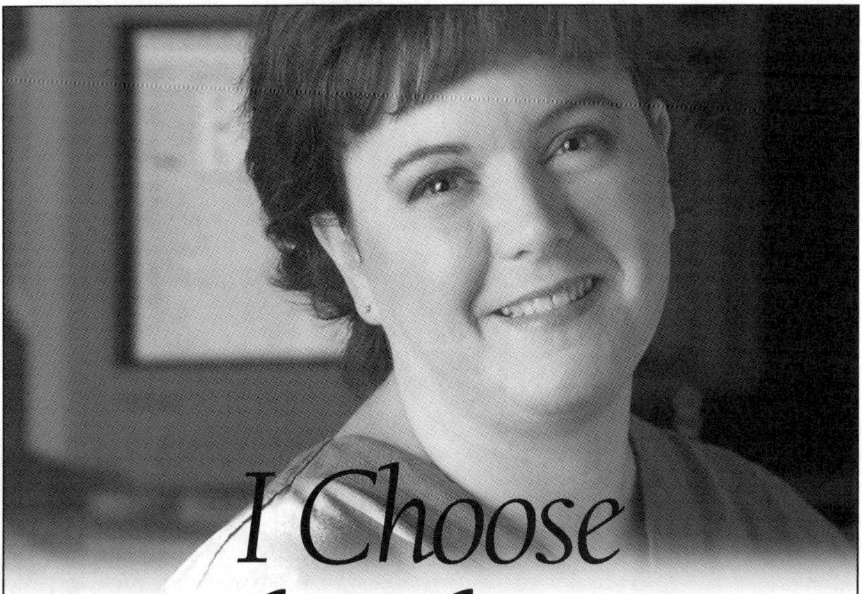

C

D

F

Q

R

S

T

Notes